AF556898

# MEDICAL RADIOLOGY

Diagnostic Imaging and Radiation Oncology

---

Springer
*Berlin*
*Heidelberg*
*New York*
*Barcelona*
*Budapest*
*Hong Kong*
*London*
*Milan*
*Paris*
*Singapore*
*Tokyo*

E.K. Lang (Ed.)

# Radiology of the Female Pelvic Organs

With Contributions by

S. M. Ascher · M. Atri · P. Baharamipour · G. Biti · C. I. Caskey · F. De Cobelli
A. Del Maschio · H. H. Dunaway Jr. · U. M. Hamper · P. Innocenti · N. G. Kasabian
K. H. Kim · E. K. Lang · G. C. Mingin Jr. · K. R. Mullangi · J. Nori · Y. D. Patel
C. Reinhold · R. Santoni · S. Sheth · A. Silva · S. Sironi · D. Spagnolo · D. B. Spring
M. Takahashi · A. Vanzulli · N. Villari · Y. Yamashita

Foreword by

J. E. Youker

With 230 Figures in 410 Separate Illustrations, Some in Color

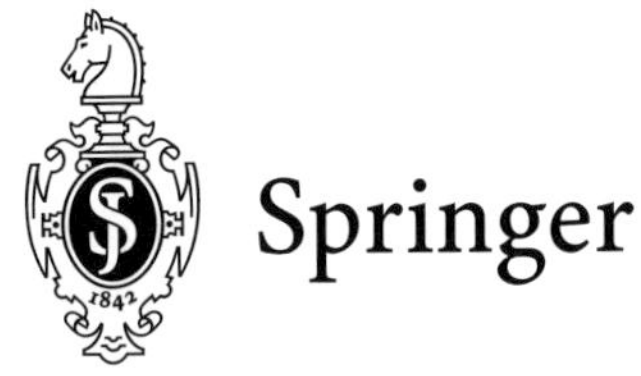

Springer

Erich K. Lang, MD
Professor of Radiology and Urology
Department of Radiology School of Medicine
Louisiana State University Medical Center
1543 Tulane Avenue
New Orleans, LA 70122-2822
USA

MEDICAL RADIOLOGY · Diagnostic Imaging and Radiation Oncology

Continuation of
Handbuch der medizinischen Radiologie
Encyclopedia of Medical Radiology

ISSN 0942-5373
ISBN 3-540-61119-3 Springer-Verlag Berlin Heidelberg New York

Library of Congress Cataloging-in-Publication Data. Radiology of the female pelvic organs / E.K. Lang (ed.) ; with contributions by S. M. Ascher ... [et al.] ; foreword by J.E. Youker. p. cm. -- (Medical radiology) Includes bibliographical references and index. ISBN 3-540-61119-3 (alk. paper) 1. Generative organs, Female--Imaging. 2. Gentiourinary organs--Imaging. 3. Pelvis--Imaging. 4. Generative organs, Female--Diseases--Diagnosis. 5. Genitourinary organs--Diseases--Diagnosis. 6. Pelvis--Diseases--Diagnosis I. Lang, Erich K. (Erich Karl), 1929- . II. Ascher Susan. III. Series. [DNLM: 1. Genital Diseases, Female--diagnosis. 2. Genital Neoplasms, Female--diagnosis. 3. Pelvis--pathology. 4. Magnetic Resonance Imaging. WP 141R129 1996] RG107.R33 1998 618.1'0754--dc21 DNLM/DLC for Library of Congress 97-50319 CIP



Printed in Germany



Typesetting: Best-set Typesetter Ltd., Hong Kong

SPIN: 10526333 21/3135 – 5 4 3 2 1 0 – Printed on acid-free paper

# Foreword

*Radiology of the Female Pelvic Organs* represents the third text in Erich K. Lang's trilogy which includes the previously published titles *Radiology of the Upper Urinary Tract* and *Radiology of the Lower Urinary Tract*. This volume provides a comprehensive review of diseases of the female pelvic organs. The clinical picture and pathology are well covered, but of course the emphasis is on imaging of the female pelvic organs and on the interventional procedures used to treat maladies of these organ systems.

The current volume departs from the preceding two works in that the major emphasis is on the new modalities of MRI, CT, and ultrasonography, including color Doppler. Professor Lang has brought together the foremost experts from around the world in each of the specific areas of radiology of the female pelvic organs. Special skills developed in each radiologic community are lucidly described. Several chapters describe the relative roles of the different new modalities and give guidance to the clinician in choosing the most appropriate imaging technique. The volume not only discusses diagnosis and staging but places a major emphasis on therapy and the evaluation of the effectiveness of various therapeutic modalities. The extensive literature citations catalog the experience of the experts worldwide and are not limited to any specific geographic area.

This volume truly confirms that medicine has become a global effort with experts from throughout the world offering their own unique contributions.

Extensive illustrations aid the reader in gaining a comprehensive view of the numerous advances that have occurred over the last several years. The book can be recommended with great enthusiasm.

Milwaukee　　　　　　　　　　　　　　　　　　　　　　　　　　　JAMES E. YOUKER

# Preface

*Radiology of the Female Pelvic Organs* completes the trilogy on radiology of the urinary tract within the *Medical Radiology* series. The three volumes – *Radiology of the Upper Urinary Tract, Radiology of the Lower Urinary Tract,* and *Radiology of the Female Pelvic Organs* – are intended to offer a comprehensive and up-to-date text on diagnosis and radiologic intervention in the genitourinary tract. However, this volume is also designed as a stand-alone text for imaging, diagnosis, and intervention pertaining to the female pelvis.

Advances in imaging and minimally invasive intervention in women with pelvic disorders have occurred at an unprecedented rate in the last two decades. This text attempts to consolidate information on innovative procedures, establish their efficacy vis-à-vis other well-established techniques, and support conclusions with an extensive up-to-date bibliography suitable for both the clinician and the researcher seeking detailed background information.

Noted authorities analyze the contributions of MRI, CT and ultrasound in the diagnosis of neoplastic disease of the uterine cervix, the endometrium, the vulva, the ovaries, and the adnexa, and in the evaluation of treatment response. The value of individual examinations, alone and in conjunction with other modalities, is established. Chapters on Doppler ultrasound highlight the use of this modality in neoplastic disease of the pelvis. Interventional radiology as germane to conditions encountered in the female pelvis is addressed in a separate chapter, as is selective salpingography and fallopian tube recanalization.

The satisfation of caring for the individual patients is one of the two principal rewards for a physician's efforts; contributing to our discipline through the dissemination of scientific knowledge and thereby earning the esteem of one's peers is the other. It is the hope of the contributors and the editor that this text will serve radiologists, urologists, gynecologists, and surgeons as a valuable reference source, and will ultimately benefit patients by way of improved diagnosis and treatment.

New Orleans

Erich K. Lang

# Contents

# 1 Introduction to Benign and Malignant Disease of the Female Pelvis

E.K. Lang

CONTENTS



## 1.1 Diseases of the Cervix Uteri

There is increasing evidence that cancer of the cervix and viral disease are related, and that benign disease and in situ neoplastic disease may coexist in many instances (Novak and Woodruff 1979, pp 111–127). While many of the inflammatory disease entities involving the cervix uteri are diagnosed at colposcopy, some lesions may present as mass lesions on endovaginal ultrasonography, computed tomography (CT), or magnetic resonance imaging (MRI).

Nabothian cysts are a classic example. These are deep-seated retention cysts of cervical glands which may cause only minor surface irregularity. When punctured they tend to yield an exudate that may be clear, mucopurulent, or plain purulent. On MRI, contrast-enhanced CT, and endovaginal ultrasonography they present in a typical fashion which should not cause confusion with malignant lesions of the cervix. While infection or preceding infection is a classic feature in the history of such patients, adenomatous hyperplasia is usually not associated with infection. Histologically there is an aggregation of cystic clefts, but the individual epithelial cells are benign. The process is probably the result of occlusion of many channels by a noninflammatory, nonneoplastic process.

Condylomata acuminata are wart-like lesions that are most commonly diagnosed by colposcopy (Novak and Woodruff 1979, pp 93–110). Occasionally endovaginal ultrasonography or MRI may suggest the presence of such lesions. Biopsy is necessary to establish a diagnosis and particularly to differentiate the lesion against in situ neoplastic processes.

Pseudoepitheliomatous hyperplasia is again a histopathologic diagnosis. However, the presence of mucous blebs and positive keratin may be heralded on MRI by signal changes on T2-weighted sequences (Novak and Woodruff 1979, pp 93–110).

Microcystic mucoid metaplasia can progress to myxoid changes and present with a pseudoadenomatous pattern (Chumas et al. 1985). Endovaginal ultrasonography, contrast-enhanced CT, and MRI may demonstrate changes similar to those seen with endocervical polyps in postmenopausal woman receiving estrogen therapy.

Acanthosis and leukoplakia are associated with condylomata acuminata and hence are likely of viral etiology (Novak and Woodruff 1979, pp 93–110). Signal changes on T1- and T2-weighted MRI scans may be observed; however, the diagnosis rests on colposcopic biopsy.

Cervical polyps are a localized proliferation of cervical mucosa. In most instances they arise from the endocervix (Novak and Woodruff 1979, pp 93–110). Their appearance on endovaginal ultrasonography, contrast-enhanced CT, and MRI is fairly characteristic, but the diagnosis again rests on histopathologic assessment. In rare instances endometrial polyps may extend through the cervical canal and mimic a cervical polyp. In a small percentage of cases epidermoid cancer may arise in the cervical polyp, which makes histopathologic assessment mandatory (Novak and Woodruff 1979, pp 111–127).

E.K. Lang, MD, Professor of Radiology and Urology, Department of Radiology School of Medicine, Louisiana State University Medical Center, 1543 Tulane Avenue, New Orleans, LA 70122-2822, USA

Leiomyomas are relatively rare in the cervix, since smooth muscle is rare in the distal uterine segments. Papillary adenofibromas usually display a quite characteristic appearance on contrast-enhanced CT, endovaginal ultrasonography, and MRI. Since they have a propensity for partially occluding the cervical canal, surgical remedy is usually indicated.

Adenomas or mesonephric tubules may be seated just lateral to the cervical duct (Gartner's duct). They represent vestigial mesonephric remnants and form cysts. Their typical location facilitates diagnosis by endocervical ultrasonography, CT, or MRI. Cytopathologically, PAS+ material of the basal lamina is the characteristic feature.

Endometriosis in the cervix is a rare lesion usually associated with adenomyosis of the uterus or other pelvic endometriosis. The diagnosis is suggested with reasonable confidence on MRI.

Mesonephric cyst remnants of the wolffian duct may occur deep in the stroma of the normal cervix. Endovaginal ultrasonography can identify such lesions but with this technique difficulty may be encountered in differentiation against deeply situated nabothian cysts.

FIGO staging of carcinoma of the cervix uteri is the basis for determining management (Novak and Woodruff 1979, pp 111–146). Stages IA1 and IA2 comprise microscopically evident stromal invasion no deeper than 5 mm, nor should the horizontal spread exceed 7 mm. These lesions will evade detection by transvaginal ultrasonography, CT, and MRI. Stage IB lesions with a greater horizontal spread likewise will usually evade detection by imaging modalities. The important contribution of imaging studies is in the differentiation of stage IIA lesions without obvious parametrial involvement and stage IIB lesions with obvious parametrial involvement. Clearly imaging studies are likewise useful for differentiation of stage IIIA lesions showing no extension to the pelvic wall from stage IIIB lesions demonstrating such extensions or resultant hydronephrosis or nonfunction of a kidney. Contiguous growth to adjacent organs, particularly the bladder or rectum, as seen with stage IV lesions, is readily assessable by imaging examinations, as is spread to distal organs (IVB lesions).

Despite the obvious contribution of imaging studies to the diagnosis and differentiation of stage II, III, and IV lesions, to date only chest x-ray, skeletal x-ray, intravenous pyelography, and barium enema have been incorporated in the official protocol for FIGO staging. In part this may reflect disenchantment with earlier efforts at staging by means of imaging examinations such as lymphography, which attained an accuracy of only about 60%. It should be emphasized that CT-guided fine-needle aspiration has improved the accuracy of diagnosis of para-aortic lymph node metastases to about 87%.

## 1.2 Benign Disorders of the Uterine Corpus

Myomas, leiomyomas, fibromyomas, and fibroids are estimated to be present in 25% of women of reproductive age women (Novak and Woodruff 1979, pp 239–259), and are 3–9 times more frequent in the black race. They are commonly multiple and may reach a large size. These lesions are usually classified by anatomic location, i.e., submucosal, intramural, or subserosal (Chumas et al. 1985). They are subject to hyaline and cystic degeneration. Deprived of their vascular supply, liquefaction necrosis may be followed by a calcific reparative phase. Calcium carbonate and calcium phosphate precipitate in a necrotic tumor. The malignant variety, leiomyosarcomas, may develop in myomas, though the incidence of this is thought to be less than 0.5%.

These lesions are readily diagnosable by transabdominal or transvaginal ultrasonography, contrast-enhanced CT, and MRI (Gross et al. 1983; Cicinelli et al. 1995). Hysterosalpingography will likewise demonstrate the majority of such lesions with ease. Hysteroscopy is particularly useful to identify submucous myomas in infertile patients and can be expanded to endoscopic surgical removal (Cicinelli et al. 1995; Novak and Woodruff 1979, pp 239–259). Large tumors or tumors interfering with gestation and/or delivery are an indication for surgical intervention. Recently selective arterial transcatheter embolization has been advocated to reduce the size of some of these tumors (Vedantham et al. 1997).

Adenomyosis is a condition in which endometrial glands and stroma are dislocated within the myometrium (Novak and Woodruff 1979, pp 280–290). The lesions display characteristic findings on MRI and are also diagnosable by transvaginal ultrasonography and contrast-enhanced CT. Clinical presentation is usually with hypermenorrhea or dysmenorrhea. The lesions must be differentiated against submucous leiomyomas and endometrial carcinoma.

Endometrial polyps are pedunculated or sessile lesions in the endometrial cavity (Novak and Woodruff 1979, pp 239–259). They tend to be benign, undergoing sarcomatous or carcinomatous degeneration only rarely. They may be single or multiple. Microscopically endometrial polyps are a mixture of dense fibrous tissue and prominent and thick-walled vascular channels lined with endometrial epithelium. They are readily identifiable on hysterosalpingography, MRI, and endovaginal, transabdominal, or endouterine ultrasonography. However, identification on contrast-enhanced CT is fraught with difficulties. Hysteroscopy is the procedure of choice for both the evaluation and the treatment of endometrial polyps (Novak and Woodruff 1979, pp 111–127).

Placental polyps consist of remnants of retained placenta. On hysteroscopy these lesions may resemble choriocarcinoma. On arteriograms and contrast-enhanced computed tomograms they tend to be very vascular. This vascularity is also shown on gradient-echo MRI sequences or on T1-weighted MRI after gadolinium enhancement. Hormonally they do not appear to be active and human chorionic gonadotropin levels are generally normal.

Pyometrium is a condition caused by an inflammatory process with concomitant stenosis of the cervix. Carcinoma of the cervix is therefore not infrequently associated with this process. The distended endometrial cavity, filled with purulent material and debris, is readily identifiable on transvaginal or transabdominal ultrasonography, CT, and MRI.

## 1.3 Carcinoma of the Endometrium

Depth of invasion and uterine size are recognized predictors of survival among patients with carcinoma of the endometrium and have been incorporated into subgroupings of particularly stage I patients (Coppleson 1992, pp 731–802). The size of the uterus appears to relate to both grade of tumor and degree of myometrial invasion. Cervical involvement (stage II lesions) has been determined in the past by fractional curettage. Transvaginal ultrasonography and MRI provide reliable data for assessing tumor extension and myometrial penetration (Fischetti et al. 1994; Smith and McCarthy 1994). Lymph node involvement is predicted with reasonable accuracy by contrast-enhanced CT and MRI, but confirmation rests on guided thin-needle biopsy. Staging lymphadenectomy, however, provides the gold standard for identification of metastatic involvement of lymph nodes, since imaging examinations such as CT and MRI incriminate only nodes larger than 1 cm and will miss microscopic involvement of nodes. Even lymphangiography, which may identify structural abnormalities in nodes of normal size, provides no criteria for identifying microscopic metastases. The incidence of node metastases is directly related to the degree of penetration of muscle. With superficial muscle penetration, pelvic node metastases are found in approximately 5% of patients, while with deep muscle penetration this figure reaches 25%. Histologic differentiation or grade of the tumor is another factor that greatly influences survival as well as the occurrence of nodal metastases. Pelvic nodal metastases have been reported in 3% of patients with grade I lesions but in 18% of those with grade II lesions (Creasmen et al. 1987; Schnall 1994).

**Table 1.1.**

| UICC | CORPUS | FIGO |
|---|---|---|
| Tis | Carcinoma in situ | 0 |
| T1 | Confined to corpus | I |
| T1a | ≤Cavity 8 cm | Ia |
| T1b | >Cavity 8 cm | Ib |
| T2 | Extension to cervix | II |
| T3 | Extension beyond uterus/within true pelvis | III |
| T4 | Extension to bladder/rectum/beyond true pelvis | IVa |
| M1 | Distant organs | IVb |

Reluctance to use surgery in the management of patients with stage III or IV endometrial carcinoma is another important reason for attaining accurate preoperative staging (Schnall 1994). The propensity for recurrence in the vaginal vault makes assessment of tumor extension into the endocervical canal of paramount importance.

Leiomyosarcomas of the myxoid or epithelioid variety (leiomyoblastoma) account for approximately 45% of nonepithelial uterine cancers. One-third to one-half of patients with leiomyosarcomas have extrauterine extension at the time of diagnosis, and their 5-year survival is only 15%. MRI and contrast-enhanced CT can accurately stage such tumors; transvaginal ultrasonography can likewise successfully assess extrauterine extension of these tumors.

## 1.4 Fallopian Tube Disease

Inflammatory disease of the fallopian tubes presents as a mass lesion (Coppelson 1992, pp. 843–862; Novak and Woodruff 1979, pp 334–354).

Salpingitis isthmica nodosa may present as a mass in the region of the isthmic segment of the fallopian tubes. It is an inflammatory process resulting in invasion by epithelium of the muscularis, similar to the process seen with adenomyosis of the uterus. Endometriosis of the tubes can present in a very similar fashion. If the inflammatory process involves the distal portion of the tubes, a pyosalpinx or, as an end stage, hydrosalpinx will result. These lesions may be diagnosed by hysterosalpingography or, better still, selective salpingography. Transabdominal or endovaginal ultrasonography, MRI, and CT will also readily identify this condition. Tubercular salpingitis has no distinguishing features on imaging studies and its definitive diagnosis rests on microscopic examination.

Perisalpingitis can result from any pelvic inflammatory disease or inflammatory disease in the abdomen with resultant contamination of the pelvis. Imaging studies provide no specific information other than to identify the possible presence of walled-off abscess cavities.

Tubal polyps (Fig. 1.1). and papillomas present as filling defects in the tubes on selective salpingograms (Novak and Woodruff 1979, pp 319–333). Histologically they are classified as adenomatoid tumors.

Carcinoma of the fallopian tubes is a rare lesion commonly misdiagnosed as an ovarian tumor or tubo-ovarian inflammatory mass (Novak and Woodruff 1979, pp 319–333). Imaging studies do not provide specific criteria for diagnosis, which is most often established by laparoscopy. The disease may extend through the open tubal orifice into the peritoneum; hence metastases to the peritoneum are common. In addition there may be lymphatic extension to the iliac, presacral, and lumbar lymph nodes.

Choriocarcinoma may occur as a primary tubal neoplasm in conjunction with either a tubal pregnancy or, in rare instances, a viable intrauterine pregnancy (Coppleson 1992, pp 1013–1046). The highly vascular lesion is best demonstrated on selective arteriograms of the uterine artery. However, contrast-enhanced CT and gradient-echo MRI sequences or T1-weighted MRI after the administration of gadolinium likewise demonstrate the characteristic findings of this neoplasm.

## Paraadnexal Lesions

Tumors of the para-adnexal structures comprise a large variety of connective tissue, vascular, mesothelial, or embryonic remnant lesions. Benign connective tissue tumors are myomas, fibromyomas, lipomas, and adenomyomas (Woodruff 1991; Novak and Woodruff 1979, pp 385–395). All of them are demonstrable by ultrasonography, CT, and MRI. Lipomas in particular are characterized by typical tissue signatures in the various examinations. Their malignant counterparts, leiomyosarcomas and fibrosarcomas, present in an identical fashion on imaging studies. Vascular tumors such as angiomas, varices, varicocele, and lymphangiomas are characterized on imaging studies on the basis of the tell-tale appearance of vascular spaces. Contrast-enhanced

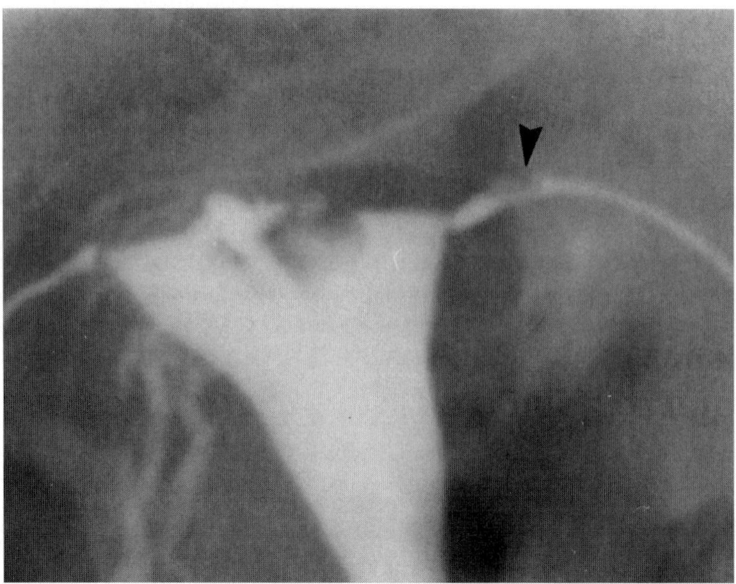

**Fig. 1.1.** Note the defect in the interstitial segment of the fallopian tube (*arrowhead*). This represents a small polyp

CT, gradient-echo MRI sequences, gadolinium-enhanced T1-weighted MRI, and arteriograms identify such lesions by their unique characteristics. In many instances color Doppler ultrasonography can likewise identify these lesions.

Mesothelial lesions such as parovarian cysts, mesonephric cysts, paramesonephric masses, and their malignant counterparts, papillary serous or endometrioid and mesonephric lesions, can be identified on imaging studies as cystic or mixed tumor masses (NOVAK and WOODRUFF 1979, pp 396–437).

Embryonic remnant masses such as hilar cell tumors or adrenal tumors present on imaging studies as a mass. Dermoid cysts, however, the definitively diagnosable on the basis of characteristic constellations of findings. Fat-fluid levels and solid tissue elements, and frequently cartilaginous or dental anlage lesions, produce a characteristic image on CT and MRI. Transvaginal ultrasonography likewise portrays the characteristic findings of this lesion.

## 1.5 Parovarian Cysts

Parovarian cysts, often described as Gartner's duct cysts, are remnants of the wolffian body and are situated in the mesosalpinx between the tubes in the hilum of the ovary (NOVAK and WOODRUFF 1979, pp 396–437). Sometimes, larger, often pedunculated cysts arise from the tip of the tube. These are of müllerian or paramesonephric origin. MRI and transvaginal ultrasonography will readily identify these structures.

## 1.6 Nonneoplastic Lesions of the Ovary

Follicular cysts, follicular hematomas, and lutein cysts are common cystic masses readily demonstrated on transvaginal or transabdominal ultrasonography. Theca or lutein cysts cause extremely large cystic ovaries and are frequently found in conjunction with hydatidiform mole. The diagnosis is again readily made on transabdominal or transvaginal ultrasonography and may be confirmed biochemically. The Stein-Leventhal ovary is significantly enlarged and studded with small cysts. Transabdominal or transvaginal ultrasonography documents multiple interfaces of these small cystic lesions. In about 10% of these patients there are coexistent dermoid cysts with characteristic manifestations best demonstrated on CT and MRI.

## 1.7 Malignant Ovarian Neoplasms

Stromoepithelial neoplasms account for 75% of all primary ovarian malignancies. The largest subgroup are serous or mucinous cysts. Simple invaginations of the celomic epithelium give rise to the classical serous papillary cystadenoma. Although these tend to be multiple, they are benign by histologic criteria. Another variation is germinal fibroadenoma. Pathologically these serous cysts have a smooth outer surface while the inner surface is studded with papillary excrescences. The cysts tend to be lobulated and multilocular, similar to those of the mucinous variety. The fluid is often chocolate colored and brownish secondary to admixture of blood. Transabdominal or transvaginal ultrasonography will readily demonstrate these lesions, as will contrast-enhanced CT and MRI (FORSTER et al. 1995). The presentation of thick septa and coexistent ascitis favors malignant lesions (MEDL et al. 1995). However, even histologically benign lesions may be associated with ascitis and massive omental "cake."

Mucinous tumors of the ovary (FIGO group II) may reach an enormous size (WOODRUFF 1991). However, they are less frequent that the serous variety. Histologically the endodermal origin is proven by the presence of argentophil granules. The tumors are intraovarian and only rarely papillary. Ultrasonography, CT, and MRI demonstrate a multilocular cyst composed of locules and compartments that appear to be separated by thin septa.

If these cysts perforate they may give rise to pseudomyxoma peritonei. The entire peritoneal cavity may then be filled with gelatinous material. The mucinous characteristic of the gelatinous material filling the peritoneum and encasing intra-abdominal organs is best appreciated on MRI using both T1- and T2-weighted scans (NOVAK and WOODRUFF 1979, pp 396–437).

**Table 1.2.**

| UICC | OVARY | FIGO |
|---|---|---|
| T1 | Limited to ovaries. | I |
| T1a | One ovary. No ascites. | Ia |
| T1b | Both ovaries. No ascites. | Ib |
| T1c | One or both ovaries. With ascites. | Ic |
| T2 | With pelvis extension. | II |
| T2a | Uterus *and/or* tubes. No ascites. | IIa |
| T2b | Other pelvic tissues. No ascites. | IIb |
| T2c | Other pelvic tissues. With ascites. | IIc |
| T3 | Extension to small bowel/omentum in true pelvis *or* intraperitoneal metastases/ intraperitoneal nodes. | III |
| M1 | Distant organs. | IV |

Endometrioid neoplasms (FIGO group III) are endometriomas that have undergone malignant degeneration. Hemorrhagic foci are frequently present.

Clear cell carcinomas (FIGO group IV) or adenosquamous carcinomas of the ovary feature cystic and solid components in the proportions dictated by the amount of stroma, the secretory activity, and the degree of degeneration. Stromal, tubal, papillary, mesothelial, and mixed histologic patterns can be found. Ultrasonography, contrast-enhanced CT, and MRI will again demonstrate the cystic, necrotic, and soft tissue elements of such tumors, as well as peritoneal implants and implants on the surface of other organs such as liver and spleen (FORSTER et al. 1995).

Stromoepithelial lesions are principally solid neoplasms, of which Brenner tumors, fibrothecomas, and sarcomas are the main representatives. The growth characteristics of Brenner tumors are similar to those of fibromas. There is little tendency to necrosis or cystic degeneration, and hemorrhage is likewise uncommon. These lesions therefore present on ultrasonography, CT, and MRI as solid masses of soft tissue density (NOVAK and WOODRUFF 1979, pp 451–460).

Fibromas are likewise solid tumors. They may cause Meig's syndrome, i.e., hydrothorax and ascitis. On ultrasonography, CT, and MRI they exhibit characteristics of a solid soft tissue tumor (NOVAK and WOODRUFF 1979, pp 451–460).

Metastases to the ovary are common and have been described as Krukenberg tumors (HA et al. 1995; COPPLESON 1992, pp 987–1002). The brisk stromal reaction to the tumor and the paucity of epithelial elements often cause a histologic misdiagnosis of sarcoma (COPPLESON 1992, pp 987–1002). The desmoblastic reaction may extend into the mesovarium and on MRI and CT may give rise to a classical spoke-wheel pattern (HA et al. 1995). The tumor metastasis itself tends to be a solid soft tissue tumor. Only rarely when it outgrows the vascular supply may there be areas of necrosis and cyst formation.

## 1.8 Benign Tumors of the Vagina

Gartner's cysts, vestigial wolffian duct remnants, are encountered in the anterior lateral wall of the vagina. They frequently form a tiny string of cysts and are readily identifiable on endovaginal ultrasonography. Vaginal inclusion cysts are found in the posterior lateral wall of the vagina near the introitus. They are again readily identifiable on transvaginal ultrasonography.

Endometriosis and adenomyomas can occur anywhere in the vagina; however, the most common site is the posterior fornix. CT, MRI, and transvaginal ultrasonography will readily identify these tumors.

Leiomyomas, fibromyomas, and neurofibromas, as well as polyps, occur in the vagina. In appearance, polyps may simulate sarcoma botryoides. The surface location of these lesions leads to their identification by visual inspection. On imaging studies they present as solid masses.

Carcinoma of the vagina, malignant melanoma, fibro- and leiomyosarcoma, and sarcoma botryoides are usually diagnosed by visual inspection and biopsy. MRI and CT, however, are useful to identify the degree of penetration and depth of invasion as well as the presence of lymph node metastases (FORSTER et al. 1995).

Choriocarcinoma of the vagina is encountered in patients with primary uterine trophoblastic neoplasms. Primary diagnosis is based on visual inspection. Presence of concomitant disease in the uterus can be assessed by imaging studies such as transvaginal ultrasonography, MRI, and contrast-enhanced CT as well as arteriography.

Metastatic carcinoma, most often to the "cuff" of the vagina, is most frequently a recurrence of cervical carcinoma. Contiguous extension of bladder or rectal neoplasms can also occur. The magnitude of penetration and extension of the neoplasm is readily assessed by MRI and CT.

## 1.9 Mass Lesions of the Vulva

Bartholin's adenitis or abscesses are a common inflammatory mass of the introitus. Their presence may be revealed on transvaginal ultrasonography, CT, and MRI (FORSTER et al. 1995). Bartholin's duct cysts present in an identical fashion but not necessarily with inflammatory manifestations. Sebaceous cysts also present in this region.

Condylomata acuminata, fibromas, fibromyomas, lipomas, angiomas, and neurofibromas are solid tumors of this region. MRI, CT, and transvaginal ultrasonography have a place in the assessment of contiguous extension and permeation, particularly in cases of condylomatous carcinoma. Carcinoma of the vulva also can be assessed by transvaginal

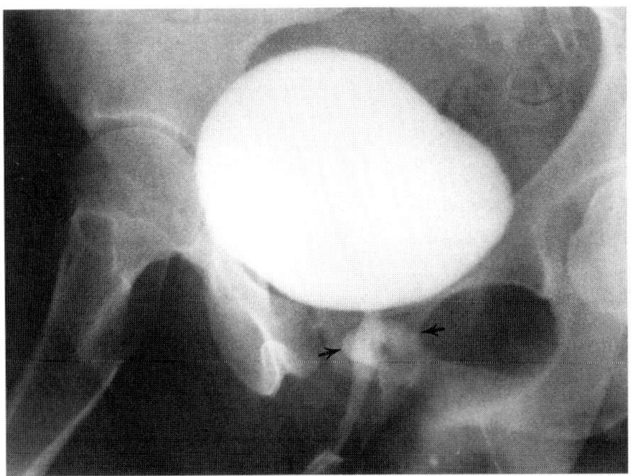

**Fig. 1.2.** A double balloon urethrogram demonstrates a compound suburethral diverticulum (arrows). Note that the intercommunicating diverticulur sacs are actually wrapped around the urethra

ultrasonography CT, and MRI for adjacent spread to the urethra, perineum, or anus or even infiltration of the bladder mucosa or rectal mucosa, as well as for the presence of enlarged regional lymph nodes (FORSTER et al. 1995).

## 1.10 Mass Lesions of the Urethra

Infected paraurethral glands (Skene's ducts) frequently present as a mass in the anterior vaginal wall. When liquefaction necrosis ensues, the abscess tends to drain into the urethra and form a suburethral diverticulum. Urethrography of the female urethra performed with a double balloon system (Lang-Davis balloon catheter) will opacify and demonstrate these often multiple interconnected saccular structures (Fig. 1.2). Transvaginal ultrasonography and voiding cystography are likewise useful for identification of this lesion.

Adenocarcinoma of the urethra is a relatively rare lesion. Contiguous penetration and extension of this tumor can be assessed by transvaginal ultrasonography, MRI, and, to a limited degree, CT.

## References


Chumas JC, Nelson B, Mann WJ, Chalos E, Kaplan CG (1985) Microglandular hyperplasia of the uterine cervix. Obstet Gynecol 66:406–409

Cicinelli E, Romano F, Anastasio PS, et al. (1995) Transabdominal sonohysterography, transvaginal sonography and hysteroscopy in the evaluation of submucous myomas. Obstet Gynecol 85:42–47

Coppleson M(ed) (1992) Gynecologic oncology: fundamental principles and clinical practice, 2nd edn, vol 2. Churchill Livingstone, Edinburgh, pp 731–802

Creasmen WT, Morrow CP, Bundy L, et al. (1987) The surgical pathologic spread pattern of endometrial cancer: a Gynecologic-Oncology Group study. 60:2035–2041

Fischetti SG, Politi G, Lomeo E, et al. (1994) Carcinoma of the uterus and cervical canal staging and biometric assessment with magnetic resonance. Radiol Med (Torino) 88:445–452

Forster R, Hricak H, White S (1995) CT and MRI of ovarian cancer. Abdom Imaging 20:228–233

Gross BH, Silver LM, Jaffe MH (1983) Sonographic features of uterine leiomyomas: analysis 41 proven cases. Gen Ultrasound Med 2:401–407

Ha HK, Baek SY, Kim HH, et al. (1995) Krukenberg's tumor of the ovary. MR imaging features. AJR 164:1435–1439

Medl M, Kulenkampff KJ, Stiskal M, et al. (1995) Magnetic Resonance imaging. Pre-operative evaluation of suspect ovarian masses. Anticancer Res 15:1123–1225

Novak ER, Woodruff JD (1979) Novak's gynecologic and obstetric pathology, 8th edn. W.B. Saunders, Philadelphia

Schnall MV (1994) Magnetic Resonance evaluation of uterine malignancies. Semin Ultrasound CT MR 15:27–37

Smith RC, McCarthy S (1994) Magnetic staging of neoplasms of the uterus. Radiol Clin North Am 32:109–131

Vedantham S, Goodman SG, McLucas B, Forno AE (1997) Uterine Artery embolization for ŭterine Fibroids: results of pilot study. A&R 168 (Suppl):41

Woodruff JD (1991) Pre-malignant and malignant disorders of the ovaries and oviduct. In: Pernoll HI (ed) Current obstetric and gynecologic diagnoses and treatment. Lange-Appleton, Norwalk, Conn., pp 974–994

# 2 Sonography in the Assessment of Benign and Malignant Conditions of the Uterus

M. ATRI

CONTENTS



## 2.1 Introduction

There has been a significant improvement in the imaging of the female pelvis over the past decade, especially with the introduction of endovaginal sonography. Ultrasound remains the primary imaging modality of the pelvis in women due to its widespread availability and low cost, despite the advances in computerized tomography and magnetic resonance imaging. Other advantages of ultrasound are that it provides high resolution, unlimited planes of examination, and the possibility of dynamic scanning. The advent of endovaginal sonography has provided a major improvement over the transabdominal approach because of the proximity to the area of interest, which permits the use of a higher frequency transducer (MENDELSON et al. 1988a; LANDE et al. 1988; LEIBMAN et al. 1988; ANDOLF and JORGENSEN 1990). High-frequency transducers significantly improve resolution. The addition of endovaginal color Doppler helps increase the accuracy of gray-scale imaging under certain circumstances. Some specific cases where endovaginal sonography is more useful than transabdominal sonography are in obese women, in women with a retroverted uterus, and when there is surgical dressing that prevents optimal access with the transabdominal approach. In addition, the fact that a full bladder is not required is considered by most patients to be a major advantage of endovaginal sonography. In fact, endovaginal sonography should be the starting examination of the pelvis when there is a clinical question of any endometrial or subendometrial pathology, such as submucosal fibroid or adenomyosis.

M. ATRI, MD, Associate Professor of Radiology, McGill University; Associate Professor, Department of Obstetrics and Gynecology; Director, Ultrasound Division, Department of Radiology, Montreal General Hospital, 1650 Cedar Avenue, Montréal, Québec H3G 1A4, Canada

## 2.2 Technique

At our institution, endovaginal sonography is the starting examination for all gynecologic pathologies, while transabdominal sonography is the initial examination only if endovaginal sonography cannot be performed because of technical difficulty or patient preference. This practice is based on the proven advantages of endovaginal sonography over transabdominal sonography (MENDELSON et al. 1988a; LANDE et al. 1988; LEIBMAN et al. 1988; ANDOLF and JORGENSEN 1990) and the low yield of transabdominal sonography following an adequate endovaginal sonographic examination (ATRI et al. 1994a). This approach is also recommended by other authors (MENDELSON et al. 1988b; TESSLER et al. 1989). We perform transabdominal sonography after endovaginal sonography if there is a large pelvic pathology (for example, large fibroids) and usually with an empty bladder. Endovaginal sonography is limited under these circumstances due to the smaller field of view and lower penetration of the high-frequency transducer. The uterus is optimally visualized by endovaginal sonography when it is either retroverted or anteverted, the latter being the normal position in most women when the bladder is empty. Visualization of the uterus is less optimal when it has a horizontal lie, since this increases the distance between the transducer and the fundus. In addition, a horizontal uterus lies parallel to the beam, whereas the endometrium is best visualized when it is perpendicular to the beam.

In sonography, we use two general principles to better assess the organ of interest:

1. The structure that is the focus of the examination should lie in the focal zone of the transducer. This is achieved by changing the transducer, modifying its focal zone, or changing the distance between the transducer and the area of interest using a different approach or by compressing the tissues between the transducer and the organ of interest.
2. Dynamic scanning helps identity the origin of a pathology by looking for concordant or discordant movement. This can be evaluated by examining the two adjacent structures while the patient is breathing or, in the case of endovaginal sonography, by bimanual examination with the probe in the vagina and one hand palpating the pelvis suprapubically.

Transabdominal sonography requires a full bladder, which causes the bowel containing gas to be displaced out of the pelvis and allows the bladder to be used as a window through which the organs of interest may be visualized. In general, adequate examination requires a full bladder that covers the fundus of the uterus. Overdistension of the bladder should be avoided because it distorts the anatomy and displaces the areas of interest beyond the focal zone of the transducer. A 3.5-MHz transducer is adequate for most pelvic examinations, whereas a 5-MHz transducer is reserved for more superficial structures.

For endovaginal sonography, the smallest possible end-fire probe increases the maneuverability of the transducer, which is crucial for the optimal visualization of pelvic organs through the vagina because of the small field of view. Endovaginal sonography transducers range from 5 to 7.5 MHz. The transducer is covered by a long condom that minimizes contamination of the probe, and a nonspermicidal lubricant, especially in the premenopausal group, is applied both inside and outside the condom.

The bladder should be empty in order to bring the pelvic structures into the focal zone of the transducer. In addition, a full bladder changes the position of the uterus from an anteverted to a horizontal lie, which is not the ideal position for endovaginal sonographic examination of the uterus. One of the disadvantages of performing endovaginal sonography following transabdominal sonography is the continuous filling of the bladder during the endovaginal sonographic examination. The examination is performed with the patient in the supine position with the knees bent and the pelvis elevated by a cushion to increase the maneuverability of the probe. Bringing the knees up over the abdomen further enhances the posterior movement of the transducer and allows better visualization of the more anteriorly located structures. The transducer lies in the anterior or posterior fornix for examination of the uterus or ovaries. Moving the probe from one fornix to the other may improve visualization of some structures. Visualization of the uterus is straightforward in most cases. However, partial withdrawal and significant anterior or posterior angulation of the probe may be necessary to visualize a uterus that is extremely anteverted or retroverted. Identification of the cervix helps localize the uterus when the latter is displaced significantly by the presence of a large pelvic mass. The cervix is best examined by endovaginal sonography after slight withdrawal of the probe.

If an endovaginal examination is not possible (for example, because the vagina is small) and transabdominal sonography is suboptimal, the transrectal approach helps visualize the uterus, especially when it is retroverted (Fig. 2.1).

The cervix and, specifically, the vagina are better visualized by the transrectal approach. The cervix

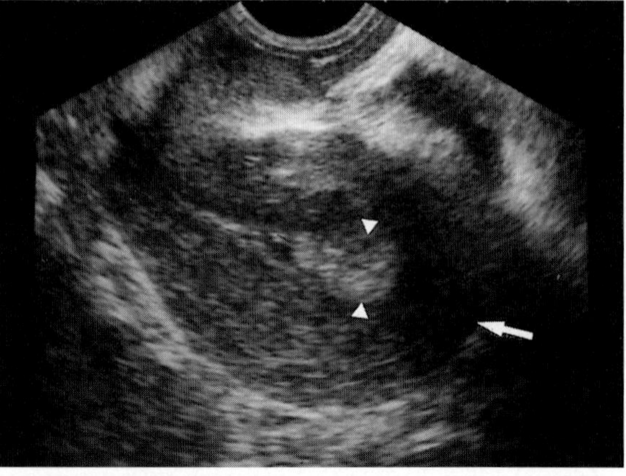

**Fig. 2.1.** Transrectal examination of a retroverted uterus. An endometrial polyp (*arrowheads*) is seen close to the fundus (*arrow*) of a retroverted uterus

of pregnant women can also be assessed by the transperineal approach (HERTZBERG et al. 1991).

## 2.3 Normal Anatomy

The vagina is a musculomembranous tube (7–9 cm in length) that descends anteroinferiorly from the rectouterine pouch. The cervix of the uterus projects into the anterior wall of the vagina. Therefore, the uterus is almost perpendicular to the vagina in its normal anteverted position when the bladder is empty. The fornices are found surrounding the cervix in the upper part of the vagina and include the anterior, posterior, and lateral fornices. The posterior fornix is the deepest part of the vagina and the only part that is covered by peritoneum. More inferiorly to the posterior fornix, the vagina is in contact with the rectum through the rectovaginal septum. Anteriorly, the vagina is in contact with the cervix, the base of the bladder, the terminal parts of the ureters, and the urethra. Laterally, the lateral fornices are attached to the broad ligaments. More inferiorly, the lateral walls are in contact with the levator ani muscles (WILLIAMS et al. 1989).

The uterus is a muscular organ 7–8 cm long, 5–7 cm wide, and 2–3 cm thick. It consists of two major parts: the expanded superior two-thirds, known as the body, and the cylindrical inferior third, called the cervix. The cervix has a vaginal and a supravaginal component. The junction of the cervix and body is a narrow transitional zone called the isthmus. The fundus of the uterus is the rounded superior part of the body that lies above the line joining the point of entrance of the fallopian tubes. This point of entrance is called the cornum. The layers of the uterus consist of a thin outer serous perimetrium, the middle thick muscular myometrium, and the inner mucous endometrium (WILLIAMS et al. 1989).

The uterus is enclosed between the layers of the broad ligament. The ligaments of the ovaries and the round ligaments of the uterus are attached to the uterus, posteroinferior and anteroinferior to the uterotubal junctions, respectively. The blood supply of the uterus is derived mainly from the uterine arteries, which are branches of the internal iliac arteries. They run in the broad ligaments and enter the uterus beside the lateral fornices. At the isthmus of the uterus, they divide into an ascending branch that supplies the body and a descending branch that supplies the cervix and vagina. The venous drainage of the uterus forms the uterine venous plexus on each side of the cervix and is a tributary of the iliac veins. They are connected with the superior rectal vein to form a portosystemic anastomosis (WILLIAMS et al. 1989).

## 2.4 Normal Sonographic Anatomy

The position of the uterus is anteverted on endovaginal sonography in most women with an empty bladder. It usually lies on the midline but may be tilted to one side. With retroversion, both cervix and body rotate counterclockwise. In an anteflexed or retroflexed uterus, the cervix is relatively constant but the body tilts; therefore, the angle between the cervix and body is accentuated. The fundus of a retroverted uterus is difficult to assess on transabdominal sonography; it may appear hypoechoic when its deep position places it outside the focal zone of the transducer. However, it is ideally located for endovaginal sonography because the probe is usually in the posterior fornix, placing it in proximity to a retroverted uterus.

The shape and size of the uterus vary with age. The cervix is longer and more prominent than the corpus in an infantile uterus. This relationship reverses in the adult uterus. Therefore, the uterus is more tubular or the cervix is wider than the fundus in infancy. The infantile uterus measures 2–3.3 cm in length and 0.5–1 cm in anteroposterior diameter. The cervix constitutes two-thirds of the length (SAMPLE et al. 1977). The uterus size and shape remain unchanged for up to 7 years, at which time the size and the ratio between the body and cervix start changing. As puberty approaches, the diameter and length of the body are double the size of the cervix (ORSINI et al. 1984). There is good correlation between the size of the uterus measured by sonography and its gross measurement at histopathology (PLATT et al. 1990; SAXTON et al. 1990). The normal postpubertal uterus varies in size with a mean maximum length of 8 cm, maximum width of 5 cm, and maximum anteroposterior diameter of 4 cm (PLATT et al. 1990). The size of the uterus is estradiol dependent, increasing slightly during the cycle and reaching its maximum size the day before ovulation (EDEN et al. 1988). This variation in size appears to be more marked in women with polycystic ovary disease (ADAMS et al. 1988). The uterus is slightly larger and the endometrium contains fluid in the immediate neonatal period because of the influence of the mother's hormonal stimulation (NUSSBAUM et al.

1986). The size of the uterus increases by 1 cm with multiple pregnancies (MILLER et al. 1977). The uterus decreases in size after the menopause, especially during the first 5–10 years. The postmenopausal uterus varies from 3.5 to 6.5 cm in length and from 1.2 to 1.8 cm in anteroposterior diameter (MILLER et al. 1977).

The endometrium is consistently seen on endovaginal sonography if the uterus is ante- or retroverted and there is no distortion of the endometrium by a uterine mass. The endometrial size and thickness vary with the menstrual cycle. The appearance of the endometrium on endovaginal sonography closely follows the histologic appearance. The endometrium consists of an outer basalis and an inner functionalis layer. The functionalis layer thickens under the influence of estrogen in the proliferative phase and undergoes changes in the secretory phase under the influence of progesterone. It makes up the major component of shedding with menstruation. The endometrium appears as a thin echogenic line representing the specular reflection of the beam immediately following menstruation. Later in the follicular phase, the endometrium takes a trilayer appearance (Fig. 2.2a,b). The central thin echogenic line corresponds to the specular reflection, the hypoechoic middle band represents an edematous functionalis layer, and an outer echogenic band corresponds to the basalis layer (Fig. 2.2a,b). The functionalis layer thickens as the follicular phase advances and reaches its maximum thickness just before ovulation (Fig. 2.2c). In addition, the functionalis layer gradually increases in echogenicity to become isoechoic to the basalis layer after ovulation, resulting in a unilayered echogenic endometrium (FLEISCHER et al. 1986a) (Fig. 2.2d). The

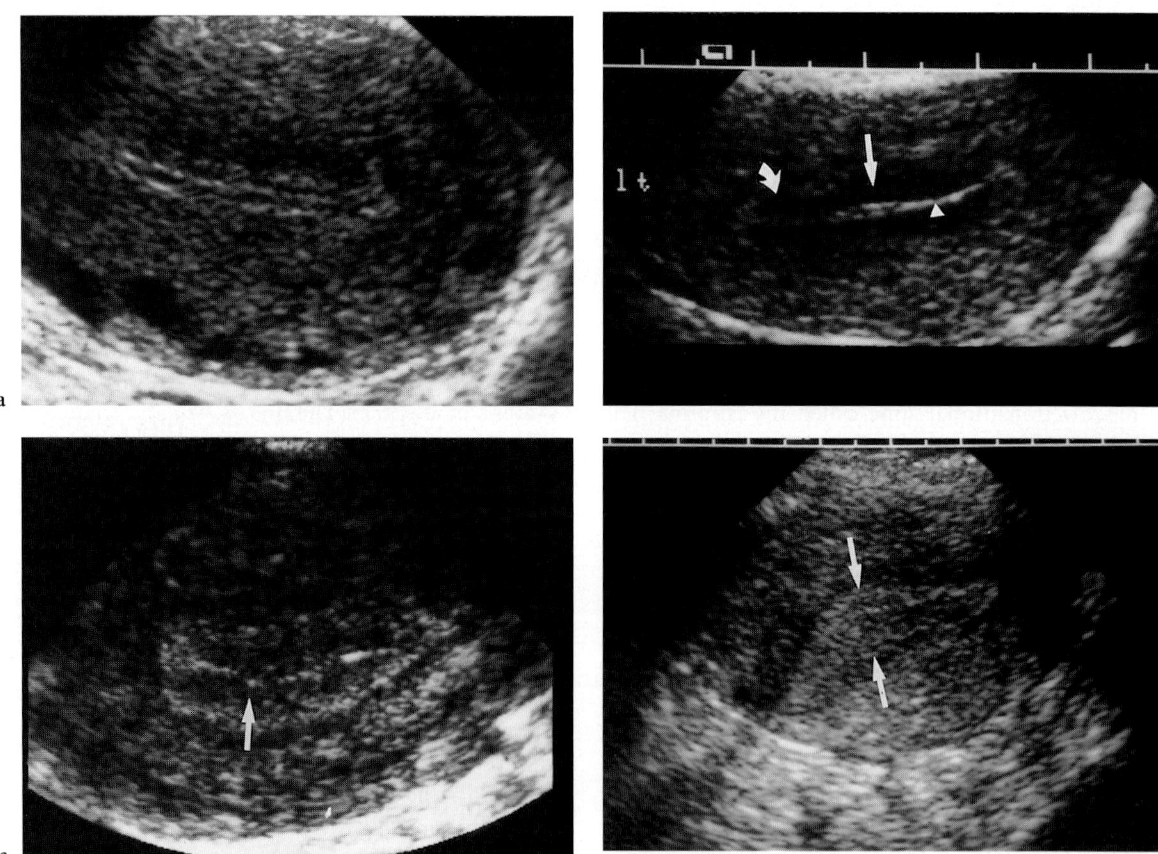


**Fig. 2.2 a–d.** Endometrial changes in a normal menstrual cycle. **a** Endometrium shortly after the termination of menstruation shows a trilayered appearance. **b** On day 7 of the cycle (early proliferative phase) increased thickness of the endometrium is seen, mostly due to thickening of the functionalis layer. The inner echogenic line corresponds to the specular reflection at the endometrial interface (*arrowhead*), the middle hypoechoic layer represents the functionalis layer (*straight arrow*), and the outer echogenic layer corresponds to the basalis layer (*curved arrow*). **c** Late profliferative phase endometrium demonstrates a further increase in the endometrial thickness and increased echogenicity of the functionalis layer (*arrow*). **d** Postovulatory secretory phase endometrium shows a single-layered echogenic endometrium (*arrows*)

increased echogenicity of the functionalis layer is likely due to a combination of an increased mucous and glycogen content of the glands and more interfaces created by increased tortuosity of the endometrial vessels. This transition from trilayered endometrium to unilayered endometrium predicts ovulation with 93% accuracy (Forrest et al. 1988). Although the endometrial thickness is generally higher in the secretory phase than in the follicular phase and a higher ultrasound grade of endometrium suggests the normal histology of the secretory phase, endovaginal sonography cannot replace endometrial biopsy for evaluating luteal phase adequacy (Doherty et al. 1993; Li et al. 1992). The endometrial thickness is best measured on a sagittal view from the myometrial–endometrial junction to the central cavity interface. If the central echo is not visible, the total anteroposterior thickness is measured and is divided by 2 for a single-layer measurement. The sonographic measurement of the endometrium is within 1 mm of the measurement at histology (Fleischer et al. 1986a). The endometrium measures 2–4 mm during the proliferative phase and 5–6 mm during the secretory phase. The endometrium atrophies with menopause and measures less than 5 mm (Fleischer et al. 1986b).

The myometrium has an intermediate echotexture, which is usually less than the endometrium. The inner myometrium is hypoechoic and forms the subendometrial hypoechoic halo. This appears to correspond to the more compact and less vascular myometrium (Fleischer et al. 1986b; Farrer-Brown et al. 1970). Arcuate arteries and veins are seen at the junction of the middle and outer thirds of the myometrium. Veins present as thin-walled distended spaces and arteries as single- or double-layered echogenic structures (Fig. 2.3). Radial and spiral vessels run perpendicular to the arcuate

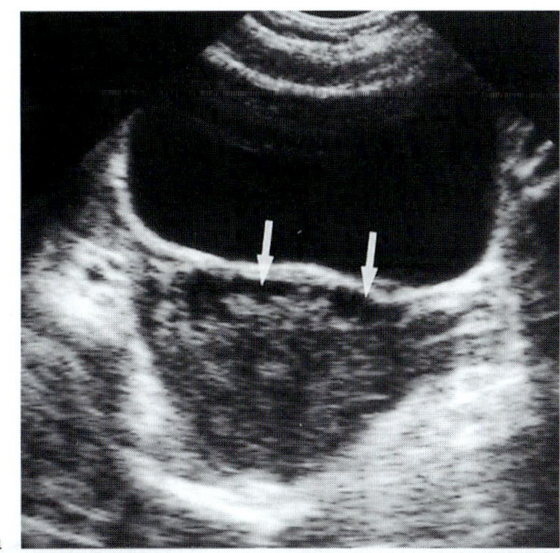

a

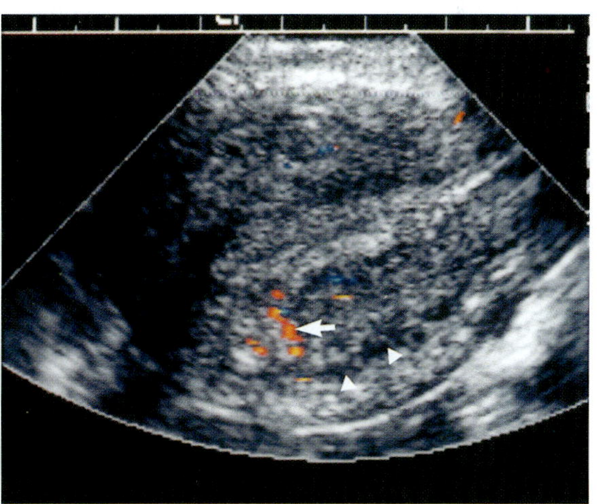

c

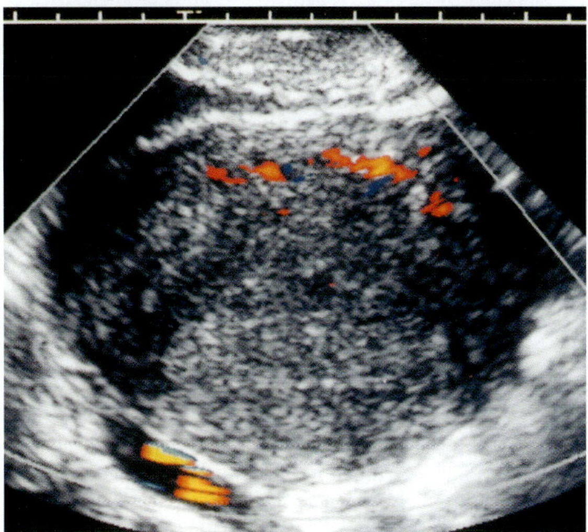

b

**Fig. 2.3 a–c.** Normal myometrial vessels. **a** Suprapubic sonographic examination shows thin-walled arcuate veins (*arrows*) in the periphery of uterus anteriorly. **b** Transverse color Doppler endovaginal sonographic examination demonstrates the arcuate vessels at the junction of the middle two-thirds and outer one-third of the myometrium. **c** Longitudinal color Doppler endovaginal sonographic examination illustrates the radial and spiral vessels (*arrow*) running perpendicular to the arcuate vessles (*arrowheads*)

vessels leading to the endometrium (Fig. 2.3c). Mönckeberg arteriosclerosis of arcuate arteries increases the echogenicity of these vessels, which may be associated with shadowing. This condition results in calcification of the medium-sized arteries and is seen more commonly in diabetic patients (Fig. 2.4) (Atri et al. 1992).

Three landmarks help identify the uterus. The best landmark is the endometrium. In the presence of significant distortion of the endometrium by multiple fibroids, the uterus can be located by following the cervix. In some postmenopausal women with a very small uterus and an atrophic endometrium, the presence of Mönckeberg calcification helps localize the uterus (Fig. 2.5).

## 2.5 Congenital Uterine Anomalies

Müllerian duct anomalies result from the following: (a) arrested development, (b) partial or complete nonfusion of the müllerian ducts, or (c) nonresorption of the median septum. They occur in 1%–5% of women (Sorensen 1988; Zanetti et al. 1978). Due to the close embryologic relationship of the müllerian and wolffian systems, müllerian duct anomalies may be associated with renal anomalies, most commonly renal agenesis or ectopia (Gilsanz et al. 1982; Fore et al. 1975; Berman et al. 1989; Rosenberg et al. 1986). These anomalies are particularly seen with vaginal agenesis, unicornuate uterus, or duplicated müllerian duct anomalies (Gilsanz et al. 1982; Fore et al. 1975; Berman et al. 1989; Rosenberg et al. 1986). The relevance of müllerian duct anomalies lies in an increased incidence of impaired fertility. Women with these disorders usually have no difficulty conceiving but do have a high frequency of spontaneous abortion, premature birth, abnormal fetal presentation, dystocia, and abnormal uterine activity during delivery (Buttram and Gibbons 1979).

### 2.5.1 Classification of Müllerian Duct Anomalies

Different terminologies and classifications for müllerian duct anomalies have been used in the past, resulting in confusion about this entity (Buttram 1983). A frequently used classification grouped these anomalies into symmetric or asymmetric double malformation. The most recent classification of müllerian duct anomalies is based upon the degree of failure of normal development and thus separates the anomalies into groups with similar clinical manifestations, treatments, and prognoses for fetal salvage (Buttram 1983; The American Fertility Society 1988). Six classes are identified (Fig. 2.6):

*Class I*, a form of bilateral arrested development, consists of different combinations of agenesis or hypoplasia of the vagina, cervix, and uterus.

*Class II*, a form of unilateral arrested development, is a unicornuate uterus either with or without

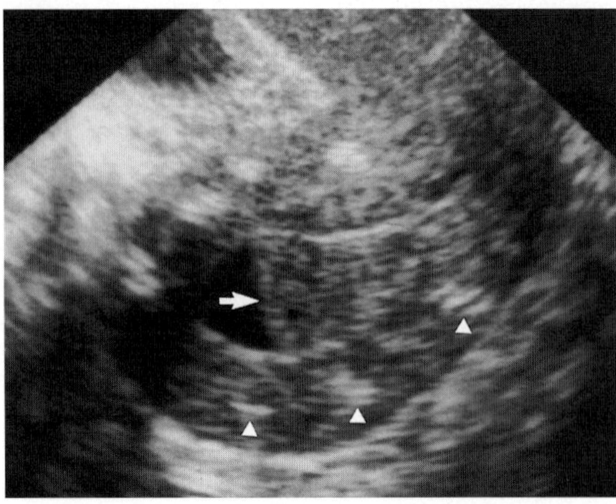

**Fig. 2.4.** Mönckeberg calcification. Longitudinal endovaginal sonography shows fluid level (*arrow*) in a distended uterine cavity in a postmenopausal woman. Benign cervical stenosis was present. Notice the small linear echogenic foci in the periphery of the uterus (*arrowheads*), consistent with Mönckeberg calcification

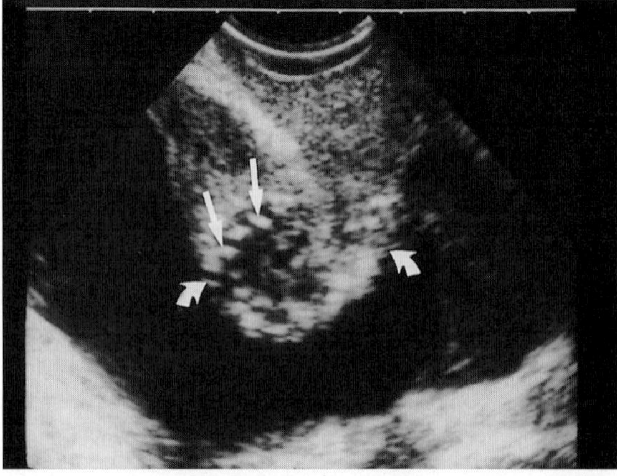

**Fig. 2.5.** Mönckeberg calcifications help identify the uterus. Multiple small peripheral linear calcifications (*straight arrows*) confirm the presence of a small atrophic uterus (*curved arrows*)

a rudimentary horn. The latter may or may not contain endometrium and may or may not be communicating with the main endometrial cavity. In a noncommunicating endometrium, no clinical symptoms occur if the endometrium is nonfunctional, but with a functional endometrium, retention of menstrual blood may occur, resulting in hematometra. Review of the literature shows a 48% abortion rate in this group (Buttram 1983).

*Class III*, a form of fusion failure, is uterus didelphys with two separate uteri with two cervices and usually a sagittal septum in the vagina. Literature review of this anomaly by Buttram (1983) shows a 43% abortion rate, similar to that of class II anomalies. Both class II and class III have a high rate of premature delivery (Buttram 1983).

*Class IV*, also a form of fusion failure, is a bicornuate uterus, which varies from a complete bicornuate uterus with two cervices (bicornuate bicolis) to an incomplete bicornuate uterus with one cervix. Although in most series the normal pregnancy rate is similar to that of the general population, Buttram (1983) found an abortion rate of 35% in his review of the literature.

*Class V*, due to failure of resorption of the median septum, is a septate uterus, which is either a complete (involving cervix) or an incomplete (subseptate, not involving cervix) septum. These anomalies are associated with a high spontaneous abortion rate, possibly because of the poor blood supply to the septum. In a series by McShane et al. (1983), 69% of pregnancies with a septate uterus resulted in abortion. The abortion rate appears to be related to the completion of the septum (Buttram 1983).

*Class VI*, an arcuate uterus, is a very mild form of bicornuate uterus that is considered a normal variant. In the original classification of müllerian duct anomalies by Buttram, an arcuate uterus is considered a mild form of class IV.

The sagittal vaginal septa, which may exist alone but usually coexist with müllerian anomalies, occur concurrently with approximately 75% of class III, less than 5% of class IV, and 25% of class V anomalies (Buttram 1983).

### 2.5.2 Sonographic Diagnosis of Müllerian Duct Anomalies

The septate uterus is the most common anomaly and is associated with the highest spontaneous abortion rate. This anomaly can be treated by hysteroscopic excision on an outpatient basis (Daly et al. 1983). A bicornuate uterus has a septum containing myometrium and, if unification is planned, its vascularity necessitates transabdominal resection. Therefore, one of the main indications for imaging is to differentiate between a septate and a bicornuate uterus. Laparoscopy is the standard of reference for making this distinction. Hysterosalpingography has been used in the past for noninvasive evaluation of congenital anomalies. However, its accuracy is low when differentiating between bicornuate and septate uteri. Reuter et al. (1989) demonstrated that hysterosalpingography alone had a diagnostic accuracy of 55% in distinguishing a septate from a bicornuate uterus. When sonography and hysterosalpingography were used together, the diagnostic

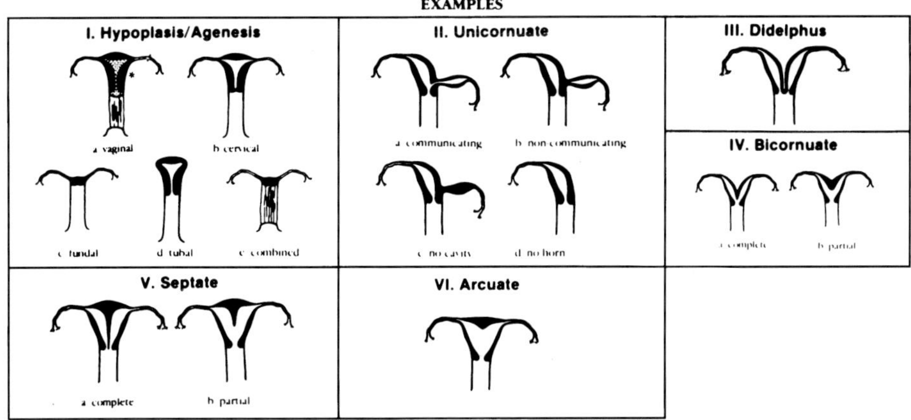


**Fig. 2.6.** The American Fertility Society classification of müllerian anomalies

accuracy improved to 90%, with all errors being noncritical. However, most reports on the use of sonography for evaluating müllerian duct anomalies are based on the use of transabdominal sonography. The differentiation between bicornuate and septate uteri is made by the detection of an external fundal notch in the bicornuate uterus and a flat or convex outer border in a septate uterus (Figs. 2.7, 2.8). In a group of 43 "bifid" uteri, FEDELE et al. (1988a) reported that the sensitivity of sonography in detecting the presence of a fundal notch was 92.3% and its specificity 100%, after excluding those cases that could not be evaluated (marked uterine retroflexion or myomas). The same investigators (FEDELE et al. 1989) could correctly predict the outcome of pregnancy in a group of 12 pregnancies in septate uteri. Eight of twelve pregnancies terminated in spontaneous abortion; all had an embryo implanted on the septum. In the remaining four that delivered live neonates, sonography demonstrated embryo implantation on the lateral wall. The differentiation of a unicornuate uterus from a normal uterus may be difficult if one does not consider this diagnosis. The clue to the diagnosis is the small narrow appearance of a uterus that is laterally positioned. A unicornuate uterus with a rudimentary horn could potentially be mistaken for a uterus with a subserosal fibroid or an adnexal mass if the central echo is not appreciated or does not exist in the rudimentary horn (Fig. 2.9). In a group of 14 infertile women with a documented unicornuate uterus with rudimentary horns, sonography demonstrated a sensitivity of 85.7% and a specificity of 100% in diagnosing the presence of a rudimentary horn and a sensitivity of 80% and a specificity of 100% in diagnosing the presence of a cavity in the rudimentary horn (FEDELE et al. 1988b). One of the horns of a bicornuate uterus may also be obstructed (Fig. 2.10).

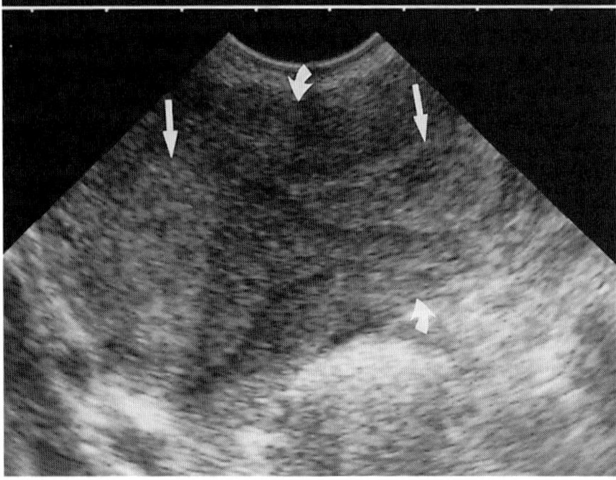

**Fig. 2.7.** Transverse endovaginal sonographic appearance of a bicornuate uterus. Two endometrical echoes (*straight arrows*) are seen in the region of fundus. Indentations (*curved arrows*) are present on the anteroposterior aspects of the fundus

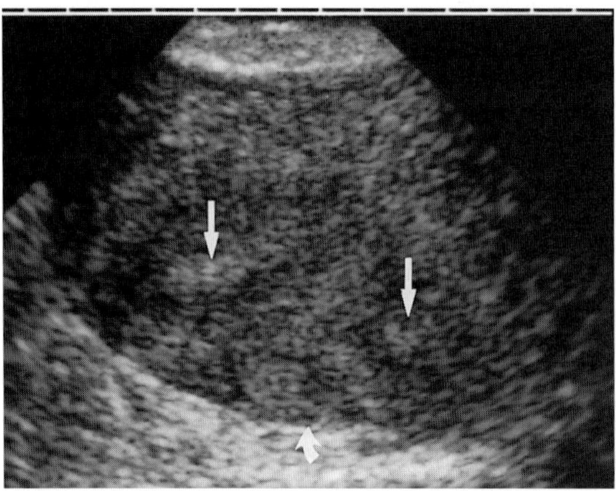

**Fig. 2.8.** Transverse endovaginal sonographic appearance of a septate uterus. Two endometrial echoes (*straight arrows*) are present. The posterosuperior aspect of the fundus is convex (*curved arrow*)

The data on the role of endovaginal sonography in the evaluation of women with müllerian duct anomalies is limited. In one series correlating endovaginal sonography and magnetic resonance imaging for the diagnosis of müllerian duct anomalies, magnetic resonance imaging had a sensitivity and specificity of 100% and endovaginal sonography had a sensitivity of 100% but a specificity of 80%. A bicornuate or didelphys uterus was differentiated from a septate uterus by the presence of bowel in the fundal notch (PELLERITO et al. 1992). The 80% specificity of endovaginal sonography was due to the presence of bowel in a fundal notch in a case of septate uterus (PELLERITO et al. 1992). Magnetic resonance imaging is being recognized as an accurate method of diagnosing müllerian duct anomalies (PELLERITO et al. 1992; CARRINGTON et al. 1990). The initial magnetic resonance imaging reports with respect to differentiation of septate and bicornuate uteri emphasized the difference in signal intensity of the tissue separating the two endometrial cavities (MINTZ et al. 1987). More recent reports show overlap between the two entities for this sign but emphasize the diagnosis based on the presence of a deep external fundal notch (PELLERITO et al. 1992; CARRINGTON et al. 1990). Since the appearance of the external contour appears to be the determining factor for distinguishing septate from bicornuate uteri, sonography should theoretically be as accurate

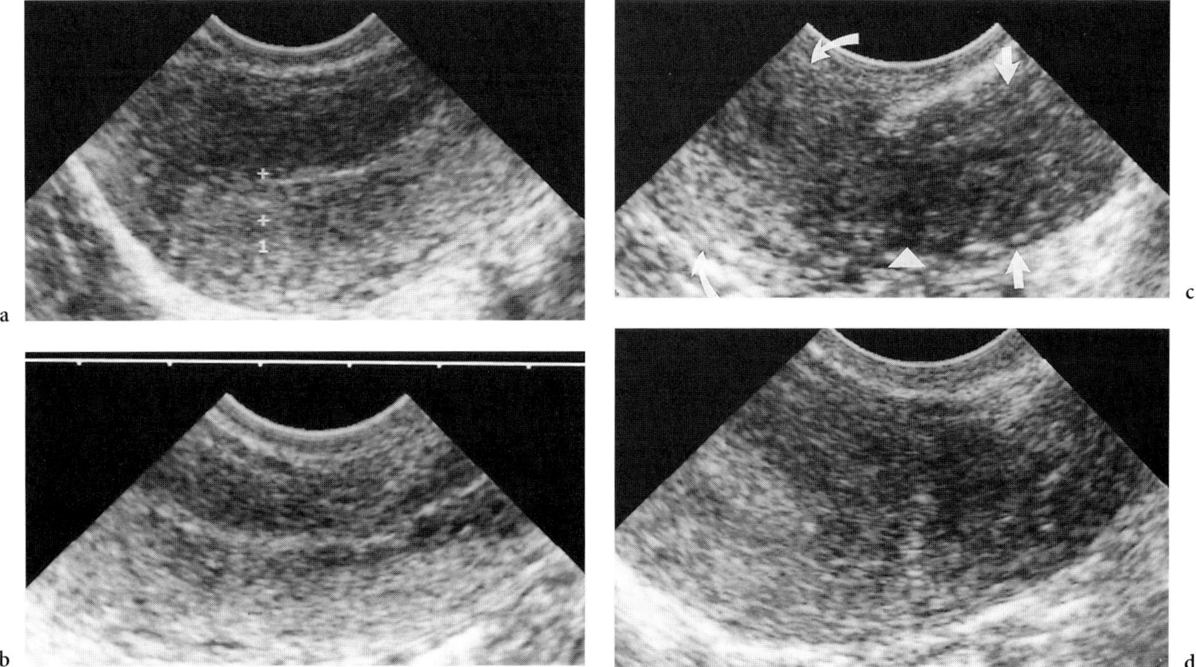

**Fig. 2.9 a–d.** Bicornuate uterus with a rudimentary horn. **a** Sagittal view of the normal horn. **b** Sagittal view of the small horn. **c** Transverse view of the lower uterine segment shows the small left horn (*straight arrows*) and normal right horn (*curved arrows*). A small indentation posteriorly (*arrowhead*) confirms the existence of a bicornuate uterus. **d** Transverse view of the upper body again demonstrates the asymmetry of the two horns

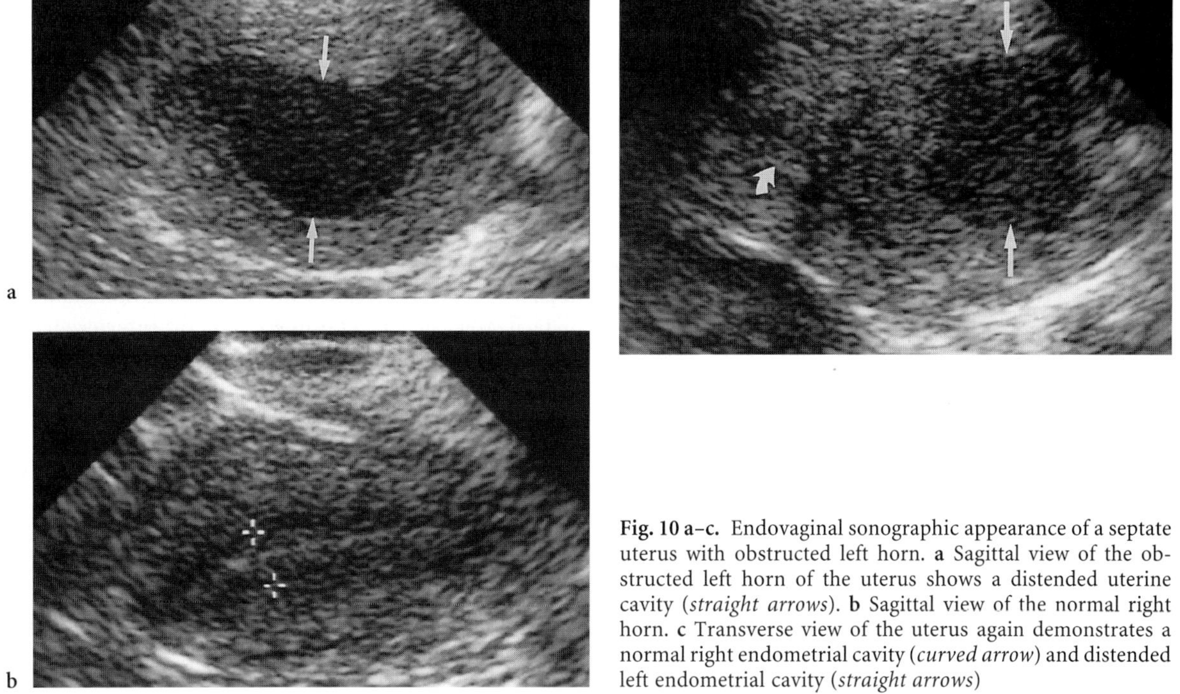

**Fig. 10 a–c.** Endovaginal sonographic appearance of a septate uterus with obstructed left horn. **a** Sagittal view of the obstructed left horn of the uterus shows a distended uterine cavity (*straight arrows*). **b** Sagittal view of the normal right horn. **c** Transverse view of the uterus again demonstrates a normal right endometrial cavity (*curved arrow*) and distended left endometrial cavity (*straight arrows*)

as magnetic resonance imaging or laparoscopy (Figs. 2.7, 2.8). However, the limitation of sonography is the difficulty in visualizing the uterus in a true coronal position, which is essential to the diagnosis. Further experience with a combination of transabdominal sonography and endovaginal sonography may increase the accuracy of sonography.

## 2.6 Uterine Abnormalities

From an imaging point of view, uterine abnormalities can be classified as myometrial, subendometrial, or endometrial.

### 2.6.1 Myometrial Abnormalities

Fibroids (leiomyomas) and adenomyosis are the two common nonmalignant conditions of the uterus. Adenomyosis is discussed in Sect. 2.6.2. Cesarean section defect is a less commonly seen abnormality of the myometrium.

#### *2.6.1.1 Leiomyoma*

Leiomyomas occur in 20%–30% of women older than 35 years and are more common in black women (Kurman 1994). They are rare in women younger than 18 years. They appear to be estrogen dependent, increasing in size in women taking oral contraceptives and in pregnant women and decreasing in size in women on the gonadotropin-releasing hormone analogs and after menopause (Scott et al. 1994).

A leiomyoma is a well-circumscribed but unencapsulated tumor, which is surrounded by a pseudocapsule representing the compressed myometrial tissue. It is mainly composed of smooth muscle but has some fibrous connective tissue elements (Kurman 1994). Multiple leiomyomas are present in two-thirds of women with these neoplasms. They show a whorled trabecular pattern on the cut surface. Leiomyomas can be subserosal, intramural, or submucosal in location. Intramural leiomyomas are the most common type and lie in the substance of the uterus. Subserosal tumors are located directly beneath the serosa and project from the external surface of the uterus. Subserosal tumors may become pedunculated, being attached to the uterus by a broad or long, thin pedicle. This pedunculated tumor may rarely become attached to the adjacent viscera, peritoneum, or omentum or lose its blood supply and develop another blood supply. Intraligamentous tumors result from the growth of a subserous tumor into the broad ligament, a not uncommon presentation. Torsion of subserosal pedunculated leiomyomas can occur, leading to presentation with an acute clinical picture. Submucosal tumors are located just beneath the endometrium. They may displace or thin the overlying endometrium or become pedunculated, bulge into the endometrial cavity, and eventually protrude into the cervical canal or the vagina. They may become the site of necrosis or infection.

Leiomyomas are subject to a variety of degenerative phenomena. Degenerative changes are usually due to alteration in their blood supply, occurring with rapid growth, pregnancy, mechanical accident, and postmenopausal atrophy. The most common type of degeneration, present in 60% of tumors, is hyalinization, where the whorled appearance is replaced by a homogeneous hyaline connective tissue. Cystic degeneration is less common, being present in 4%, and is due to liquefaction and myxomatous change in the tumor. Edema (in 50%), significant hemorrhage (in 10%), and calcification (in 4%) are other degenerative changes. The last-mentioned is more common in postmenopausal women (Kurman 1994). Necrosis occurs because of torsion of a pedunculated leiomyoma or as a red degeneration during pregnancy (Scott et al. 1994). Rosati et al. (1992) observed an increase in the volume of leiomyomas during pregnancy in 31.6% of cases. The greatest increase in their volume occurred before the 10th week of gestation. The larger leiomyomas showed a higher rate of complications.

Most leiomyomas are asymptomatic. Submucous leiomyomas may produce excessive bleeding because of congestion, necrosis, ulceration, increasing surface area of the endometrium, or interference with the ability of the uterus to contract. Pain is gradual and intermittent and is due to the degeneration of the leiomyoma. Acute pain occurs with torsion of a pedunculated tumor. Rarely, leiomyomas cause a pressure sensation due to their size, and uncommonly they result in hydronephrosis because of compression of the ureters (Scott et al. 1994). Infertility can occur because of occlusion of the endocervical canal, distortion of the isthmic portion of the fallopian tube, or impairment of proper implantation (Scott et al. 1994).

The *sonographic appearance* of leiomyomas consists of well-defined masses, which are generally hypoechoic but also include iso- and hyperechoic tumors. They characteristically cause attenuation of the ultrasound beam, presumably due to their fibrous component, or result in edge shadows because of their whorled appearance (Fig. 2.11) (Kliewer et al. 1995). Atypical tumors are nonattenuating and may be partly or completely cystic (Figs. 2.12, 2.13). Endovaginal sonography reveals more leiomyomas and is more likely to reveal the typical attenuating appearance of the tumor than transabdominal sonography because of the higher frequency of the beam, which increases the resolution but is more likely to be attenuated. Also, the fundus of the uterus is better assessed by endovaginal sonography; therefore, a pseudomass appearance of the fundus on transabdominal sonography can be resolved and the true masses identified. Some fibroids may be poorly defined, even on endovaginal sonography, and can be suspected by the indication of a mass effect presenting as a bulge of the external contour or indentation of the endometrium or as a displacement of the uterine vessels. Differentiation should be made from the uterine contraction by the presence of normal echotexture and the transient nature of the "mass." Diffuse leiomyomatosis is a rare condition presenting as symmetrical global enlargement of the uterus, which results from diffuse nodular myometrial hypertrophy (Kurman 1994). The majority of pedunculated

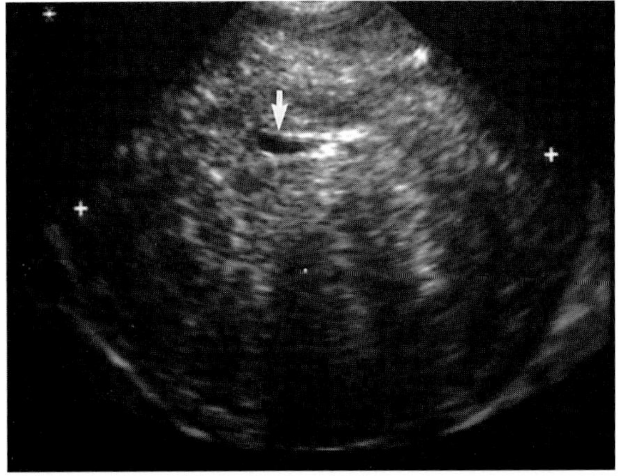

**Fig. 2.11.** Typical attenuating fibroid. Transverse endovaginal sonography shows a large fibroid (between the calipers) posterior to the fluid-containing endometrium (*arrow*), causing attenuation of sound and multiple edge shadows

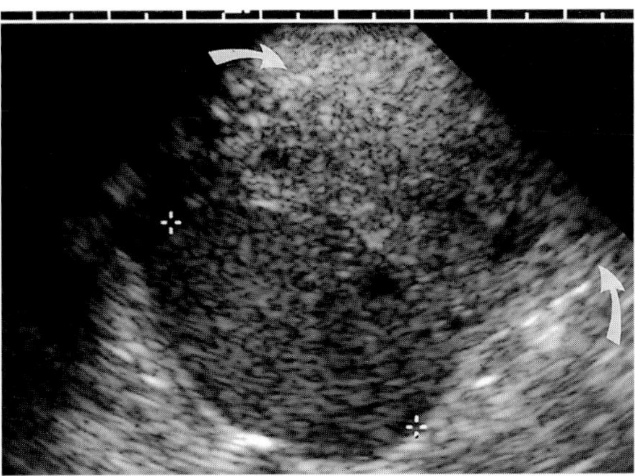

**Fig. 2.12.** Nonattenuating fibroid. Endovaginal sonography shows a relatively homogeneous nonattenuating subserosal fibroid (between the calipers) arising from the right posterior aspect of the uterus (*arrows*)

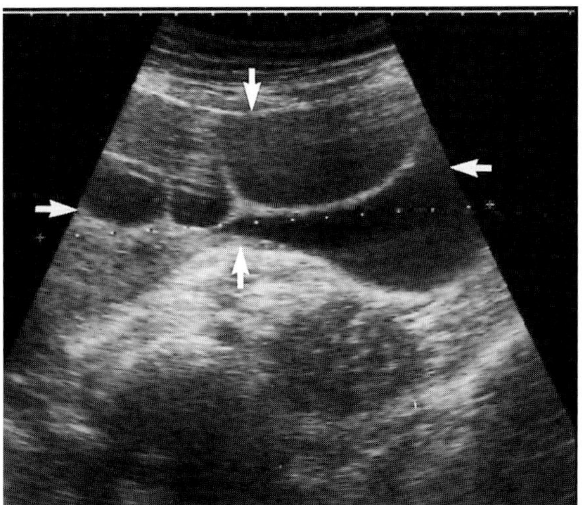

a

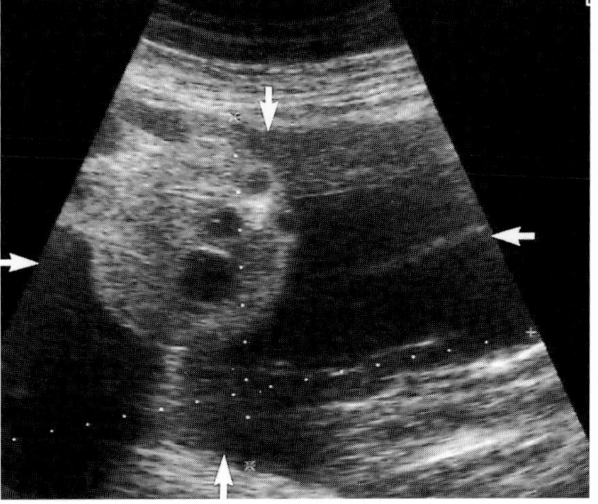

b

**Fig. 2.13 a,b.** Cystic degeneration of a benign fibroid. A large, partly cystic, partly solid subserosal fibroid (*arrows*) is seen on transabdominal sonography

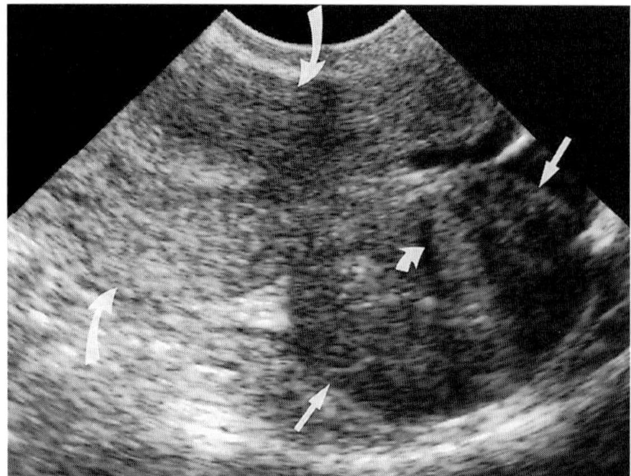

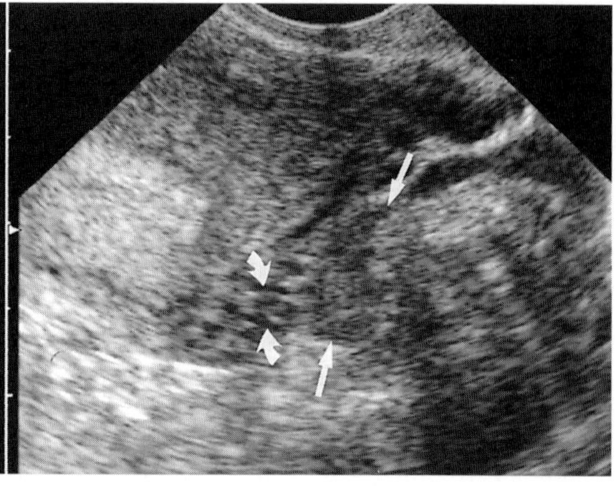

**Fig. 2.14 a,b.** Pedunculated subserosal fibroid. **a** A hypoechoic mass (*straight arrows*) with edge shadows (*small curved arrow*) is seen adjacent to the uterus (*large curved arrows*) on endovaginal sonography. **b** A broad pedicle (*arrows*) connects this mass to the serosal aspect of the uterus. Uterine vessels (*curved arrows*) are seen feeding this mass

subserosal fibroids are in general easily recognized by the presence of a broad-based attachment (Fig. 2.14). The uterine vessels leading to these masses may also be a clue to their diagnosis (Fig. 2.14b). On rare occasions, the pedicle is thin, in which case it may not be evident, even on endovaginal sonography; the mass may, therefore, be mistaken for an adnexal mass. In this case, visualization of a separate ovary and the attenuating nature of the mass help suggest this diagnosis. Minimal or significant calcification, which may be clumpy or linear, may be seen. Myolipoma, a variant of leiomyoma, contains fat, which generally occurs in circumscribed areas within a leiomyoma but may be present diffusely (Kurman 1994). These fat-containing tumors may attenuate the ultrasound beam and present as partly or completely echogenic masses, an appearance similar to some dermoids (Fig. 2.15) (Pham et al. 1993; Dodd and Budzik 1990).

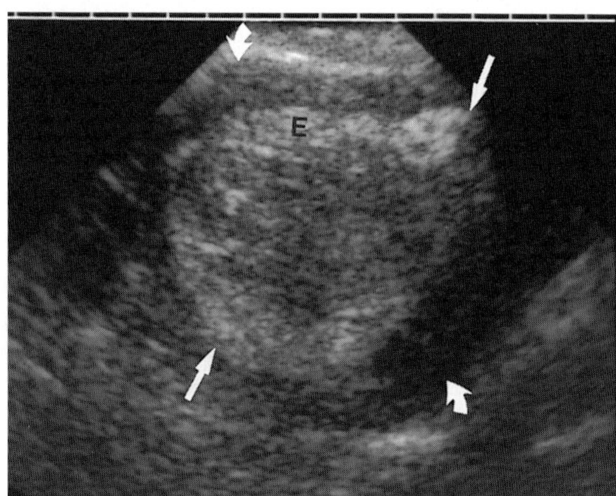


**Fig. 2.15.** Fibrolipoma. Endovaginal sonography shows an inhomogeneous mass (*straight arrows*) of the uterus (*curved arrows*) containing echogenic areas (*E*) corresponding to fat at pathology

Leiomyosarcomas represent 1.3% of uterine malignancies and about one-quarter of uterine sarcomas (Kurman 1994). The mean age of detection is approximately one decade older than the mean age for leiomyomas. There is no consistent racial predisposition. They are usually large at the time of detection, with an average diameter of 9 cm. They tend to be larger and softer than leiomyomas, and to have more irregular margins, more hemorrhage, and more necrosis. Since leiomyomas tend to stabilize or decrease in size after the menopause, a rapid increase in the size of the tumor after menopause should raise the suspicion of malignancy. The sonographic appearance is similar to a degenerated fibroid, and this diagnosis can only be suspected if there is invasion of the adjacent structures or distant metastases.

### 2.6.1.2 Cesarean Section Defect

A cesarean section scar is seen as a transverse linear band of hypo- or hyperechogenicity at the lower uterine segment and is associated with thinning of the myometrium, asymmetric isthmal structures, and ventral ballooning of the isthmus (Kirkinen 1990).

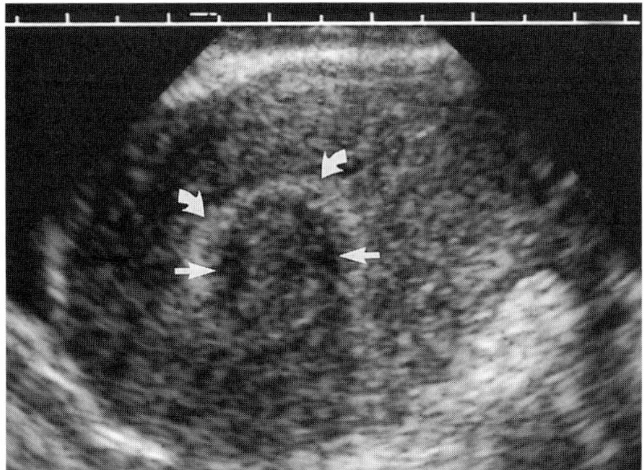

**Fig. 2.16.** Endovaginal sonography of a submucosal fibroid. A well-defined hypoechoic mass (*straight arrows*) with attenuation is seen indenting the adjacent endometrium (*curved arrows*)

### 2.6.2 Subendometrial Abnormalities

Two conditions present as a subendometrial abnormality: adenomyosis and submucosal leiomyoma.

#### 2.6.2.1 *Submucosal Leiomyoma*

Submucosal leiomyomas are generally easily diagnosed by the lack of myometrial tissue between them and the endometrium, the latter being displaced by the mass (Fig. 2.16). Occasionally, the tumor can appear completely inside the endometrial cavity or even extend through the cervical canal into the vagina (Fig. 2.17). The latter type can potentially be mistaken for an endometrial mass. However, the hypoechoic nature of the mass and attenuation (Fig. 2.18), if present, help to distinguish them from endometrial polyp or carcinoma. These masses can be vascular, like other leiomyomas (Fig. 2.18b). The extensive vascularity accompanying these masses is occasionally seen in the subendometrial location.

#### 2.6.2.2 *Adenomyosis*

Adenomyosis is a benign disease of the uterus characterized by areas of endometrial glands and stroma in the myometrium separated from the basalis layer of endometrium by more than half of a low-power

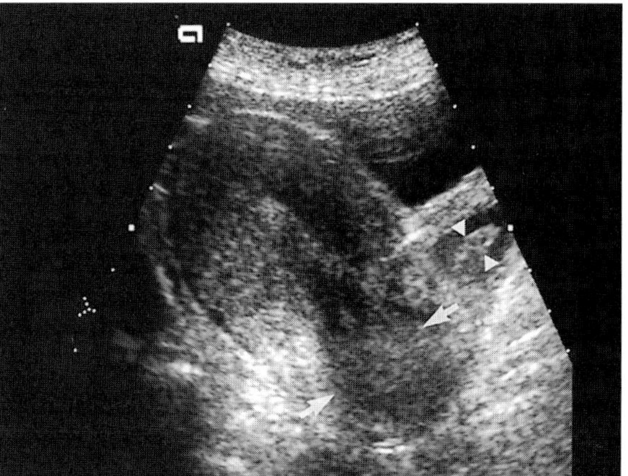

a

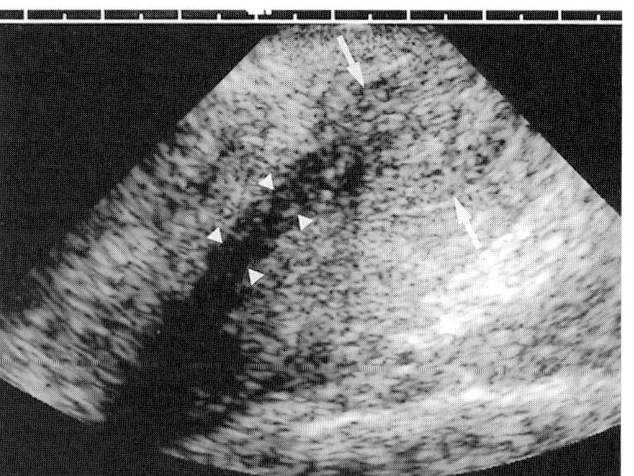

b

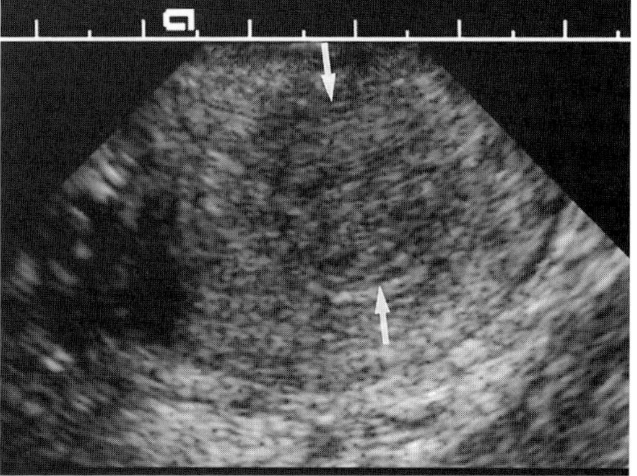

c

**Fig. 2.17 a–c.** Submucosal fibroid protruding into the endocervical canal. **a** Transabdominal sonography shows a mass expanding the endocervical canal (*arrows*) and extending to the vagina surrounded by fluid (*arrowheads*). **b** Longitudinal and **c** transverse endovaginal sonography views of the lower uterine segment and cervix illustrate the mass (*arrows*) in the endocervical canal. *Arrowheads* point to the pedicle of the mass

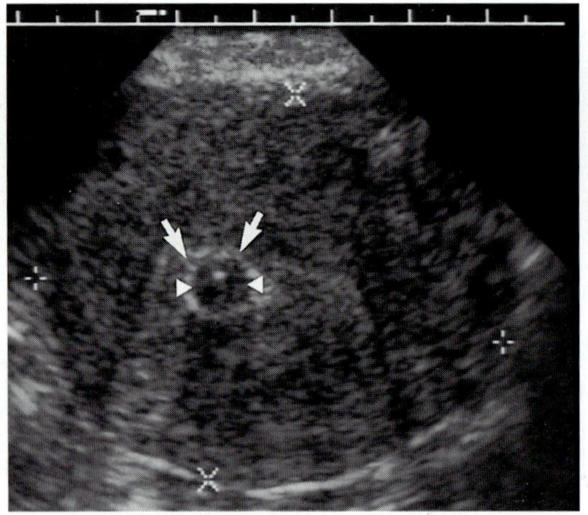

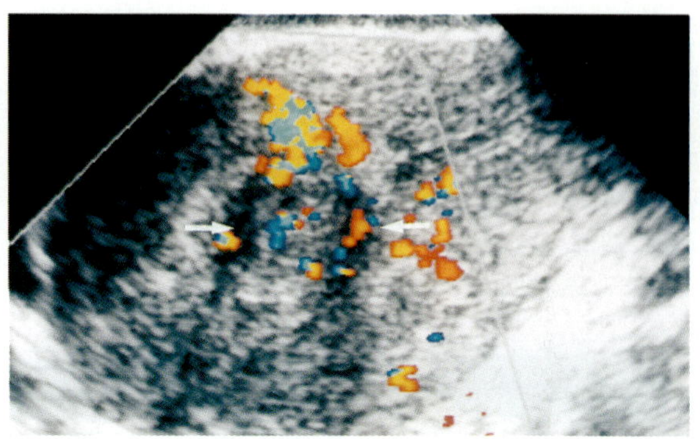

**Fig. 2.18 a,b.** Hypoechoic attenuating intraluminal submucosal fibroid. **a** Endovaginal sonography demonstrates a small hypoechoic attenuating mass (*arrowheads*) lying in the uterine cavity surrounded by endometrium (*arrows*). **b** A vascular submucosal fibroid (*arrows*) in a different patient

field (KURMAN 1994). It primarily affects women of the reproductive age group. Adenomyosis has been reported to occur in 10%–47% of hysterectomy specimens, with the higher figures being associated with hysterectomy specimens performed for ovarian endometriosis (EGGER and WEIGMAN 1982). However, adenomyosis is generally considered unrelated to endometriosis (SCOTT et al. 1994). Adenomyosis and uterine leiomyomas frequently coexist, and some authors believe that endometrial hyperplasia commonly occurs in the same uterus (EMGE 1962). In the late reproductive years, symptomatic adenomyosis is characterized by menorrhagia, dysmenor-rhea, or both (SCOTT et al. 1994). Menorrhagia is attributed to a lack of adequate myometrial contraction and dysmenorrhea, to irritation and contractility of uterine muscles (SCOTT et al. 1994).

At gross pathology, the uterus is grossly enlarged, especially the posterior wall, and has a somewhat globular appearance.

Data on the *sonographic evaluation* of the uterus to diagnose adenomyosis are limited. Transabdominal sonography has proven inaccurate in the assessment of the uterus for adenomyosis (BOHLMAN et al. 1987; BULI et al. 1986). The advent of endovaginal sonography has significantly improved the accuracy of sonography for diagnosing adenomyosis. FEDELE et al. (1992a), using endovaginal sonography, achieved an 87% sensitivity and a 99% specificity for diagnosing adenomyosis in 405 patients who underwent hysterectomy for symptomatic uterine masses. The positive predictive value was 74.1% and the negative predictive value, 98.6%. The same investigators evaluated 43 patients with menorrhagia who had no endometrial abnormality on curettage or leiomyomas on trasabdominal sonography. Twenty had hysterectomy confirmation of adenomyosis. The sensitivity of endovaginal sonography in diagnosing adenomyosis in this group of patients was 80% and the specificity was 74% (FEDELE et al. 1992b). They used poorly defined heterogeneous area(s) containing 1- to 3-mm round anechoic lakes within the myometrium as the criterior for diagnosing adenomyosis.

More recently, we reported on the accuracy of endovaginal sonography in diagnosing adenomyosis in 100 unselected consecutive patients who underwent hysterectomy for different indications. The criteria we used included poorly defined zone(s) of decreased (Fig. 2.19), increased and coarse (Fig. 2.20), or heterogeneous (Fig. 2.21) echotexture in the myometrium with or without small myometrial cysts (Fig. 2.22). With these criteria, endovaginal sonography had a sensitivity of 86%, a specificity of 86%, a positive predictive value of 71%, and a negative predictive value of 94% (REINHOLD et al. 1995). Endometrial cysts ranging in size from 2 to 7 mm were present in approximately half of the true-positive cases. Vascular calcification and muscular hypertrophy were the most common explanations for the false-positive cases. There were no false-positive diagnoses when a myometrial cyst was identified.

The uterus may acquire a globular shape (Fig. 2.20). The subendometrial myometrium is generally

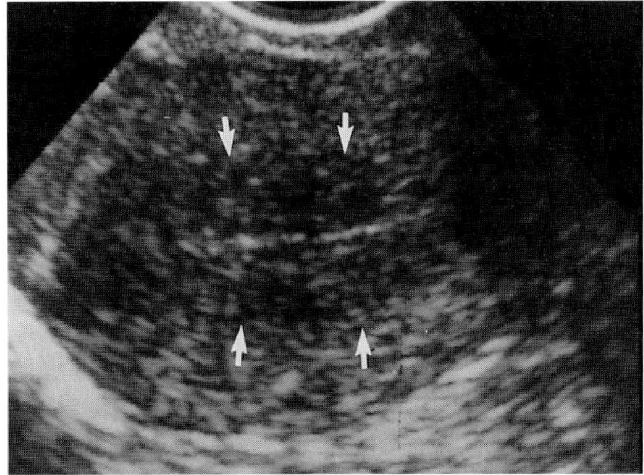

**Fig. 2.19.** Adenomyosis. Longitudinal endovaginal sonography shows a predominantly hypoechoic inner half of the myometrium (*arrows*)

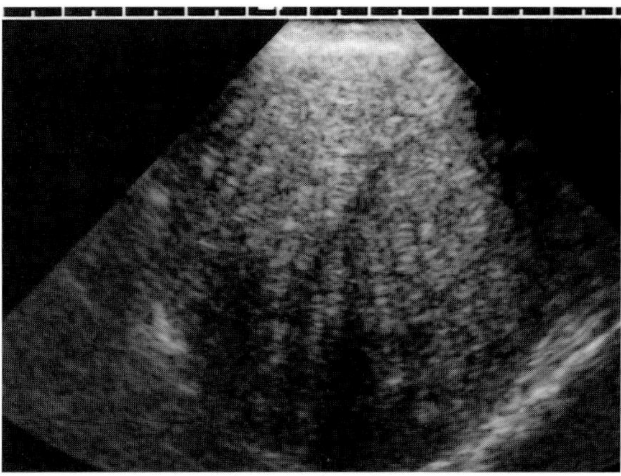

**Fig. 2.20.** Adenomyosis. Endovaginal sonographic appearance of diffuse adenomyosis, which is predominantly hyperechoic and coarse, obliterating the endometrium. The uterus is enlarged with a globular shape

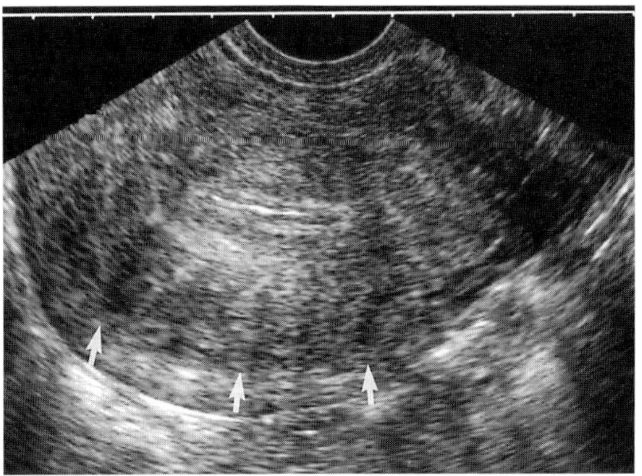

**Fig. 2.21.** Adenomyosis. Mixed hyper- and hypoechoic appearance of the inner two-thirds of myometrium (*arrows*) on endovaginal sonography

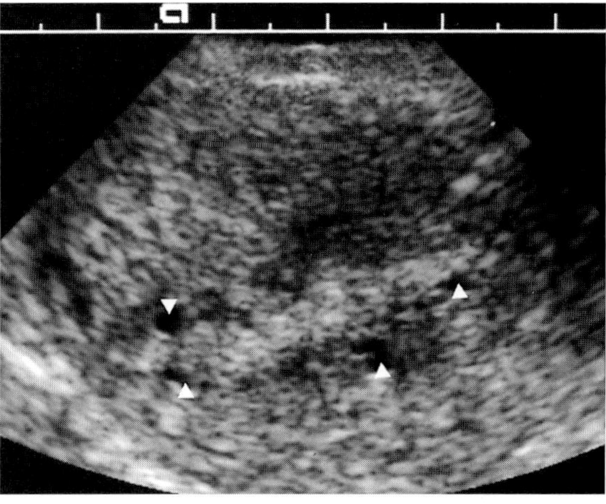

**Fig. 2.22.** Adenomyosis. Longitudinal endovaginal sonographic examination of the uterus illustrates mild hypoechoic adenomyosis of the inner third of myometrium with multiple subendometrial cysts (*arrowheads*)

involved, but the disease may extend to the middle or outer third of the myometrium, depending on the severity of disease. In addition, endovaginal sonography appears to be accurate in showing the extent of the disease (Reinhold et al. 1995; Damirov et al. 1994). Adenomyosis may less commonly present in a more localized fashion (Fig. 2.23). However, the endovaginal sonographic features of adenomyosis are subtle and the learning period may be longer than for other gynecologic pathologies. Also, since the findings are often echotexture abnormalities, real-time diagnosis is required, especially in less severe cases.

### 2.6.3 Endometrial Abnormalities

Endovaginal sonography is now considered the sonographic standard for endometrial assessment (Mendelson 1988b). Endovaginal sonography should be the starting examination when there is a question of endometrial abnormality.

The main indications for sonographic assessment of the endometrium are postmenopausal and abnormal premenopausal bleeding. Endometrial hyper-

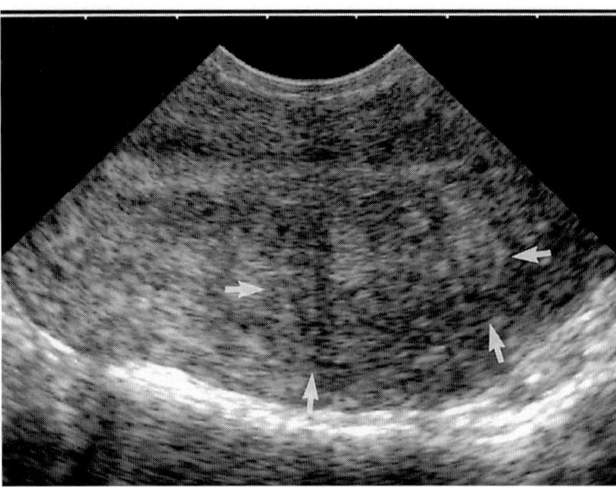

Fig. 2.23. Localized adenomyosis. Longitudinal endovaginal sonography demonstrates a more localized form of adenomyosis of the posterior aspect of the uterus (*arrows*)

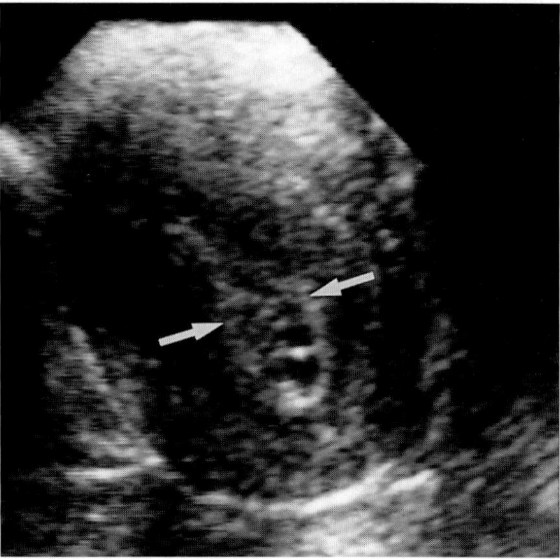

Fig. 2.24. Endometrial cystic atrophy. Endovaginal sonographic examination of a postmenopausal woman with apparent thickening of the endometrium (*arrows*) mostly due to the presence of cystic changes. (From Atri et al. 1994b)

plasia, polyps, and, less commonly, endometrial carcinoma are the organic causes of premenopausal bleeding. The same etiologies, as well as endometrial atrophy, are the causes in the postmenopausal age group, with the cancer being more common in this group. The individual endometrial features evaluated include thickness of the endometrium, echotexture relative to the myometrium, homogeneity of the endometrium, definition and smoothness of the endometrial contour, and the presence of an endometrial mass or endometrial cysts.

#### 2.6.3.1 Endometrial Cystic Atrophy

Endometrial cystic atrophy is a variant of endometrial atrophy that has cystically dilated glands. It may, in fact, represent the atrophic variant of cystically dilated glands that are present in the lower functionalis layer in women older than 35 years of age (Kurman et al. 1994). An atrophic endometrium measures less than 4–5 mm (Fleischer et al. 1986b; Granberg et al. 1991; Verner et al. 1991). However, associated cysts may cause apparent thickening (Fig. 2.24). Cystic atrophy can be differentiated from cystic endometrial hyperplasia by the lack of a thick endometrium between the cystic changes (Atri et al. 1994b). The absence of a mass helps to differentiate this condition from a cystic endometrial polyp.

#### 2.6.3.2 Endometrial Hyperplasia

The different terminologies used for endometrial hyperplasia are confusing. The new classification of endometrial hyperplasia, proposed by the International Society of Gynecological Pathologists, includes simple hyperplasia, complex adenomatous hyperplasia without atypia, and complex adenomatous hyperplasia with atypia (Kurman 1994). Simple hyperplasia is the most common type and is usually cystic (Fig. 2.25). However, endometrial cystic and adenomatous hyperplasia have a similar appearance on endovaginal sonography and demonstrate well-defined echogenic endometria with or without cystic changes (Atri et al. 1994b).

#### 2.6.3.3 Endometrial Polyp

Endometrial polyps are common lesions often encountered between 40 and 50 years of age and frequently after menopause. They start as focal hyperplasia and develop into a variable amount of glands, stroma, and blood vessels covered by epithelium (Kurman 1994). They are benign lesions that may be broad-based, pedunculated, or attached to the endometrium by a thin stalk. The most

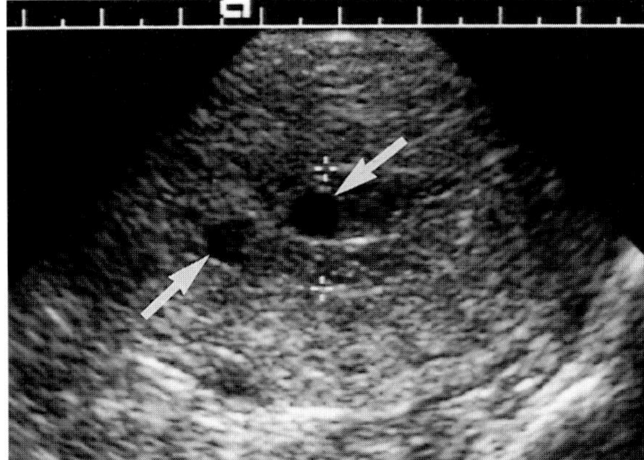

**Fig. 2.25.** Endometrial cystic hyperplasia. Endovaginal sonography of a premenopausal woman demonstrates a thickened, slightly echogenic, well-defined endometrium (between calipers) with cystic spaces (*arrows*). (From ATRI et al. 1994b)

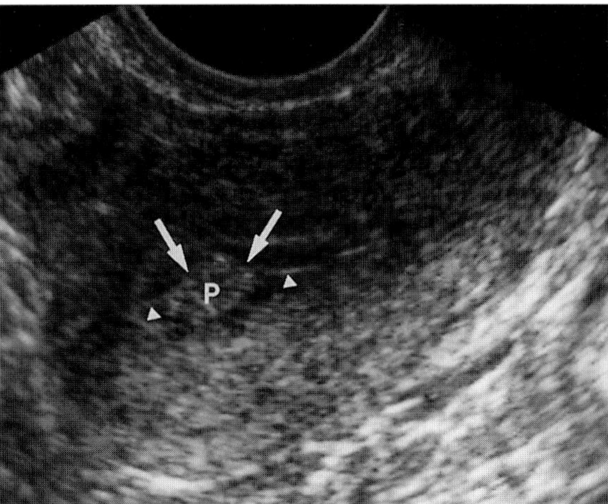


**Fig. 2.26.** Longitudinal endovaginal sonographic examination of a small endometrial polyp in a premenopausal woman. A small endometrial polyp is recognized by the presence of a well-defined echogenic nodule (*P*) surrounded by a complete functionalis layer of the endometrium (*arrows*), expanding the endometrial cavity (*arrowheads*)

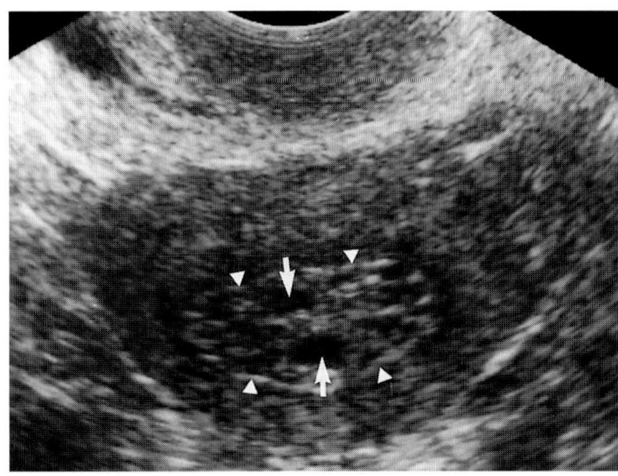

**Fig. 2.27.** Endovaginal sonographic examination of an endometrial polyp in a postmenopausal woman. The endometrium is thickened by a mass containing multiple cystic spaces (*arrows*). Note the complete thin endometrium surrounding this mass (*arrowheads*)

common site of origin is the cornum, but they may extend down and through the endocervix. They may also arise from the endocervix or have a mixed endometrial-endocervical origin (KURMAN 1994). There are three categories of endometrial polyps: hyperplastic, functional, and atrophic. The hyperplastic type is estrogen dependent and resembles endometrial hyperplasia. The functional type, the least frequent, is similar to the surrounding endometrium, and responds to the hormones of the menstrual cycle. The atrophic type shows atrophic glandular epithelium and probably represents regressive changes of the other two types; it is most frequently seen in the postmenopausal age group and is often cystic (KURMAN 1994). Malignancy in a benign polyp is rare and probably occurs in no more than 0.5% of cases (KURMAN 1994). Polyps may be difficult to recognize on dilatation and curettage specimens. The endometrial polyp should always be considered if abnormal bleeding persists after curettage. Polyps present with intermenstrual bleeding, menometrorrhagia, postmenopausal bleeding, or may be the cause of infertility. The diagnostic feature of an endometrial polyp on endovaginal sonography is a well-defined mass, usually echogenic, in the endometrial cavity that can be identified separately from the overlying intact endometrium (Figs. 2.26, 2.27). It may contain cystic areas (Fig. 2.27); this feature was present in 91% of 11 surgically confirmed polyps that we recently reported (ATRI et al. 1994b). Endometrial polyps tend to be vascular on color Doppler. The presence of a single vascular pedicle is very suggestive of a polyp (Fig. 2.28), although it is also seen in other causes of endometrial thickening (e.g., endometrial carcinoma and protruding submucosal leiomyoma).

### 2.6.3.4
### Endometrial Malignancy

Endometrial carcinoma is the most common invasive neoplasm of the female genital tract. Endometrioid carcinoma accounts for three-quarters of endometrial carcinomas, the remaining

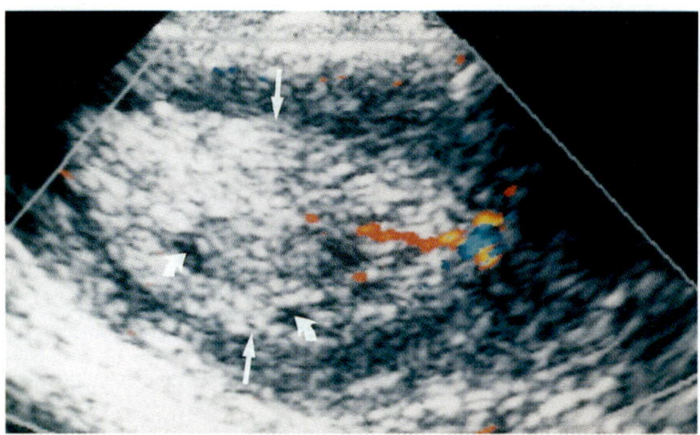

Fig. 2.28. Color Doppler endovaginal sonographic examination of an endometrial polyp with a single pedicle. A large echogenic mass (*straight arrows*) with cystic spaces (*curved arrows*) thickens the endometrium. A single vascular pedicle supplies this mass

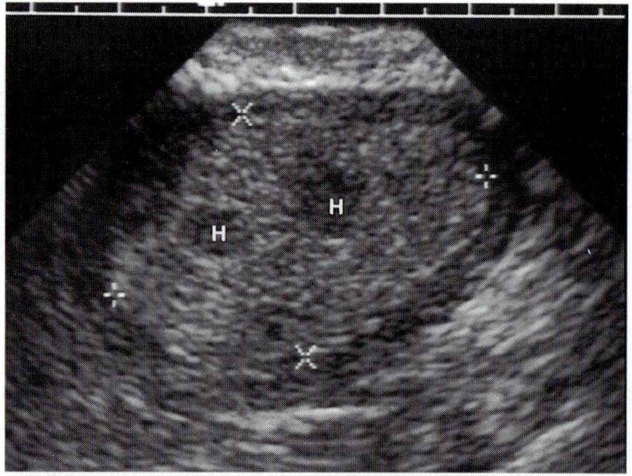


a

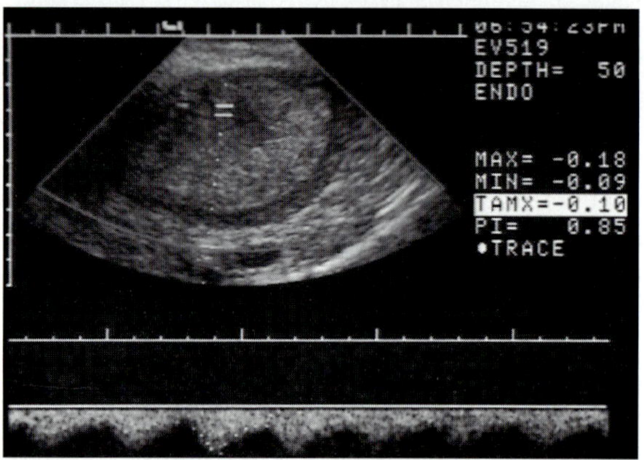


b

Fig. 2.29 a,b. Endometrial carcinoma. **a** Endovaginal sonographic examination shows a relatively well-defined mass (between the calipers) that is predominantly echogenic but contains two hypoechoic zones (*H*). **b** Doppler examination reveals low-impedance flow

tumors being squamous, serous, mucinous, or clear-cell tumors. The squamous category is rare and is strongly associated with cervical stenosis, pyometra, and chronic inflammation. The median age of patients is 61; only 5% of endometrial cancers are seen before 40 years of age and 25% before menopause (Scott et al. 1994).

There is a strong association between estrogen replacement therapy and the development of endometrial cancer. Other risk factors are obesity, hypertension, diabetes mellitus, nulliparity, and late menopause (Kurman 1994). Endometrial cancer has been reported to occur in 25% of patients with polycystic ovary syndrome because of exposure to unopposed estrogen (Scott et al. 1994). Endometrial cancer developing because of estrogen replacement has an excellent prognosis, with a 5-year survival rate of 90%. The addition of progestin has a protective effect against the development of endometrial cancer (Scott et al. 1994).

Mixed mesodermal tumors contain both epithelium and mesenchymal elements. They include adenofibromas, adenosarcomas, and mixed müllerian tumors, which range from benign to malignant tumors (Kurman 1994). A mixed müllerian tumor is the most common uterine sarcoma, exceeding leiomyosarcomas in frequency. A disproportionate number of uterine tumors developing after radiation are mixed müllerian tumors.

The gross appearance of endometrial carcinoma on endovaginal sonography is variable. In our review of 25 surgically confirmed endometrial cancers, the maximum thickness ranged from 0.7 to 7 cm (mean, 2.7 cm) (Atri et al. 1994b). The majority (76%) were hyperechoic, 12% were isoechoic, and 12% contained both hyper- and hypoechoic components (Fig. 2.29). Sixty percent showed an irregular contour, 86% of which were poorly defined. An endometrial mass may be identified. Although this mass may be polypoid, its broad base helps differentiate it from a benign polyp (Fig. 2.30) (Atri et al. 1994b). However, it was found that 40% presented as well-defined simple endometrial thickening. Cystic area(s) were present in 24% of these cancers (Fig. 2.31). In one patient, the tumor contained calcification (Atri et al. 1994b).

Mixed mesodermal tumors tend to be polypoid neoplasms that usually fill the endometrial cavity and may protrude through the external os. The cut surface generally shows areas of hemorrhage and necrosis that may contain bone or cartilage (Kurman 1994).

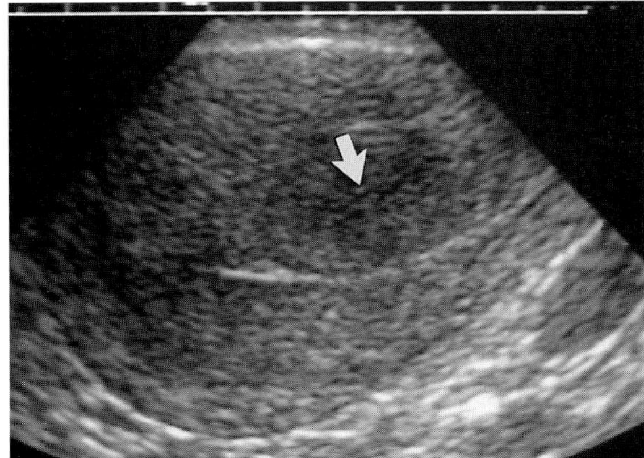

a

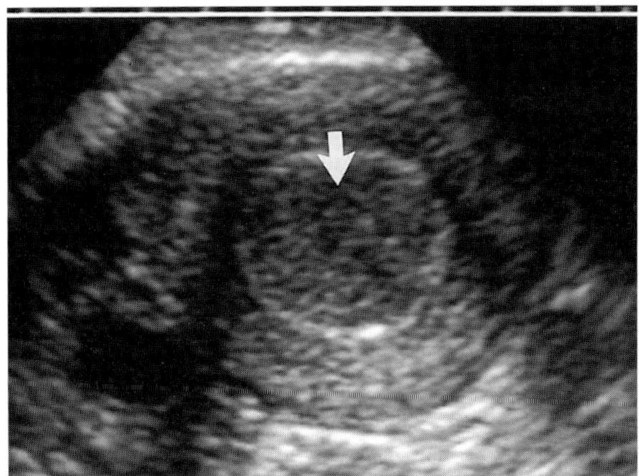

b

Fig. 2.30 a,b. Broad-based polypoid endometrial carcinoma. Sagittal (a) and transverse (b) endovaginal sonographic images demonstrate an isoechoic polypoid mass (*arrow*) expanding the uterine cavity with no defined stalk. The mass is completely surrounded by endometrium on the transverse view, but the sagittal view confirms its broad-based nature. (From Atri et al. 1994b)

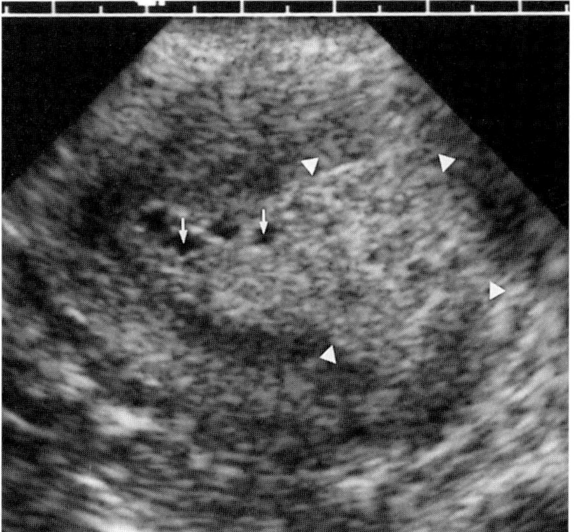

Fig. 2.31. Endometrial carcinoma with cystic changes. Endovaginal sonography illustrates endometrial thickening with more localized expansion of the endometrium (*arrowheads*) by a poorly defined echogenic mass. Cystic spaces are seen in this endometrium (*arrows*)

### 2.6.3.5 Differential Diagnosis of Endometrial Abnormalities on Endovaginal Sonography

Efforts are generally made to differentiate between the more serious endometrial carcinoma and benign conditions. The following features are used to help their differentiation on endovaginal sonography.

#### 2.6.3.5.1 Endometrial Thickness

Endometrial thickness less than or equal to 4–5 mm in postmenopausal women who are not on hormone replacement has been shown to correspond to endometrial atrophy in a number of studies (Fleischer et al. 1986b; Granberg et al. 1991; Verner et al. 1991; Atri et al. 1994b; Osmers et al. 1990; Botsis et al. 1992; Karlsson et al. 1995; Sheth et al. 1993; Goldstein et al. 1990). In a Nordic study of 1168 women with postmenopausal bleeding, no cancer was found when the endometrium was less than 5 mm. Use of this threshold as a cutoff value to triage patients with postmenopausal bleeding would have prevented 70%–82% of dilatation and curettage procedures (Botsis et al. 1992; Karlsson et al. 1995). The risk of developing other endometrial abnormalities with an endometrium of less than or equal to 4 mm was 5.5% in one series (Karlsson et al. 1995).

In women who are on unopposed estrogen or sequential estrogen and progesterone hormone replacement therapy, the endometrium is reported to increase in thickness by 1–3 mm (Granberg et al. 1991; Lin et al. 1991; Pirhonen et al. 1993; Levine et al. 1995). Maximum increase reaching statistical significance occurs in women receiving sequential estrogen and progesterone (Levine et al. 1995). It is recommended that women with postmenopausal bleeding who have an endometrial thickness greater than or equal to 5 mm undergo endometrial biopsy (Levine et al. 1995). However, if the postmenopausal women are asymptomatic, with or without hormone replacement, endometrial biopsy is recommended only if the endometrium measures more than 8 mm

(Levine et al. 1995; Bonilla-Musoles et al. 1995a; Aleem et al. 1995; Malpani et al. 1990; Shipley et al. 1994). Because of significant variation in the endometrial thickness during the hormone cycle of women with sequential hormone replacement, with the peak between days 13 and 23, the endometrium should be evaluated at the beginning or end of the cycle in these women (Levine et al. 1995).

### 2.6.3.5.2 ENDOMETRIAL DOPPLER

The initial results of endometrial Doppler used to differentiate between benign and malignant endometrial thickening were highly accurate, with a resistive index threshold of 0.4 (Kurjak et al. 1993) and a pulsatility index of 1 (Bourne et al. 1991) used as a cutoff value. However, more recent reports show an overlap between the values of endometrial cancer and those of benign causes of endometrial thickening, although in general resistive index and pulsatility index values are lower in malignant endometrial thickening (Fig. 2.29) (Chan et al. 1994; Sladkevicius et al. 1994; Sheth et al. 1995). Also, arterial flow may not be detectable in some endometrial carcinomas (Fig 2.32). However, the combination of a well-defined echogenic mass that is separate from the endometrial echo and a single vascular pedicle is strongly suggestive of an endometrial polyp. The single vascular pedicle alone is not diagnostic because a single pedicle is also seen in endometrial malignancy, and multiple pedicles may represent multiple polyps. Uterine arterial and intramyometrial arterial impedance increase following menopause, with a positive correlation between the years from menopause and increasing impedance (Bonilla-Musoles et al. 1995b; Kurjak and Kupesic 1995). A similar effect is seen with the administration of gonadotropin-releasing hormone agonists, causing chemical castration (Battaglia et al. 1995). Opposite changes are shown with hormone replacement therapy because of the estrogenic effect (Bonilla-Musoles et al. 1995a; Kurjak and Kupesic 1995). The addition of a progestogen does not appear to alter the effect of estrogen alone (Bonilla-Musoles et al. 1995b). The presence of vascularity in an endometrial mass helps differentiate true pathologies from a blood clot in a patient who has vaginal bleeding (Fig. 2.33).

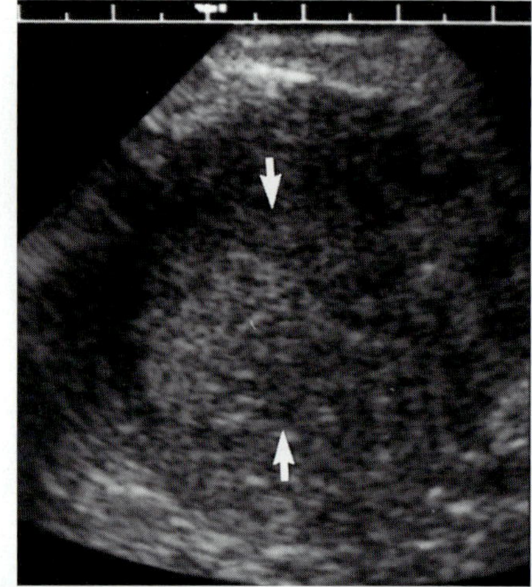

a

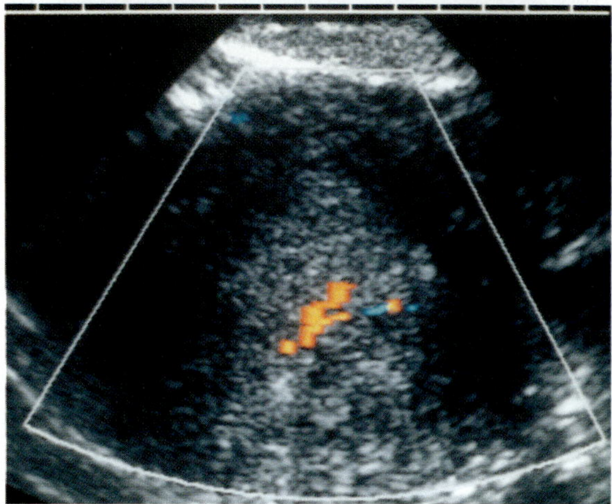

b

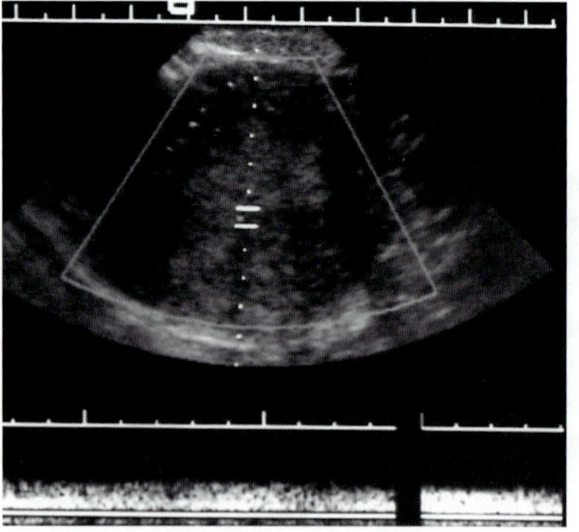

c

**Fig. 2.32 a,b.** Malignant-appearing endometrial carcinoma with no arterial flow. **a** Poorly defined thick endometrium (*arrows*) strongly suggestive of endometrial cancer. **b** Color Doppler shows slight vascularity. **c** Pulsed Doppler only revealed venous flow

### 2.6.3.5.3 ENDOMETRIAL FLUID

Fluid in the endometrial cavity in postmenopausal women is a nonspecific finding and is frequently be-

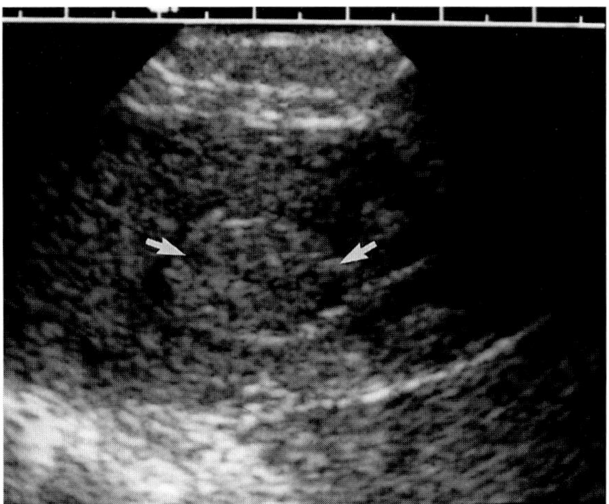

Fig. 2.33. Blood clot in the uterine cavity of a postmenopausal woman with vaginal bleeding. Endovaginal sonographic image shows a well-defined mass (*arrows*), which was avascular on Doppler; such a mass can mimic an endometrial pathology. However, this mass disintegrated during the examination, confirming its nature

nign in cause (Levine et al. 1995; Goldstein 1994a). It may be related to the associated cervical stenosis (Fig. 2.4) (Goldstein 1994a).

2.6.3.5.4
ENDOMETRIAL APPEARANCE

The presence of cystic areas in a thick endometrium is suggestive of a benign process (Figs. 2.24, 2.25, 2.27) (Atri et al. 1994b; Sheth et al. 1993) although they may also be seen in association with endometrial cancer, presumably due to a combination of cystic hyperplasia and malignancy (Fig. 2.31) (Atri et al. 1994b). An intact endometrial echo completely surrounding an echogenic endometrial mass is diagnostic of an endometrial polyp (Figs. 2.26, 2.27) (Atri et al. 1994b). Irregular inhomogeneous endometrium is seen with endometrial malignancy and complex hyperplasia is seen with atypia (Atri et al. 1994b; Sheth et al. 1993). Most submucosal leiomyomas can be correctly diagnosed by real-time imaging by the presence of a hypoechoic mass with or without attenuation that is closely related to and compresses overlying endometrium (Atri et al. 1994b). Endometrial appearance appears to be most helpful in the differential diagnosis of endometrial thickening.

### 2.6.3.6 Endovaginal Sonography Versus Endometrial Biopsy, Dilatation and Curettage, and Hysteroscopy

Endometrial biopsy is generally considered accurate in diagnosing endometrial cancer (Stovall et al. 1991a) and assessing the endometrium in premenopausal patients (Kaunitz et al. 1988; Eddowes et al. 1990; Check et al. 1989; Henig et al. 1989; Hill et al. 1989; Silver et al. 1991; Stovall et al. 1991b; Koonings et al. 1990). However, the results are less accurate for diagnosing benign causes of endometrial thickening in postmenopausal women (Shipley et al. 1994; Karlsson et al. 1993, 1994; Van Den Bosch et al. 1995). Endometrial biopsy is insensitive to the detection of endometrial hyperplasia, endometrial polyp, and submucosal leiomyoma. Even dilatation and curettage is known to be inaccurate for diagnosing endometrial polyps and submucosal leiomyomas (Karlsson et al. 1994). In fact, in the series of Karlsson et al. (1994), the presence of endometrial atrophy on dilatation and curettage with an endometrial thickness greater than or equal to 8 mm always corresponded to an endometrial polyp or submucosal leiomyoma on hysteroscopy. Emanuel et al. (1995) have shown a significant decrease in the number of invasive tests such as diagnostic hysteroscopy and histologic examination if endovaginal sonography is used for screening women with abnormal uterine bleeding. Whereas the pretest probability (prevalence) of a uterine abnormality was 0.42, the post-test probability was 0.03 in the case of a normal sonogram and 0.87 for an abnormal sonogram (Emanuel et al. 1995). Therefore, endovaginal sonography appears to be an effective tool for screening women with postmenopausal bleeding. It can eliminate a number of unnecessary invasive procedures and is also useful in performing a guided targeted dilatation and curettage by showing the site of origin of the pedicle of an endometrial polyp.

### 2.6.3.7 Endometrial Cancer Staging

The local extent of endometrial carcinoma is an important prognostic factor for the disease. Both tumor differentiation (grade) and local extent of the disease (stage) determine the incidence of lymph node metastasis. According to the FIGO (Fédération Internationale de Gynécologie et d'obstétrique) staging system (SHEPHERD 1989), stage I disease is limited to the uterine corpus and stage II extends to the cervix. Stage IA is limited to the endometrium, IB invades the myometrium but is limited to the inner half, and IC involves the outer half of the myometrium. Stage II disease is divided into IIA, which involves only the endocervix, and IIB, which extends to the cervical stroma (SCOTT et al. 1994). With the same grade of disease, the incidence of lymph node metastasis increases when the disease invades the outer half of the myometrium (LEWIS et al. 1970) or extends to the cervix (MORROW et al. 1973).

Endovaginal sonography is shown to be accurate in local staging of endometrial cancer (CACCIATORE et al. 1989; CONTE et al. 1990; SAHAKIAN et al. 1991; GORDON et al. 1990; ARTNER et al. 1994; BIDZINSKI and LEMIESZCZUK 1993). Reported accuracies for depth of myometrial invasion range from 84% to 98.6% (Fig. 2.34) (CACCIATORE et al. 1989; CONTE et al. 1990; SAHAKIAN et al. 1991; GORDON et al. 1990; ARTNER et al. 1994; BIDZINSKI and LEMIESZCZUK 1993) and for cervical invasion, from 93.5% to 95.6% (Fig. 2.35) (ARTNER et al. 1994; BIDZINSKI and LEMIESZCZUK 1993). In general, the larger the tumor, the more likely the invasion of the myometrium (CACCIATORE et al. 1989). False-positive cases of deep invasion are more common with the large polypoid masses, which cause thinning of overlying

a

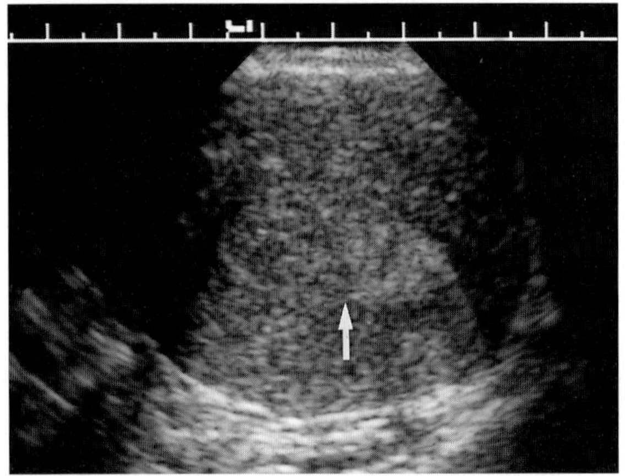

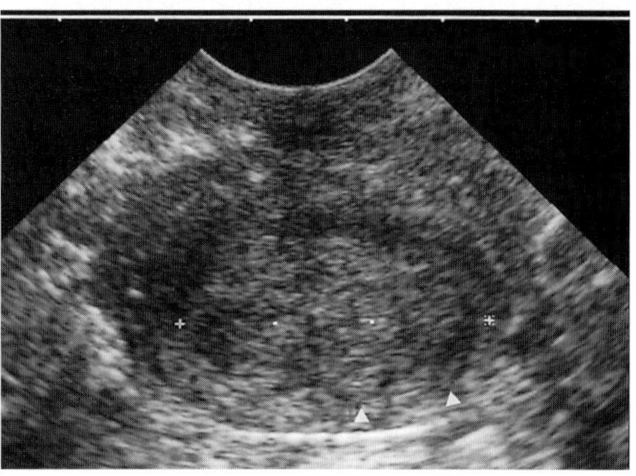

b

**Fig. 2.34 a,b.** Two endometrial carcinomas with different degrees of myometrial invasion. **a** Endovaginal sonography illustrates endometrial thickening with localized poor definition (*arrow*) indicating superficial invasion. **b** Endovaginal sonography shows a poorly defined mass (between calipers) thickening the endometrium with evidence of deep myometrial invasion posteriorly (*arrowheads*)

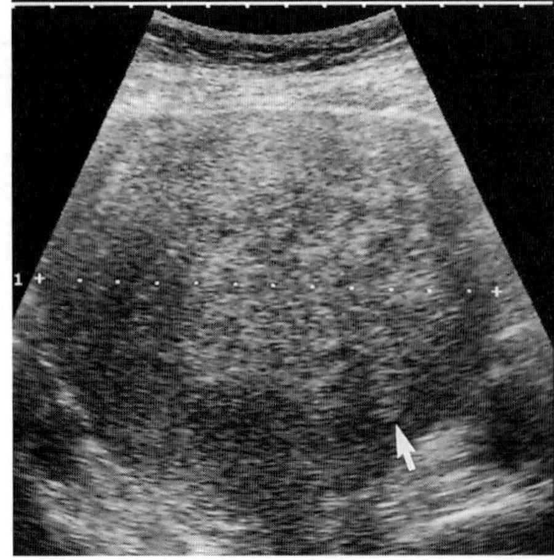

a

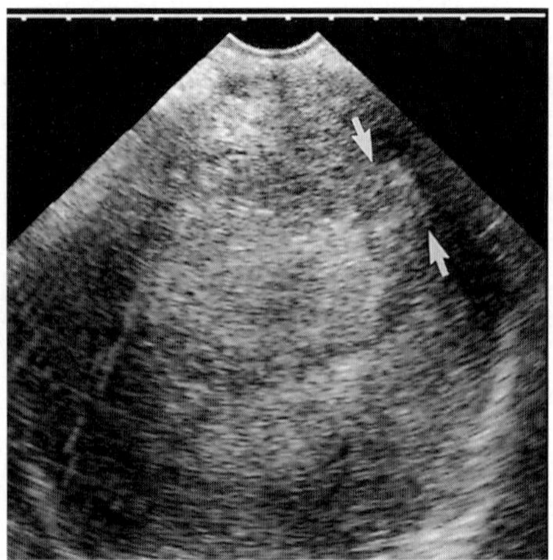

b

**Fig. 2.35 a,b.** Endometrial carcinoma with deep myometrial and cervical invasion. **a** Transverse endovaginal sonographic view of the uterus shows an echogenic, poorly defined mass extending to the outer half of myometrium (*arrow*). **b** Sagittal endovaginal sonographic view illustrates extension of the mass to the cervical rigion (*arrows*)

myometrium that can be mistaken for myometrial invasion (Fig. 2.36a) (CACCIATORE et al. 1989). Associated leiomyomas and adenomyosis are other causes of false-positive diagnosis of myometrial invasion (Fig. 2.36b) (SAHAKIAN et al. 1991; BIDZINSKI and LEMIESZCZUK 1993). In a series correlating endovaginal sonography and magnetic resonance imaging for staging of endometrial carcinoma, endovaginal sonography was 69% accurate and magnetic resonance imaging was 74% accurate, with no significant difference between the two (DELMASCHIO et al. 1993).

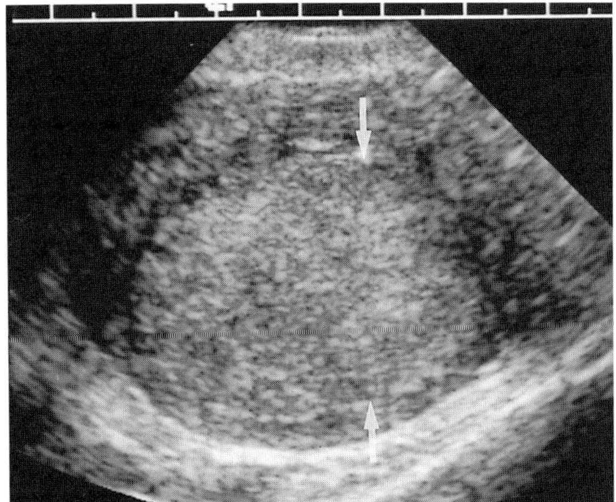

a

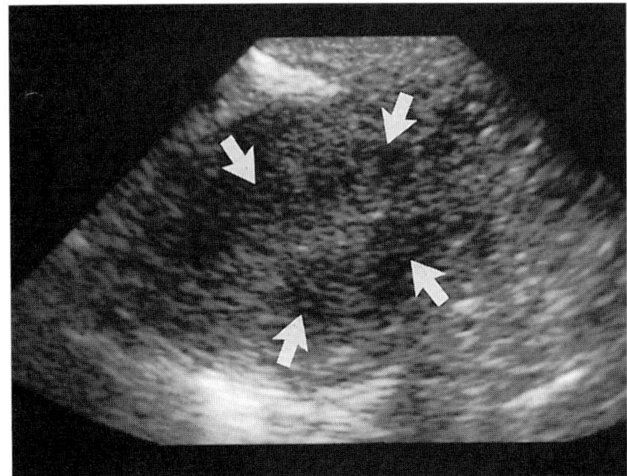

b

**Fig. 2.36 a,b.** Causes of false-positive diagnosis of myometrial invasion. **a** Endovaginal sonography shows a large endometrial mass (*arrows*) with significant thinning of posterior myometrium, falsely suggesting deep invasion. **b** Sagittal endovaginal sonography examination of the uterus demonstrates a poorly defined endometrium in a patient with a proven endometrial cancer without myometrial invasion. Hypoechoic subendometrial changes of adenomyosis (*arrows*) are responsible for poor definition of the endometrium

#### *2.6.3.8*
#### *Tamoxifen Endometrium*

Tamoxifen citrate is a nonsteroidal estrogen antagonist used as an adjuvant therapy for breast cancer and is suggested as a prophylactic against cancer development in women with hereditary cancer. Tamoxifen may act as a partial estrogen agonist on the reproductive tract. Proliferative endometrium, endometrial hyperplasia, endometrial polyp with cystically dilated glands, and endometrial carcinoma have been reported in postmenopausal patients receiving tamoxifen (WOLF and JORDAN 1992). Endovaginal sonographic confirmation of thickening of the endometrium has been shown with the use of tamoxifen (ROSEN et al. 1994). Endovaginal sonographic changes of tamoxifen endometrium range from homogeneous echogenic thick endometrium, to homogeneous or heterogeneous thick endometrium with cystic spaces, to heterogeneous solid endometrium (HULKA and HALL 1993). The endometrium tends to be irregular and cystic changes may have a band-like appearance (Fig. 2.37) (ATRI et al. 1994b). Although endovaginal sonographic endometrial changes are shown to correspond to proliferative and hyperplastic endometrium as well as endometrial polyps at histology (Fig. 2.38) (HULKA and HALL 1993; LAHTI et al. 1994), repeated dilatation and curettage or endometrial biopsy may show atrophic changes in others (ACHIRON et al. 1995a; GOLDSTEIN 1994b). Sonohysterographic studies with instillation of normal saline in the endometrial cavity (see Sect.

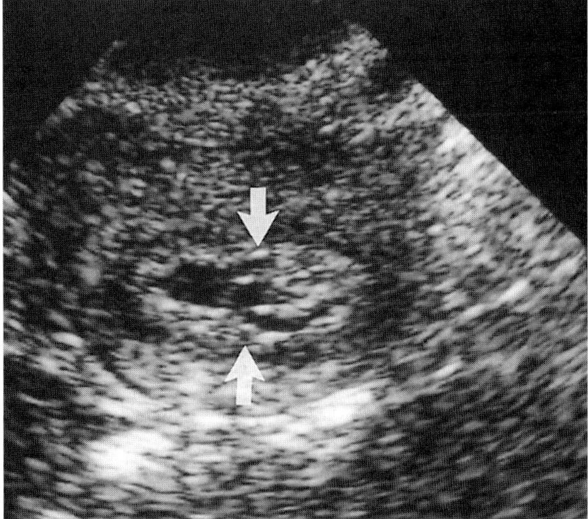

**Fig. 2.37.** Tamoxifen endometrium. There is thickening of the endometrium (*arrows*) with a band-like appearance

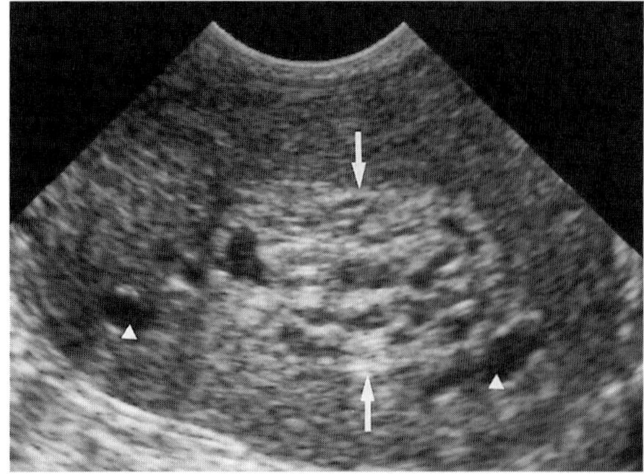

a

b

Fig. 2.38 a,b. Tamoxifen endometrium with a large polyp. Oblique (a) and longitudinal (b) endovaginal sonographic images of the uterus of a postmenopausal woman with breast cancer on tamoxifen. There is thickened, expanded endometrium (*arrows*), which is suggestive of an endometrial polyp since it is partly surrounded by fluid in the lower uterine segment (*F*). Subendometrial myometrial cysts are present (*arrowheads*)

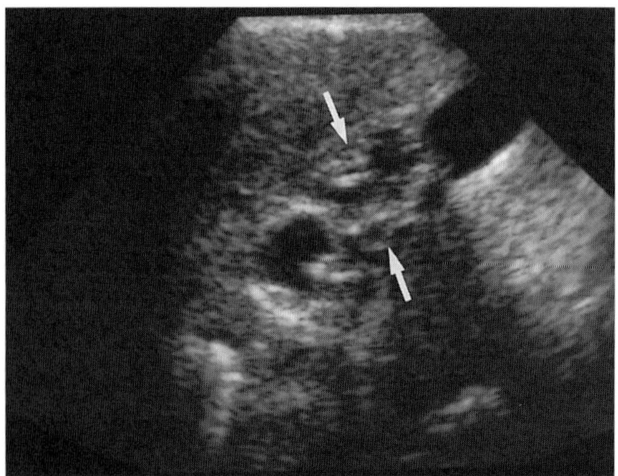

a

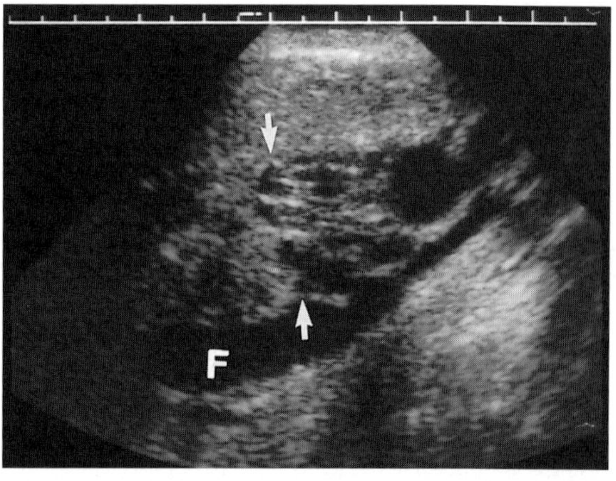


b

**Fig. 2.39 a,b.** Sonohysterography of a tamoxifen endometrium in a patient with negative dilatation and curettage. **a** Endovaginal sonographic examination shows thickened endometrium with multiple cystic areas (*arrows*). **b** On sonohysterography there is no abnormality of the endometrial cavity but cystic changes (*arrows*) appear to be subendometrial in location. Fluid is present in the distended uterine cavity (*F*)

2.6.5) have shown no endometrial abnormalities but cystic changes at the endometrial–myometrial junction in the latter group (Fig. 2.39) (Achiron et al. 1995a; Goldstein 1994b). These changes may represent adenomyosis (Fig. 2.38a). There may be increased fluid in the uterine cavity in these patients (Figs. 2.38, 2.40).

Doppler studies of the endometrium of women on tamoxifen have shown lower impedance of the uterine and endometrial flow compared with that of the control groups (Kedar et al. 1994; Achiron et al. 1995b). Achiron et al. (1995c) compared two groups of breast cancer patients on tamoxifen, one with thick irregular cystic endometrium measuring greater than or equal to 5 mm and the other with an endometrium measuring less than 5 mm. The first group had a significantly lower endometrial resistive index than the second group. Although the true incidence of endometrial cancer in women receiving tamoxifen is not known, increased incidence has been suggested (Kedar et al. 1994; Ismail 1994; Segna et al. 1992), which necessitates close monitoring of these women. In this way, endovaginal sonography may play a role in the triage of patients

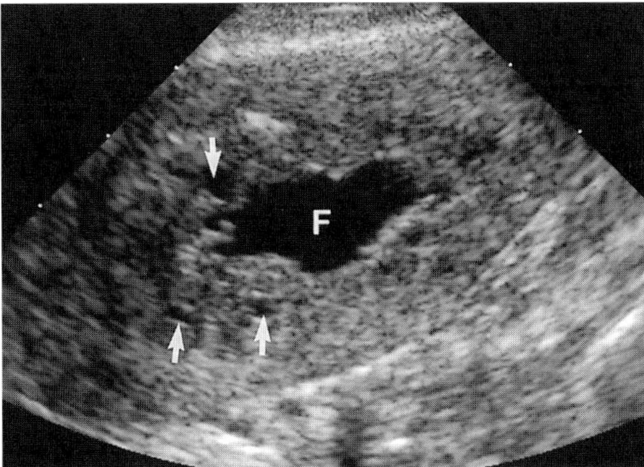


**Fig. 2.40.** Tamoxifen endometrium with fluid in the uterine cavity. Endovaginal sonographic image demonstrates an irregular endometrial thickness with fluid retention in the uterine cavity (*F*) and subendometrial myometrial cysts (*arrows*)

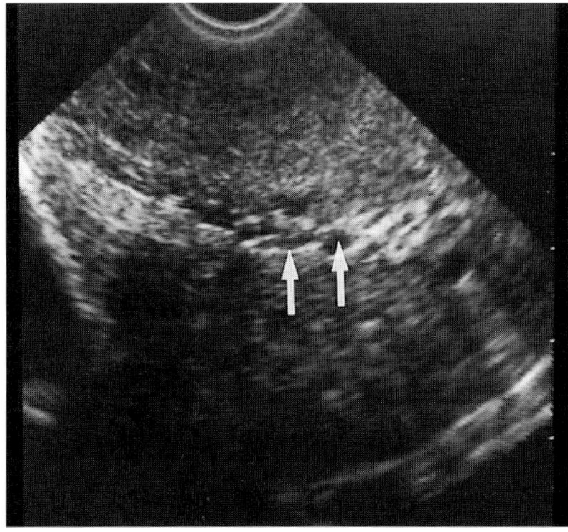

**Fig. 2.41.** Asherman syndrome. A 40-year-old patient with a history of dilatation and curettage complicated by infection. Endovaginal sonographic image demonstrates an echogenic endometrium with cystic changes and endometrial bands (*arrows*). (From Atri et al. 1994b)

for endometrial biopsy by confirming endometrial thickening.

#### 2.6.3.9 *Other Benign Endometrial Conditions*

##### 2.6.3.9.1 ASHERMAN SYNDROME

Intrauterine adhesions (Asherman syndrome) may present with varying degrees of hypomenorrhea, amenorrhea, infertility, and early pregnancy loss. Vigorous and repeat curettage performed in the postabortion or postpartum period, particularly if a uterine infection is present, is an inciting factor (Kurman 1994). The diagnosis is made by hysterosalpingography or hysteroscopy, which demonstrates bands of tissue traversing but rarely obliterating the endometrial cavity (Foix et al. 1966). No significant inflammation is present in these synechiae that consist of fibrous or smooth muscle tissue. On endovaginal sonography, Asherman syndrome demonstrates thickened endometrium with cystic changes due to the presence of multiple adhesive bands (Fig. 2.41) (Atri et al. 1994b). However, these findings are nonspecific. The addition of sonohysterography can be diagnostic for this condition (see Sect. 2.6.5).

##### 2.6.3.9.2 HETEROTOPIC BONE OR CARTILAGE

Heterotopic bone or cartilage in the endometrium is frequently associated with a history of repeated abortions and endometritis (Newton and Abell 1973; Roth and Taylor 1966). The strong association with pregnancy and the rarity of osseous metaplasia in other types of endometritis suggest that heterotopic bone or cartilage may represent implantation of fetal parts (Roth and Taylor 1966). The presence of endometrial calcification on endovaginal sonography is suggestive of this diagnosis (Fig. 2.42).

##### 2.6.3.9.3 ENDOMETRITIS

Endometritis occurs in the following situations: postpartum, chlamydial or gonococcal infection, after instrumentation or surgery, secondary to cervical stenosis, after radium insertion, in the presence of intrauterine devices, and in tuberculous patients (Scott et al. 1994). The diagnosis is made by the presence of plasma cells or a specific causative factor in the uterine secretions (Scott et al. 1994). Sonographic features of endometritis are nonspecific and include different degrees of regular or irregular endometrial thickening with or without fluid in the endometrial cavity. Gas bubbles may be present.

### 2.6.4 Abnormalities of the Uterine Cavity

#### 2.6.4.1 *Hydrometrocolpos or Hematometrocolpos*

Retention of fluid or blood occurs when there is a blockage to the flow of uterine or cervical secretion

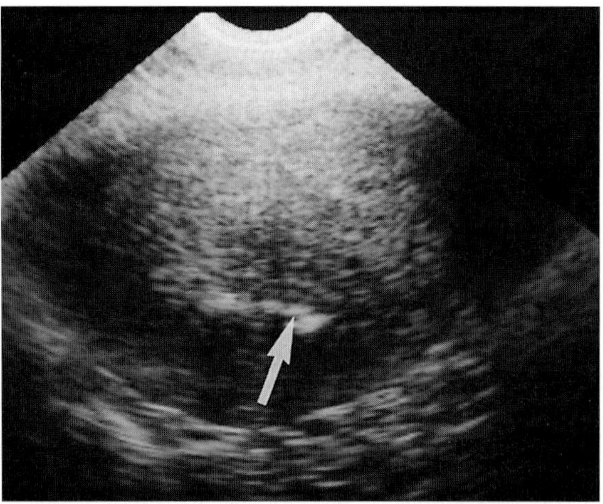

**Fig. 2.42.** Calcified endometrium in a 38-year-old woman with a history of repeated abortions. Endovaginal sonographic image shows calcification (*arrow*) in the endometrium. (From ATRI et al. 1994b)

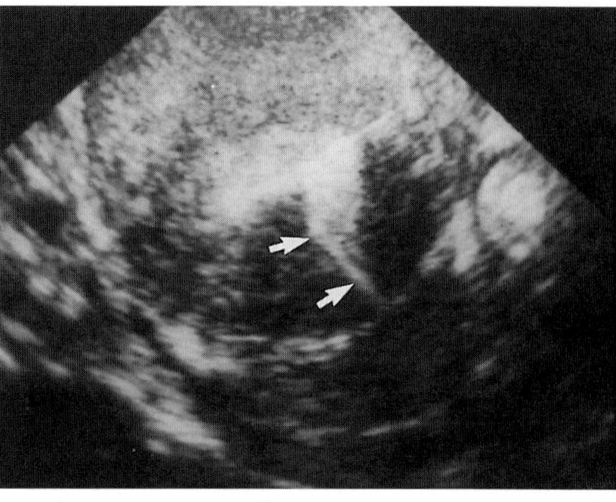

**Fig. 2.43.** Pierced intrauterine device. Longitudinal image of the uterus illustrates an intrauterine device penetrating the posterior myometrium (*arrows*)

or blood in the uterus. Blockage at the level of the cervix causes distention of the uterine cavity with fluid (hydrometra), blood (hematometra), or exudate (pyometra). The causative factors include endometrial or cervical tumors or cervical fibrosis (Fig. 2.4) (SCOTT et al. 1981). Obstruction at the level of the vagina results in hydro- or hematometrocolpos (distention of the uterus and vagina) or hydro- or hematocolpos (distention limited to the vagina). The obstruction is usually congenital and results from a vaginal septum, vaginal atresia, or rudimentary uterine horn (WILSON et al. 1978).

On sonography the uterine cavity is ballooned by the fluid, and the surrounding myometrium may be thin or thick depending on the chronicity of the obstruction and the age of the patient. The echotexture of the fluid is related to its nature, with hydrometra being clear and hemato- and pyometra being echogenic. A fluid level may be present because of the precipitation of the debris (Fig. 2.4). Continuity with the cervix helps in the differentiation of this condition from a cystic adnexal mass.

#### *2.6.4.2 Intrauterine Contraceptive Device*

Intrauterine contraceptive devices are clearly seen with sonography as very bright echogenic structures that present as a single or double line (entrance–exit reflections). The majority of IUDs cause shadowing (CALLEN et al. 1980). A problem with localization may arise in late pregnancy or when there is a large uterine mass that distorts the endometrial cavity. Sonography can be used to determine the proper position of the intrauterine device in the upper body or fundus. Myometrial penetration of the intrauterine device can be accurately assessed by endovaginal sonography (Fig. 2.43). When the string of the intrauterine device is not visible, sonography can confirm its intrauterine location. If the intrauterine device is not seen in the uterus, a plain x-ray confirms or excludes an intra-abdominal or pelvic location.

### 2.6.5 Sonohysterography

Sonohysterography is a technique used to improve the accuracy of endovaginal sonography for differentiating among subendometrial, endometrial, and uterine cavity abnormalities and to visualize the endometrial cavity to a better advantage (VAN ROESSEL et al. 1987). Sonohysterography has the potential to decrease the number of invasive procedures and triage the patients for the proper procedure.

The procedure is generally performed without premedication of antibiotics (CULLINAN et al. 1995). However, women with a history of chronic pelvic inflammatory disease are premedicated with antibiotics (CULLINAN et al. 1995). Catheters ranging from 5F to 8F, with or without a balloon at the end, are used. The straight catheter can be left anywhere in

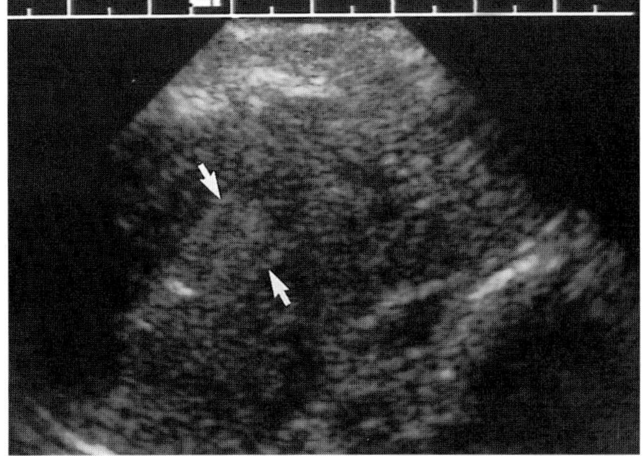

a

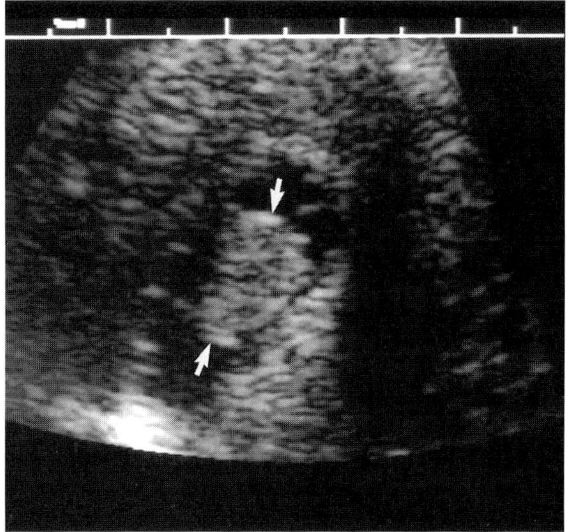

b

**Fig. 2.44 a,b.** Sonohysterography of an endometrial polyp. **a** Initial endovaginal sonography shows nonspecific endometrial thickening (*arrows*). **b** A polyp (*arrows*) completely surrounded by fluid is demonstrated following instillation of normal saline

the cavity, but the balloon-ended catheter is pulled back to the region of the cervix to block the uterine cavity and prevent interference with interpretation of the examination. The balloon can be deflated at the end of the examination to better assess the lower uterine segment. A straight catheter may be adequate in most cases but an inflated balloon is essential in the presence of a patulous uterine cavity, seen in multiparous women and in women with multiple uterine fibroids. The catheter is filled with normal saline before it is inserted to reduce the chance of introducing air into the cavity. A total of 5–10 ml of normal saline is usually sufficient to demonstrate the uterine cavity but volumes as high as 60 ml may be required.

Sonohysterography confirms the presence of an endometrial polyp by showing an intraluminal mass completely surrounded by fluid with or without a thin stalk (Fig. 2.44). In the rare form of a broad-based polyp, differentiation from an endometrial cancer is difficult. Submucosal fibroids, in general, indent the endometrial cavity (Fig. 2.16). However, different degrees of the intraluminal component, including a broad-based mass protruding into the uterine cavity, may be demonstrated. The combination of the presence of a broad base and the hypoechoic nature with or without an attenuating component help to differentiate them from endometrial polyps (Figs. 2.16, 2.18, 2.45). Endometrial hyperplasia demonstrates diffuse or focal thickening of the endometrium, which is better appreciated once the uterine cavity is distended (Fig. 2.46a,b). Endometrial wrinkles may be seen in the proliferative phase of the endometrial cycle (Parsons and Lense 1993). Endovaginal sonography alone is inaccurate for evaluating women for the presence of uterine synechiae. Sonohysterography confirms the existence of uterine synechiae by showing complete or incomplete bands in the uterine cavity (Fig. 2.46c) (Cullinan et al. 1995).

In a series by Cicinelli et al. (1995), endovaginal sonography had a sensitivity of 90% and a specificity of 98% in diagnosing submucosal leiomyomas. The sensitivity and specificity of sonohysterography were 100% and were similar to the results for hysteroscopy. However, sonohysterography was more accurate than hysteroscopy in showing the size and depth of submucosal leiomyomas. The same group correlated endovaginal sonography and transabdominal and transvaginal sonohysterography results with hysteroscopy for diagnosing endometrial polyps in a group of 50 women who underwent hysterectomy. The sensitivity and specificity of endovaginal sonography were 33.3% and 100%, respectively, as compared with 91.7% and 100% for a combination of transabdominal and transvaginal sonohysterography. Hysteroscopy had 100% sensitivity and specificity (Cicinelli et al. 1994).

Sonohysterography has been shown to be accurate to triage women on tamoxifen who had an abnormal endometrium for further invasive pro-

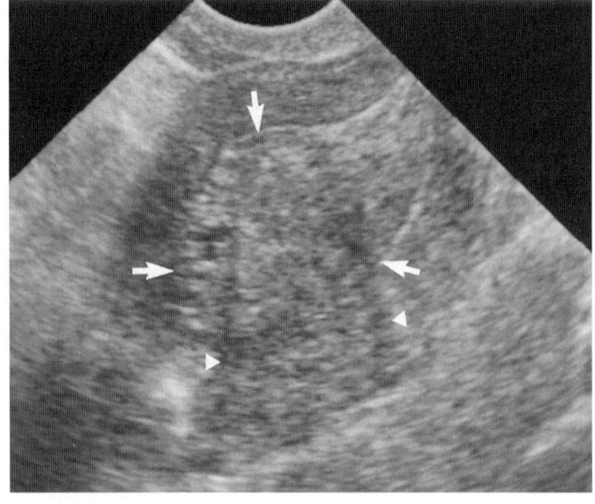

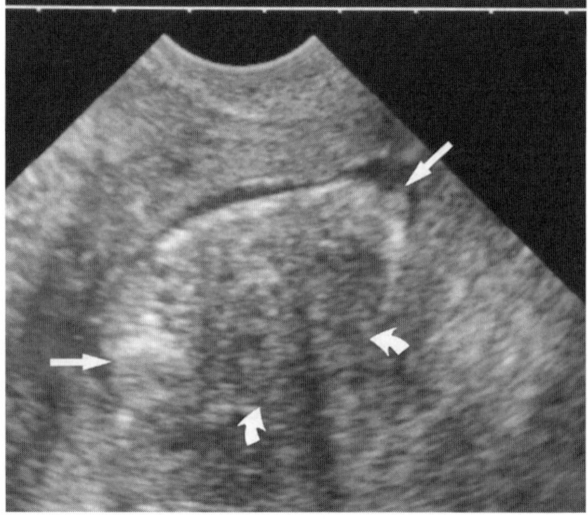

**Fig. 2.45 a,b.** Sonohysterography of a submucosal fibroid. **a** Initial endovaginal sonography illustrates thickening of endometrium with an apparent mass in the uterine cavity (*arrows*). Notice that there is a suggestion of sound attenuation (*arrowheads*). **b** Sonohysterography reveals a polypoid mass (*straight arrows*) with a broad base (*curved arrows*) protruding into the uterine cavity. The mass remains attenuating

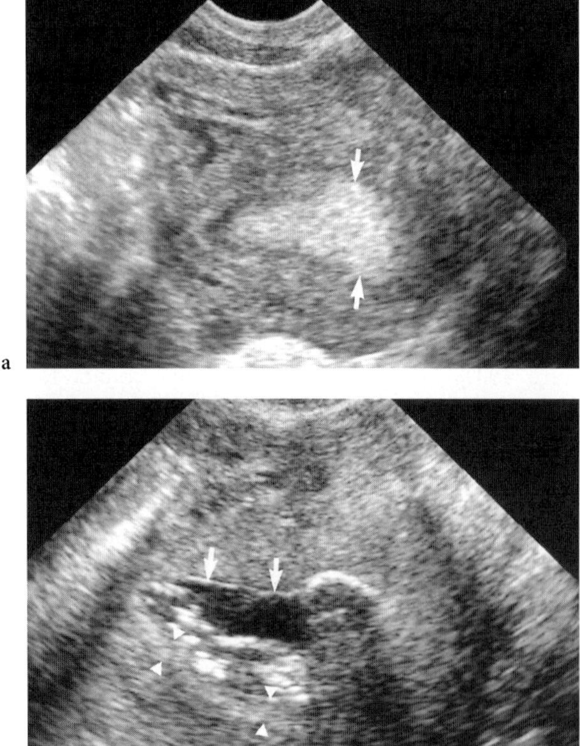

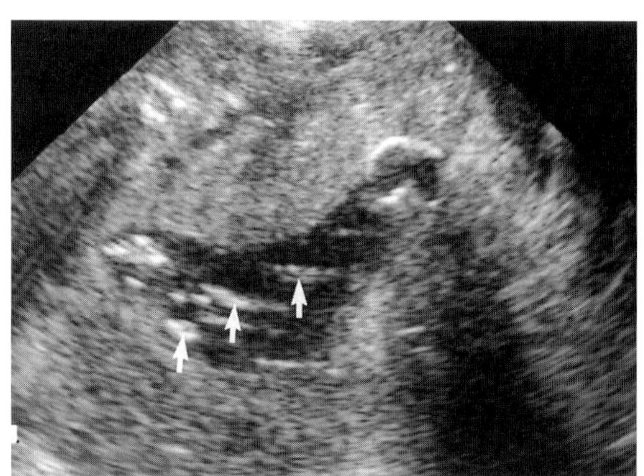

**Fig. 2.46 a–c.** Focal hyperplasia and uterine synechiae. **a** Endovaginal sonography shows echogenic thickening of the endometrium (*arrows*). **b** With instillation of normal saline, the anterior endometrial lining is very thin (*arrows*) but the posterior wall remains thick (*arrowheads*). **c** Numerous echogenic bands are demonstrated in the uterine cavity (*arrows*), consistent with synechiae

cedures. In a group of 20 women with an abnormal endometrium, ACHIRON et al. (1995a) identified eight women with endometrial polyps that were confirmed and treated by hysteroscopy and 12 women with normal endometrium but cystic changes at the endomyometrial junction that showed no significant pathology on dilatation and curettage (Fig. 2.39). GOLDSTEIN (1994c) has suggested the use of sonohysterography for the triage of women with perimenopausal bleeding, those with minimal tissue whose bleeding may be of anovulatory origin and who are best treated with hormonal therapy, and those with significant thickening of the endometrium requiring formal curettage. Furthermore, polyps may be distinguished from submucosal myomas, which allows appropriate preoperative triage for operative hysteroscopy. Also, larger fibroids can be triaged for laparotomy resection.

Further studies are required to compare endovaginal sonography and sonohysterography to determine the exact role of sonohysterography for triage of patients with abnormal endometrium for more invasive procedures.

### 2.6.6 Abnormalities of the Cervix

Gynecologic abnormalities of the cervix are diagnosed clinically, and sonography is not usually used for this purpose. Nebothian cysts are the most common recognizable abnormality of the cervix on sonography. They are the result of retention of mucus and other fluid within blocked endocervical glands secondary to chronic cervicitis, which is a common condition in parous women and is usually asymptomatic (SCOTT et al. 1994). They may be single or multiple and reach large proportions (Fig. 2.47). They are usually clear but may be echogenic. They may get infected.

Leiomyomas of the cervix are rare but have the same three origins as those in the corpus. They may be intramural, subserosal, or submucosal and may pedunculate through the endocervical canal.

Cervical carcinomas are not usually diagnosed by sonography. However, sonography has been used for their staging with mixed results (AOKI et al. 1990; YAMAMOTO and KITAO 1989). Overall, computed tomography and magnetic resonance imaging are more accurate for the staging of cervical carcinomas. Gynecologic problems of the cervix and vagina are best assessed by the transrectal approach. Cervical carcinoma rarely causes obstruction of the uterus (Fig. 2.48).

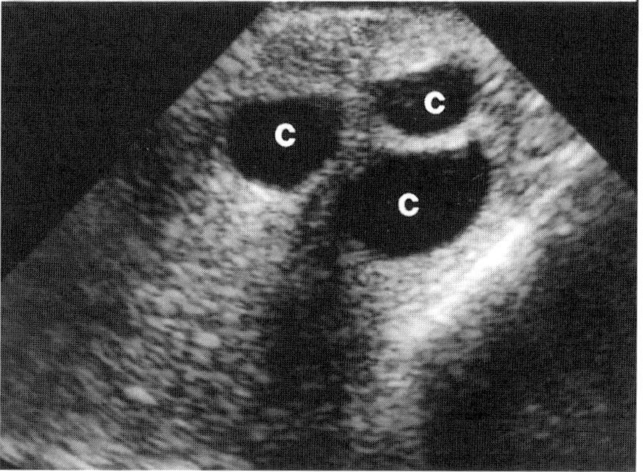


**Fig. 2.47.** Multiple nabothian cysts. Endovaginal sonographic image of the cervix demonstrates multiple thin-walled cysts of the cervix (*c*)

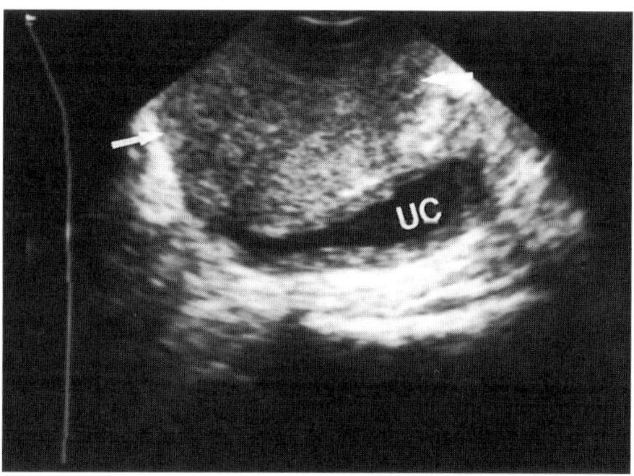


**Fig. 2.48.** Obstructed uterus due to the presence of cervical carcinoma. Endovaginal sonographic examination reveals a retroverted small uterus with significant atrophy of the corpus, distension of the uterine cavity (*UC*), and a large cervical solid mass (*arrows*)

## References

Achiron R, Lipitz S, Frenkel Y, Mashiach S (1995a) Endometrial blood flow response to estrogen replacement therapy and tamoxifen in asymptomatic, postmenopausal women: a transvaginal Doppler study. Ultrasound Obstet Gynecol 5:411–414

Achiron R, Lipitz S, Sivan E, et al. (1995b) Changes mimicking endometrial neoplasia in postmenopausal, tamoxifen-treated women with breast cancer: a transvaginal Doppler study. Ultrasound Obstet Gynecol 6:116–120

Achiron R, Lipitz S, Sivan E, Goldenberg M, Mashiach S (1995c) Sonohysterography for ultrasonographic evaluation of tamoxifen-associated cystic thickened endometrium. J Ultrasound Med 14:685–688

Adams JM, Tan SL, Wheeler MJ, et al. (1988) Uterine growth in the follicular phase of spontaneous ovulatory cycles and during luteinizing hormone-releasing hormone-induced cycles in women with normal or polycystic ovaries. Fertil Steril 49:52–55

Aleem F, Predanic M, Calame R, Moukhtar M, Pennisi J (1995) Transvaginal color and pulsed Doppler sonography of the endometrium: a possible role in reducing the number of dilatation and curettage procedures. J Ultrasound Med 14:139–145

Andolf E, Jorgensen C (1990) A prospective comparison of transabdominal and transvaginal ultrasound with surgical findings in gynecologic disease. J Ultrasound Med 9:71–75

Aoki S, Hata T, Senoh D, et al. (1990) Parametrial invasion of uterine cervical cancer assessed by transrectal ultrasonography: preliminary report. Gynecol Oncol 36:82–89

Artner A, Bosze P, Gonda G (1994) The value of ultrasound in preoperative assessment of the myometrial and cervical invasion in endometrial carcinoma. Gynecol Oncol 54: 147–151

Atri M, de Stempel J, Senterman MK, et al. (1992) Diffuse peripheral uterine calcification (manifestation of Mönckeberg's arteriosclerosis) detected by ultrasonography. J Clin Ultrasound 20:211–216

Atri M, Leduc C, Aldis AE, Kintzen G, Thibodeau M, Reinhold C, Bret PM (1994a) Can endovaginal ultrasound be the starting examination of the pelvis? (abstract). American Institute of Ultrasound in Medicine 38th Annual Convention. Baltimore, MD, March 20–23, 1994

Atri M, Nazarnia S, Aldis AE, et al. (1994b) Transvaginal US appearance of endometrial abnormalities. Radiographics 14:483–492

Battaglia C, Artini PG, Bencini S, Bianchi R, D'Ambrogio G, Genazzani AR (1995) Doppler analysis of uterine blood flow changes in spontaneous and medically induced menopause. Gynecol Endocrinol 9:143–148

Berman L, Stringer DA, St. Onge O, et al. (1989) Unilateral haematocolpos in uterine duplication associated with renal agenesis. Clin Radiol 40:577–581

Bidzinski M, Lemieszczuk B (1993) The value of transvaginal ultrasonography (TVS) in the assessment of myometrial and cervical invasion in corpus uterine neoplasms. Eur J Gynaecol Oncol 14:86–91

Bohlman ME, Ensor RE, Sanders RC (1987) Sonographic findings in adenomyosis of the uterus. Am J Roentgenol 148:765–766

Bonilla-Musoles F, Ballester MJ, Marti MC, Raga F, Osborne NG (1995a) Transvaginal color Doppler assessment of endometrial status in normal postmenopausal women: the effect of hormone replacement therapy. J Ultrasound Med 14:503–507

Bonilla-Musoles F, Marti MC, Ballester MJ, Raga F, Osborne NG (1995b) Normal uterine arterial blood flow in postmenopausal women assessed by transvaginal color Doppler ultrasonography. J Ultrasound Med 14:491–494

Botsis D, Kassanos D, Pyrgiotis E, et al. (1992) Vaginal sonography of the endometrium in postmenopausal women. Clin Exp Obstet Gynecol 19:189–192

Bourne TH, Campbell S, Steer CV, et al. (1991) Detection of endometrial cancer by transvaginal ultrasonography with color flow imaging and blood flow analysis: a preliminary report. Gynecol Oncol 40:253–259

Buli CM, Kasnar V, Dukovic I (1986) Use of ultrasound in the diagnosis of genital endometriosis. Jugosl Ginekol Perinatol 26:33–34

Buttram VC Jr (1983) Müllerian anomalies and their management. Fertil Steril 40:159–163

Buttram VC, Gibbons WE (1979) Müllerian anomalies: a proposed classification (an analysis of 144 cases). Fertil Steril 32:40–46

Cacciatore B, Lehtovirta P, Wahlstrom T, Ylostalo P (1989) Preoperative sonographic evaluation of endometrial cancer. Am J Obstet Gynecol 160:133–137

Callen PW, Filly RA, Munyer TP (1980) Intrauterine contraceptive devices: evaluation by sonography. Am J Roentgenol 135:797–800

Carrington BM, Hricak H, Nuruddin RN, et al. (1990) Müllerian duct anomalies: MR imaging evaluation. Radiology 176:715–720

Chan FY, Chau MT, Pun TC, Lam C, Ngan HY, Leong L, Wong RL (1994) Limitations of transvaginal sonography and color Doppler imaging in the differentiation of endometrial carcinoma from benign lesions. J Ultrasound Med 13:623–628

Check JH, Chase JS, Nowroozi K, Wu CH, Chern R (1989) Clinical evaluation of the Pipelle endometrial suction curette for timed endometrial biopsies. J Reprod Med 34:218–220

Cicinelli E, Romano F, Anastasio PS, Blasi N, Parisi C (1994) Sonohysterography versus hysteroscopy in the diagnosis of endouterine polyps. Gynecol Obstet Invest 38:266–271

Cicinelli E, Romano F, Anastasio PS, et al. (1995) Transabdominal sonohysterography, transvaginal sonography, and hysteroscopy in the evaluation of submucous myomas. Obstet Gynecol 85:42–47

Conte M, Guariglia L, Benedetti Panici P, Scambia G, Cento R, Mancuso S (1990) Transvaginal ultrasound evaluation of myometrial invasion in endometrial carcinoma. Gynecol Obstet Invest 29:224–226

Cullinan JA, Fleischer AC, Kepple DM, Arnold AL (1995) Sonohysterography: a technique for endometrial evaluation. Radiographics 153:501–514

Daly DC, Walter CA, Soto Albors CE, Riddick DH (1983) Hysteroscopic metroplasty: surgical technique and obstetric outcome. Fertil Steril 39:623–628

Damirov MM, Bakuleva LP, Shabanov AM, Sliusar' NN (1994) A clinico-morphological comparison of the ultrasonic criteria of adenomyosis. Akusherstvo i Ginekologiia 2:40–43

DelMaschio A, Vanzulli A, Sironi S, Spagnolo D, Belloni C, Garancini P, Taccagni GL (1993) Estimating the depth of myometrial involvement by endometrial carcinoma: efficacy of transvaginal sonography vs MR imaging. Am J Roentgenol 160:533–538

Dodd GD III, Budzik RF Jr (1990) Lipomatous uterine tumors: diagnosis by ultrasound, CI and MR. J Comput Assist Tomogr 14:629–632

Doherty CM, Silver B, Binor Z, et al. (1993) Transvaginal ultrasonography and the assessment of luteal phase endometrium. Am J Obstet Gynecol 168:1702–1707

Eddowes HA, Read MD, Codling BW (1990) Pipelle: a more acceptable technique for outpatient endometrial biopsy. Br J Obstet Gynaecol 97:961–962

Eden JA, Place J, Carter GD, et al. (1988) What are the ultrasound and biochemical features of impending ovulation? Aust NZJ Obstet Gynecol 28:225–227

Egger H, Weigman P (1982) Clinical and surgical aspects of ovarian endometriotic cysts. Arch Gynecol 233:37–45

Emanuel MH, Verdel MJ, Wamsteker K, Lammes FB (1995) A prospective comparison of transvaginal ultrasonography and diagnostic hysteroscopy in the evaluation of patients with abnormal uterine bleeding: clinical implications. Am J Obstet Gynecol 172:547–552

Emge LA (1962) Elusive adenomyosis of the uterus: its historic past and its present state of recognition. Am J Obstet Gynecol 83:1541

Farrer-Brown G, Beilby JOW, Tarbit MH (1970) The blood supply of the uterus. II. Venous pattern. Br J Obstet Gynecol Comm 77:682–689

Fedele L, Ferrazzi E, Dorta M, Vercellini P, Candiani GB (1988a) Ultrasonography in the differential diagnosis of "double" uteri. Fertil Steril 50:361–364

Fedele L, Dorta M, Vercellini P, Brioschi D, Candiani GB (1988b) Ultrasound in the diagnosis of subclasses of unicornuate uterus. Obstet Gynecol 71:274–277

Fedele L, Dorta M, Brioschi D, Giudici MN, Candiani GB (1989) Pregnancies in septate uteri: outcome in relation to site of uterine implantation as determined by sonography. Am J Roentgenol 152:781–784

Fedele L, Bianchi S, Dorta M, Arcaini L, Zanotti F, Carinelli S (1992a) Transvaginal ultrasonography in the diagnosis of diffuse adenomyosis. Fertil Steril 58:94–97

Fedele L, Bianchi S, Dorta M, Zanotti F, Brioschi D, Carinelli S (1992b) Transvaginal ultrasonography in the differential diagnosis of adenomyoma versus leiomyoma. Am J Obstet Gynecol 167:603–606

Fleischer AC, Kalemeris GC, Entmann SS (1986a) Sonographic depiction of the endometrium during normal cycles. Ultrasound Med Biol 12:271–277

Fleischer AC, Kalemeris GC, Machin JE, Entman SS, James AE Jr (1986b) Sonographic depiction of normal and abnormal endometrium with histopathologic correlation. J Ultrasound Med 5:445–452

Foix A, Bruno RO, Davison T, et al. (1966) The pathology of postcurettage intrauterine adhesions. Am J Obstet Gynecol 96:1027–1033

Fore SR, Hammond CB, Parker RT, Anderson EE (1975) Urologic and genital anomalies in patients with congenital absence of vagina. Obstet Gynecol 46:410–415

Forrest TS, Elyaderani MK, Muilenburg MI, et al. (1988) Cyclic endometrial changes: US assessment with histologic correlation. Radiology 167:233–237

Gilsanz V, Cleveland RH, Reid BS (1982) Duplication of the müllerian ducts and genitourinary malformations. Radiology 144:791–801

Goldstein SR (1994a) Postmenopausal endometrial fluid collections revisited: look at the doughnut rather than the hole. Obstet Gynecol 83:738–740

Goldstein SR (1994b) Unusual ultrasonographic appearance of the uterus in patients receiving tamoxifen. Am J Obstet Gynecol 170:447–451

Goldstein SR (1994c) Use of ultrasonohysterography for triage of perimenopausal patients with unexplained uterine bleeding. Am J Obstet Gynecol 170:565–570

Goldstein SR, Nachtigall M, Snyder JR, Nachtigall L (1990) Endometrial assessment by vaginal ultrasonography before endometrial sampling in patients with postmenopausal bleeding. Am J Obstet Gynecol 163:119–123

Gordon AN, Fleischer AC, Reed GW (1990) Depth of myometrial invasion in endometrial cancer: preoperative assessment by transvaginal ultrasonography. Gynecol Oncol 39:321–327

Granberg S, Wikland M, Karlsson B, et al. (1991) Endometrial thickness as measured by endovaginal sonography for identifying endometrial abnormality. Am J Obstet Gynecol 164:47–52

Henig I, Chan P, Tredway DR, Maw GM, Gullett AJ, Cheatwood M (1989) Evaluation of the Pipelle curette for endometrial biopsy. J Reprod Med 34:786–789

Hertzberg BS, Bowie JD, Weber TM, et al. (1991) Sonography of the cervix during the third trimester of pregnancy: value of the transperineal approach. Am J Roentgenol 157:73–76

Hill GA, Herbert GM III, Parker RA, Wentz AC (1989) Comparison of late luteal phase endometrial biopsies using the Novak curette or Pipelle endometrial suction curette. Obstet Gynecol 73:443–445

Hulka CA, Hall DA (1993) Endometrial abnormalities associated with tamoxifen therapy for breast cancer: sonographic and pathologic correlation. Am J Roentgenol 160:809–812

Ismail SM (1994) Pathology of endometrium treated with tamoxifen. J Clin Pathol 47:827–833

Karlsson B, Granberg S, Wikland M, Ryd W, Norstrom A (1993) Endovaginal scanning of the endometrium compared to cytology and histology in women with postmenopausal bleeding. Gynecol Oncol 50:173–178

Karlsson B, Granberg S, Hellberg P, Wikland M (1994) Comparative study of transvaginal sonography and hysteroscopy for the detection of pathologic endometrial lesions in women with postmenopausal bleeding. J Ultrasound Med 13:757–762

Karlsson B, Granberg S, Wikland M, et al. (1995) Transvaginal ultrasonography of the endometrium in women with postmenopausal bleeding: a Nordic multicenter study. Am J Obstet Gynecol 172:1488–1494

Kaunitz AM, Masciello A, Ostrowski M, Bovira EZ (1988) Comparison of endometrial biopsy with the endometrial Pipelle and Vabra. J Peprod Med 33:427–431

Kedar RP, Bourne TH, Powles TJ, Collins WP, Ashley SE, Cosgrove DO, Campbell S (1994) Effects of tamoxifen on uterus and ovaries of postmenopausal women in a randomized breast cancer prevention trial. Lancet 343:1318–1321

Kirkinen P (1990) Ultrasonography of the lower uterine segment after multiple cesarean sections. Ann Med 22:137–139

Kliewer MA, Hertzberg BS, George PY, McDonald JW (1995) Acoustic shadowing from uterine leiomyomas: sonographic-pathologic correlation. Radiology 196:99–102

Koonings PP, Moyer DL, Grimes DA (1990) A randomized clinical trial comparing Pipelle and Tis-u-trap for endometrial biopsy. Obstet Gynecol 75:293–295

Kurjak A, Kupesic S (1995) Ovarian senescence and its significance on uterine and ovarian perfusion. Fertil Steril 64:532–537

Kurjak A, Shalan H, Sosic A, et al. (1993) Endometrial carcinoma in postmenopausal women: evaluation by transvaginal color Doppler ultrasonography. Am J Obstet Gynecol 169:1597–1603

Kurman RJ (ed) (1994) Blaustein's pathology of the female genital tract. Springer, Berlin Heidelberg New York

Lahti E, Vuopala S, Kauppila A, Blanco G, Ruokonen A, Laatikainen T (1994) Maturation of vaginal and endometrial epithelium in postmenopausal breast cancer patients receiving long-term tamoxifen. Gynecol Oncol 55:410–414

Lande IM, Hill MC, Cosco FE, et al. (1988) Adnexal and cul-de-sac abnormalities: transvaginal sonography. Radiology 166:325–332

Leibman AJ, Kruse B, McSweeney MB (1988) Transvaginal sonography: comparison with transabdominal sonography in the diagnosis of pelvic masses. Am J Roentgenol 151:89–92

Levine D, Gosink BB, Johnson LA (1995) Change in endometrial thickness in postmenopausal women undergoing hormone replacement therapy. Radiology 197:603–608

Lewis B, Stallworthy JA, Cowdell R (1970) Adenocarcinoma of the body of the uterus. Br J Obstet Gynaecol Comm 77:343–348

Li TC, Nuttall L, Klentzeris L, et al. (1992) How well does ultrasonographic measurement of endometrial thickness predict the results of histological dating? Hum Reprod 7:1–5

Lin MC, Gosink BB, Wolf SI, et al. (1991) Endometrial thickness after menopause: effect of hormone replacement. Radiology 180:427–432

Malpani A, Singer J, Wolverson MK, Merenda G (1990) Endometrial hyperplasia: value of endometrial thickness in ultrasonographic diagnosis and clinical significance. J Clin Ultrasound 18:173–177

McShane PM, Peilly RJ, Schiff I (1983) Pregnancy outcomes following Tompkins metroplasty. Fertil Steril 40:190–194

Mendelson EB, Bohm-Velez M, Joseph N, et al. (1988a) Gynecologic imaging: comparison of transabdominal and transvaginal sonography. Radiology 166:321–324

Mendelson EB, Bohm-Velez M, Joseph N, et al. (1988b) Endometrial abnormalities: evaluation with transvaginal sonography. Am J Roentgenol 50:139–141

Miller EI, Thomas RH, Lines P (1977) The atrophic postmenopausal uterus. J Clin Ultrasound 5:261–263

Mintz MC, Thickman DI, Gussman D, Kressel HY (1987) MR evaluation of uterine anomalies. Am J Roentgenol 148:287–290

Morrow CP, DiSaia PJ, Townsend DE (1973) Current management of endometrial carcinoma. Obstet Gynecol 42:399–406

Newton CW III, Abell MR (1973) Iatrogenic fetal implants. Obstet Gynecol 40:686–691

Nussbaum AR, Sanders RC, Jones MD (1986) Neonatal uterine morphology as seen on real-time US. Radiology 160:641–643

Orsini LF, Salardi S, Pilu G, et al. (1984) Pelvic organs in premenarcheal girls: real-time ultrasonography. Radiology 153:113–116

Osmers R, Volksen M, Schauer A (1990) Vaginosonography for early detection of endometrial carcinoma? Lancet 335:1569–1571

Parsons AK, Lense JJ (1993) Sonohysterography for endometrial abnormalities: preliminary results. J Clin Ultrasound 21:87–95

Pellerito JS, McCarthy SM, Doyle MB, Glickman MG, DeCherney AH (1992) Diagnosis of uterine anomalies: relative accuracy of MR imaging, endovaginal sonography, and hysterosalpingography. Radiology 183:795–800

Pham CA, Atri M, Senterman MK (1993) Ultrasonographic appearance of uterine lipoleiomyoma. J Can Assoc Radiologists 44:463–465

Pirhonen JP, Vuento MH, Makinen JI, Salmi TA (1993) Long-term efects of hormone replacement therapy on the uterus and on uterine circulation. Am J Obstet Gynecol 168:620–630

Platt JF, Bree RL, Davidson D (1990) Ultrasound of the normal nongravid uterus: correlation with gross and histopathology. J Clin Ultrasound 18:15–19

Reinhold C, Atri M, Mehio A, et al. (1995) Diffuse uterine adenomyosis: morphologic criteria and diagnostic accuracy of endovaginal sonography. Radiology 197:609–614

Reuter KL, Daly DC, Cohen SM (1989) Septate versus bicornuate uteri: errors in imaging diagnosis. Radiology 172:749–752

Rosati P, Exacoustos C, Mancuso S (1992) Longitudinal evaluation of uterine myoma growth during pregnancy. A sonographic study. J Ultrasound Med 11:511–515

Rosen DJ, Shapira J, Cordoba M, et al. (1994) Endometrial changes with tamoxifen: comparison between tamoxifen-treated and nontreated asymptomatic, postmenopausal breast cancer patients. Gynecol Oncol 52:185–190

Rosenberg HK, Sherman NH, Tarry WF, et al. (1986) Mayer-Rokitansky-Küster-Hauser syndrome: US aid to diagnosis. Radiology 161:815–819

Roth E, Taylor HB (1966) Heterotopic cartilage in uterus. Obstet Gynecol 27:838–844

Sahakian V, Syrop C, Turner D (1991) Endometrial carcinoma: transvaginal ultrasonography prediction of depth of myometrial invasion. Gynecol Oncol 43:217–219

Sample WF, Lippe BM, Gyepes MT (1977) Gray-scale ultrasonography of the normal female pelvis. Radiology 125:477–483

Saxton DW, Farquhar CM, Rae T et al. (1990) Accuracy of ultrasound measurements of female pelvic organs. Br J Obstet Gynecol 97:695–699

Scott JR, Disaia PJ, Hammond CB, Spellacy WN (1994) Danforth's obstetrics and gynecology, 7th edn. Lippincott, Philadelphia

Scott WW Jr, Rosenshein NB, Siegelman SS, et al. (1981) The obstructed uterus. Radiology 141:767–770

Segna RA, Dottino PR, Deligdisch L, Cohen CJ (1992) Tamoxifen and endometrial cancer. Mt Sinai J Med 59:416–418

Shepherd JH (1989) Revised FIGO staging for gynecological cancer. Br J Obstet Gynaecol 96:889–892

Sheth S, Hamper UM, Kurman RJ (1993) Thickened endometrium in the postmenopausal woman: sonographic-pathologic correlation. Radiology 187:135–139

Sheth S, Hamper UM, McCollum ME, Caskey CI, Rosenshein NB, Kurman RJ (1995) Endometrial blood flow analysis in postmenopausal women: can it help differentiate benign from malignant causes of endometrial thickening? Radiology 195:661–665

Shipley CF 3rd, Simmons CL, Nelson GH (1994) Comparison of transvaginal sonography with endometrial biopsy in asymptomatic postmenopausal women. J Ultrasound Med 13:99–104

Silver MM, Miles P, Rosa C (1991) Comparison of Novak and Pipelle endometrial biopsy instruments. Obstet Gynecol 78:828–830

Sladkevicius P, Valentin L, Marsal K (1994) Endometrial thickness and Doppler velocimetry of the uterine arteries as discriminators of endometrial status in women with postmenopausal bleeding: a comparative study. Am J Obstet Gynecol 171:722–728

Sorensen SS (1988) Estimated prevalence of müllerian anomalies. Acta Obstet Gynecol Scand 67:441–445

Stovall TG, Photopulos GJ, Poston WM, et al. (1991a) Pipelle endometrial sampling in patients with known endometrial carcinoma. Obstet Gynecol 77:954–956

Stovall TG, Ling FW, Morgan PL (1991b) A prospective, randomized comparison of the Pipelle endometrial sampling device with the Novak curette. Am J Obstet Gynecol 165:1287–1290

Tessler FN, Schiller VL, Perrella RR, et al. (1989) Transabdominal versus endovaginal pelvic sonography: prospective study. Radiology 170:553–556

The American Fertility Society (1988) Classification of adnexal adhesions, distal tubal occlusion, tubal occlusion secondary to tubal ligation, tubal pregnancies, müllerian anomalies and intrauterine adhesions. Fertil Steril 49:944–955

Van Den Bosch T, Vandendael A, Van Schoubroeck D, Wranz RAB, Lombard CJ (1995) Combining vaginal ultrasonography and office endometrial sampling in postmenopausal women. Obstet Gynecol 85:349–352

Van Roessel J, Wamsteker K, Exalto N (1987) Sonographic investigation of the uterus during artifical uterine cavity distension. J Clin Ultrasound 15:439–450

Verner RE, Sparks JM, Cameron CD, et al. (1991) Transvaginal sonography of endometrium in postmenopausal women. Obstet Gynecol 78:195–199

Williams PL, Warwick ••, Dyson ••, Bannister •• (eds) (1989) Gray's anatomy. Churchill Livingstone, New York

Wilson DA, Stacy TM, Smith EI (1978) Ultrasound diagnosis of hydrocolpos and hydrometrocolpos. Radiology 128: 451–454

Wolf DM, Jordan VC (1992) Gynecologic complications with long-term adjuvant tamoxifen therapy for breast cancer. Gynecol Oncol 45:118–128

Yamamoto K, Kitao M (1989) The evaluation of transrectal radial ultrasonography on parametrial infiltration in untreated cervical carcinoma for more accurate staging. Acta Obster Gynaecol Jpn 41:487–494

Zenetti BE, Ferrari LR, Rossi G (1978) Classification and radiographic features of uterine malformations: hysterosalpingographic study. Br J Radiol 51:161–170

# 3 Magnetic Resonance Imaging Versus Ultrasound in the Assessment of Benign Uterine Lesions

A. Silva, S. Ascher, and C. Reinhold

CONTENTS




A. Silva, MD, Clinical Instructor, Department of Radiology, Georgetown University Medical Center, 3800 Reservoir Road NW, Washington, DC 20007-2197, USA
S.M. Ascher, MD, Associate Professor of Radiology, Director of Body MRI, Department of Radiology, Georgetown University Medical Center, 3800 Reservoir Road NW, Washington, DC 20007-2197, USA
C. Reinhold, MD, Assistant Professor of Radiology, Director of Body MRI, Montreal General Hospital, McGill University, 1650 Cedar Ave., Montréal, Québec H3G 1A4, Canada


## 3.1 Introduction

Recent developments in magnetic resonance imaging (MRI), including the advent of fast pulse sequences and phased-array multicoil technology, have increased the role of MRI in evaluating benign pathology of the uterus (Hricak 1993). Although ultrasound remains the procedure of choice for the initial evaluation of patients with suspected uterine disease, MRI is an important adjunct due to its excellent soft tissue differentiation (Chang and Hricak 1989; Hricak 1986). MRI is indicated in patients for whom the ultrasound examination is technically suboptimal or nondiagnostic. This is true, for example, in cases where the origin of a pelvic mass is uncertain and further tissue characterization is required. Patients with complex uterine congenital anomalies may also benefit from MRI, particularly when transvaginal ultrasound is not feasible. Similarly, in patients undergoing uterus-sparing surgery, MRI can be performed to accurately localize uterine leiomyomas for preoperative planning in selected cases. In addition, for patients receiving hormonal therapy in the treatment of leiomyomas or adenomyosis, MRI is ideal for monitoring the evolution of disease because standard and reproducible images can be obtained. This chapter will address the role of MRI in the evaluation of benign uterine pathology with an emphasis on its merits compared with ultrasound.

## 3.2 Normal Anatomic Structures

### 3.2.1 Uterine Corpus

The uterus is divided into three major segments: (1) the fundus, which consists of that portion of the uterus cephalad to the cornua, (2) the body or corpus, and (3) the cervix. In women of reproductive age the uterus measures 6–9 cm in length, of which the corpus measures 4–6 cm and the cervix 2.5–3.2 cm. The uterus measures approximately 4 cm in thickness and 6 cm in its maximal transverse dimension (Lee et al. 1985; Demas et al. 1986; McCarthy et al. 1986; Langlois 1970; Jones and Jones 1982a). Histologically, the uterine corpus is divided into three tissue layers: (1) the serosa, which consists of the peritoneum; (2) the myometrium, which is largely made up of involuntary smooth muscle; and (3) the endometrium, composed of the mucosal stratum functionalis (responsive to hormonal stimuli) and the stratum basale (responsible for growth and regeneration of the endomtrium) (Jones and Jones 1982b). The inner third of the myometrium is composed of densely packed smooth muscle bundles with an orientation that is parallel to the stratum basale of the endometrium (Schwalm and Dubrauszky 1966). On the other hand, the outer myometrium or myometrium proper consists of randomly oriented and loosely packed smooth muscle bundles. This difference in the orientation and density of smooth muscle bundles between the inner and outer myometrium is of interest because it may be one of the factors contributing to the MRI appearance of the myometrium (Brown et al. 1991).

### 3.2.2
### Cervix

The cervix is separated from the corpus of the uterus by the internal os, which corresponds to a slight constriction visible externally, and by the entrance of the uterine vessels. The cervical canal is lined by the endocervix, which is composed of columnar epithelium. Small folds in the mucous membrane called plicae palmatae are present (Bloom and Fawcett 1975). Surrounding the endocervix is the fibrous stroma. The outermost layer of the cervix is composed of a muscular coat that becomes increasingly thin in the lower portion of the cervix. The external os marks the opening between the cervix and vagina and is defined histologically by the squamocolumnar junction. The portion of the cervix protruding into the vagina is called the pars or portio vaginalis and is covered by stratified squamous epithelium (Jones and Jones 1982a).

### 3.2.3
### Parametrium and Ligaments of the Uterus

It is important to be familiar with the ligaments of the uterus because they may serve as pathways for local spread of disease. The parametrium is located between the layers of the broad ligament adjacent to the lateral margins of the uterine corpus and cervix (Jones and Jones 1982a). It is composed largely of loose connective and areolar tissue. The broad ligament consists of a double sheet of peritoneum that reflects off the ventral and dorsal surfaces of the uterus and extends to the pelvic side wall. The lower border of the broad ligament is thickened, with a condensation of connective tissue and smooth muscle fibers forming the paired cardinal ligaments (Jones and Jones 1982a). The paired uterosacral ligaments fuse anteromedially with the cardinal ligaments, as well as with the fascia surrounding the upper vagina and cervix, before coursing posteriorly to the sacrum. The paired round ligaments are muscular bands (5–6 mm in diameter) that arise from the lateral aspect of the uterine fundus, slightly below and anterior to the insertion of the fallopian tubes (Jones and Jones 1982a). They pass through the inguinal canal to fuse with the subcutaneous tissue of the labia majora. The uterovesical ligaments extend from the cervix to the base of the urinary bladder (Jones and Jones 1982a). The cardinal, uterosacral, and uterovesical ligaments are the main suspensory ligaments of the uterus. The main function of the round ligaments is to prevent retrodisplacement (Jones and Jones 1982a).

## 3.3
## MR Technique

### 3.3.1
### General Guidelines

#### *3.3.1.1*
#### *Patient Preparation*

No special patient preparation is required for MRI of the uterus; however, it is preferable that patients fast for a minimum of 6 h in order to minimize bowel peristaltism. Immediately prior to the examination, patients should be asked to void. This limits phase ghost artifacts of the distended urinary bladder induced by patient motion. In addition, an overly distended bladder may result in uterine compression, which may alter the appearance of normal and pathologic structures.

Although examinations are usually performed in the supine position, placing patients with claustrophobia in the prone position often obviates the need for administering a sedative.

#### 3.3.1.2 Surface/Endoluminal Coils

A phased-array pelvic multicoil should be routinely used if available. Pelvic multicoils markedly increase the signal-to-noise ratio (S/N) of the image and permit the use of a small field of view (FOV), ranging from 20 to 26 cm, depending on the size of the patient (Hricak 1993). In addition, in conjunction with T2-weighted echo-train spin-echo (SE) sequences, higher matrix sizes of 256–512 in the frequency encode direction and 256 in the phase encode direction become feasible (Smith et al. 1992b). The combination of a small FOV and a large matrix size results in high-resolution T2-weighted images of the uterus.

Although a larger FOV is usually prescribed for *body coil* imaging due to S/N considerations, the FOV should be maintained as small as possible, usually on the order of 28–32 cm, depending on the patient's size.

### 3.3.2 Imaging Protocol

#### 3.3.2.1 Pulse Sequences

We routinely perform a localizing sequence using a fast T2-weighted sequence such as a breath-hold echo-train SE sequence. This localizing sequence can be acquired in less than 24 s. We recommend using a fast T2-weighted sequence over a gradient-echo sequence because pelvic structures are better defined on T2-weighted sequences, allowing technologists to readily identify the uterus and other important landmarks.

T2- and T1-weighted sequences are standard techniques for evaluating the uterine corpus and cervix. The uterine and cervical zonal anatomy is best defined on *T2-weighted* sequences (Fig. 3.1). In the pelvis, T2-weighted echo-train SE sequences have largely replaced conventional SE sequences because

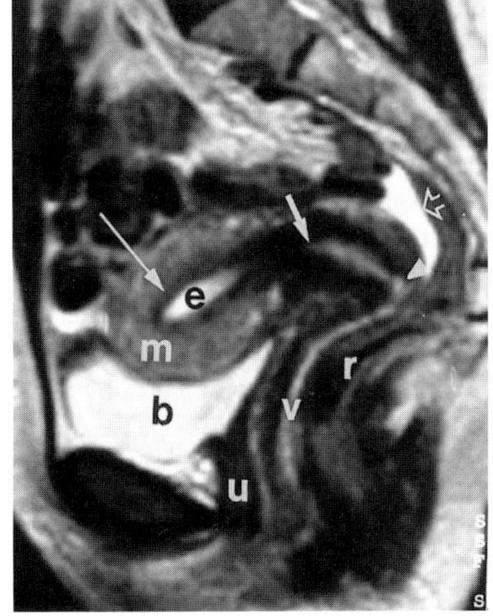


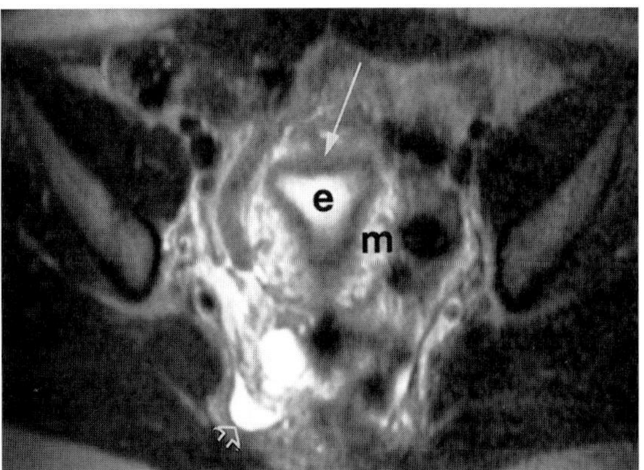


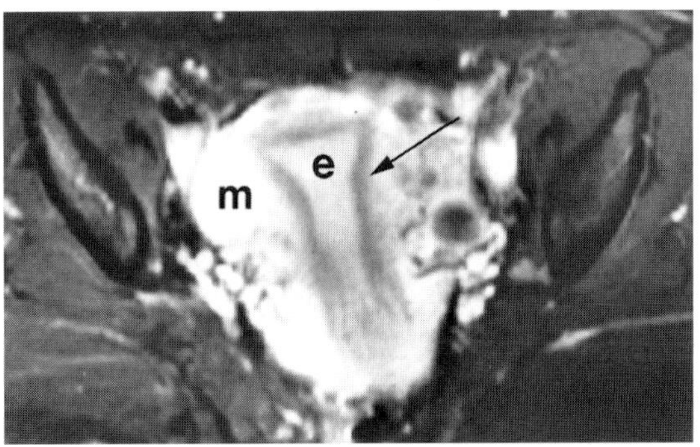


**Fig. 3.1 a–c.** Normal uterus and cervix. **a** Sagittal T2-, **b** axial T2-, and **c** postcontrast T1-weighted MR images from three different patients show that the endometrium (*e*) of the uterine corpus is separated from the myometrium (*m*) by the junctional zone (*long arrow*, a–c). The cervix extends from the internal os (*short arrow*, **a**) to the external os (*arrowhead*, **a**), which protrudes into the vagina (*v*). The vagina is positioned between the bladder (*b*) and urethra (*u*) anteriorly and the rectum (*r*) posteriorly. Fluid is seen in the cul-de-sac (*open arrow*). Note that, after contrast, uterine zonal anatomy normally not seen on T1-weighted images becomes apparent. (From Ascher et al. 1997)

of shortened acquisition times (Nghiem et al. 1992). The imaging time with echo-train SE sequences is inversely proportional to the number of 180° pulses applied, or the echo-train length (ETL). In the pelvis, where only a single-echo (T2-weighted) image is acquired, an ETL of 16 can potentially decrease the acquisition time by a factor of 16, if all other imaging parameters remain constant (Smith et al. 1992a). The shorter acquisition time achievable with echo-train SE sequences is partially offset by the use of higher matrix sizes, which would not be feasible with T2-weighted conventional SE sequences, and longer repetition times (TR), which are needed to cover the desired anatomic region. We routinely use a T2-weighted echo-train SE sequence with a TR in the range of 3000–5000 ms and an effective TE of 90–120 ms. The T2 contrast of this sequence approximates that of a conventional T2-weighted SE sequence; however, the contrast of certain tissues is altered with echo-train SE imaging. For example, fat is of a higher signal intensity on echo-train SE sequences due to altered J-coupling between neighboring protons in the hydrocarbon chains, while muscle shows lower signal intensity due to magnetization transfer effects (Constable et al. 1992; Jolesz and Jones 1993).

*T1-weighted* sequences maximize the image contrast between muscle and fat (Fig. 3.2). In addition, the presence of hemorrhage or fat within a lesion is best depicted on T1-weighted images. Since acquisition times are considerably shorter for T1-weighted images, conventional SE sequences (TR = 500–800 ms; TE = 10–30 ms) may be performed. Alternatively, breath-hold T1-weighted spoiled gradient-echo (SGE) sequences (TR = 140 ms; TE = 4 ms; flip angle = 80°) can be obtained with a saving in acquisition time, and without a loss of spatial resolution.

Gadolinium-enhanced (.1 mmole/kg) studies are primarily reserved for evaluating the endometrium and for tumor staging.

#### 3.3.2.2
#### Imaging Planes

Three orthogonal planes (transverse, sagittal, and coronal), as well as off-axis imaging, can be performed with MRI. Each plane of section has distinct advantages for imaging uterine and cervical pathology. Only general guidelines will be presented here; more detail will be provided in the various sections dealing with specific disease processes.

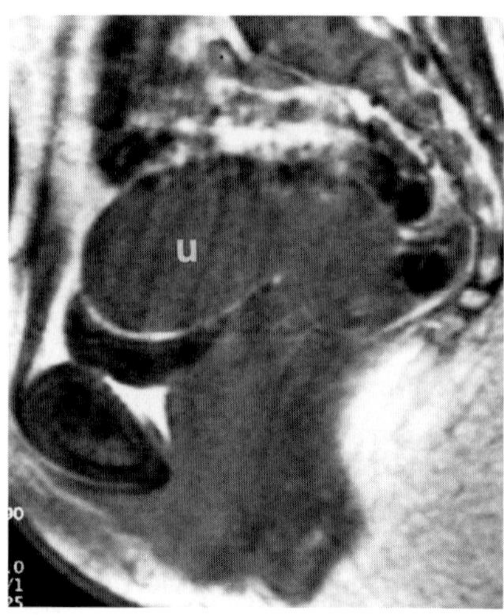


**Fig. 3.2.** Normal uterus. Sagittal T1-weighted MR image shows the uterus (*u*) to be of homogeneous intermediate signal intensity. Uterine zonal anatomy cannot be discerned. (From Ascher et al. 1997)

Transverse and sagittal planes are most commonly used to image the uterus and cervix. *Sagittal sections* image the uterus parallel to its long axis. In addition, the cervix, including the pars vaginalis, and the posterior vaginal fornix are well demonstrated on T2-weighted sequences (Fig. 3.3). On sagittal images, the bladder, rectum, and anterior and posterior cul de sac are all visualized in a single plane of section. *Transverse sections* demonstrate the uterus and cervix, as well as the parametrium. Transverse sections are also most commonly used to detect the presence of lymphadenopathy. *Coronal sections* are supplementary and provide an additional view of the parametrium. In specific instances, *off-axis imaging planes* may be helpful. For example, an oblique transverse section parallel to the endometrium results in a "long-axis view" and is ideal for imaging the fundal contour in congenital uterine anomalies. A coronal oblique section, obtained perpendicular to the endometrium, results in a "short-axis" view and allows accurate assessment of zonal anatomy, such as in the diagnosis of adenomyosis.

### 3.3.3
### Artifacts

#### 3.3.3.1
#### Motion Artifact Reduction

To minimize motion artifacts from intestinal peristaltism, patients should ideally have been

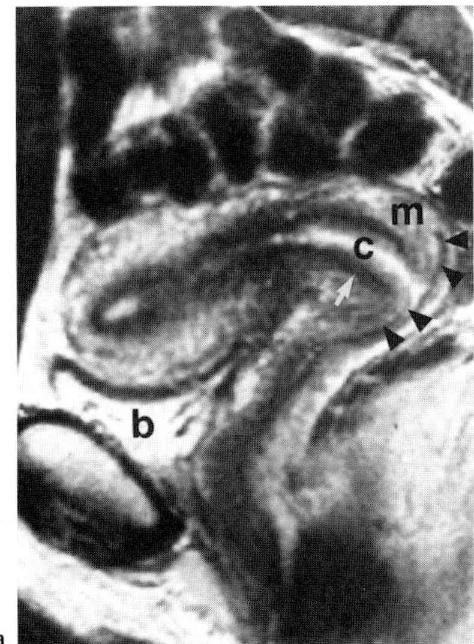


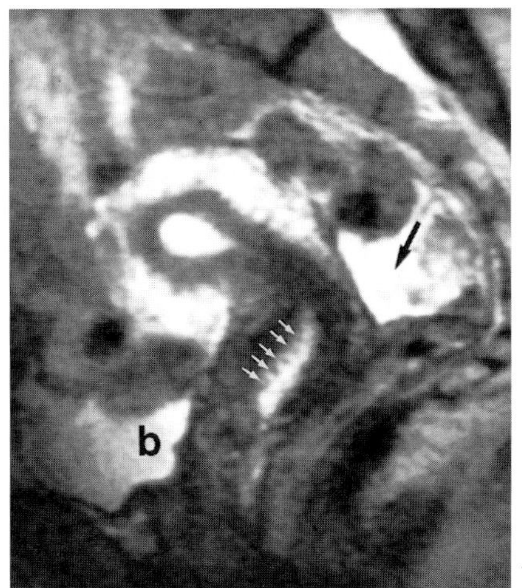


**Fig. 3.3 a,b.** Normal cervix. **a** Sagittal body coil T2- and **b** sagittal surface coil T2-weighted MR images demonstrate cervical zonal anatomy. The body coil image shows the high-signal-intensity endocervical canal (*c*) surrounded by both the low-signal-intensity fibrocervical stroma (*arrow*) and intermediate-signal-intensity myometrium (*m*). The anterior and posterior cervical lips (*arrowheads*) are seen protruding into the vaginal fornices. With the aid of a pelvic surface coil, improved spatial resolution highlights the intermediate-signal-intensity mucosal plicae palmatae (*short arrows*). Note is made of free fluid in the cul-de-sac (*long arrow*). Urine in the bladder has high signal intensity (*b*). (From Ascher et al. 1997)

fasting for a minimum of 6h. In addition, an antispasmodic can be administered, provided no medical contraindications are present. Immediately prior to the examination, patients should be asked to void.

Respiratory motion artifacts are frequently accentuated with multicoil imaging for two reasons: (1) superficial structures that generate artifact (for example, subcutaneous fat, bladder, and bowel) are in close proximity to the coils and therefore have relatively high signal when compared to the uterus, which is typically located farther from the coils; (2) the intensity of phase ghost artifacts generated by respiration is greater with a small voxel size (McCauley et al. 1992). The following steps can be taken to minimize respiratory motion with multicoil imaging. Motion of the coil itself is restricted by binding the coil firmly to the patient's abdomen. In-field-of-view saturation bands are placed over the subcutaneous fat anteriorly and posteriorly to decrease the signal of the fat immediately adjacent to the coils. For conventional SE sequences, respiratory-ordered phase encoding is used where available; however, this option is not compatible with fast imaging sequences. Therefore, in patients who are unable to cooperate, consideration should be given to using the HASTE (half-Fourier single-shot turbo spin echo) sequence for T2-weighted imaging, since it is relatively breathing independent. SGE sequences, where possible, are best performed during a breath-hold.

#### 3.3.3.2 Metallic Artifacts

The usual contraindications to MRI also apply to examinations of the uterus. The presence of orthopedic devices, although not hazardous to the patient, can seriously impair image quality. Extensive signal loss is usually present at the site of a metallic device. In patients with a hip prosthesis, the signal loss may extend across, as far as the mid pelvis. Most intrauterine contraceptive devices do not cause sufficient signal loss to render the examination of the uterus nondiagnostic (Mark and Hricak 1987). Surgical clips and certain types of surgical suture may also result in areas of signal loss (Haramati et al. 1994). Magnetic susceptibility artifacts can be minimized by utilizing HASTE sequences and are most accentuated with gradient-echo sequences (Jolesz and Jones 1993).

## 3.4 MR Imaging Considerations

The uterus is optimally depicted with MRI using T2-weighted sagittal sequences. In women of reproductive age, three different zones can be identified within the uterine corpus on T2-weighted images (see Fig. 3.1) (LEE et al. 1985; LANGE et al. 1991; MCCARTHY et al. 1989). A high-signal-intensity stripe representing the normal endometrium and secretions within the endometrial cavity is present centrally. The width of the endometrial stripe varies with the menstrual cycle, being thinnest at the time of menstruation. The endometrium increases in width rapidly during the follicular or proliferative phase and continues to increase during the secretory phase, although at a slower rate (HAYNOR et al. 1986). The reported thickness of the endometrial stripe varies widely but averages 3–6 mm in the follicular phase and 5–13 mm during the secretory phase (DEMAS et al. 1986; MCCARTHY et al. 1986; WICZYK et al. 1988; KASAI 1990).

Immediately subjacent to the endometrial stripe, a band of low signal intensity referred to as the junctional zone (JZ) is seen. Histologic studies have demonstrated that this zone corresponds to the innermost layer of the myometrium (BROWN et al. 1991; MITCHELL et al. 1990). The histologic basis for the low signal of the JZ has not yet been established; however, a number of factors likely contribute to this imaging appearance. BROWN et al. (1991) hypothesized that the compact smooth muscle bundles, as well as the orientation of the fibers within the JZ, may contribute to its low signal on T2-weighted images. MCCARTHY et al. (1989) found that the water content of the JZ was significantly lower than that of the endometrium and outer myometrium. SCOUTT et al. (1991) found an increase in the percentage of nuclear area in the JZ in comparison with that of the outer myometrium. How these differences in cellular composition result in T2 shortening of the JZ can only be subject to speculation. Further study will be needed to fully elucidate the basis for the lower signal intensity. The outer layer of the myometrium is of intermediate signal intensity on T2-weighted images. During the menstrual cycle, the thickness of the myometrium increases slightly and is greatest during the secretory phase (HAYNOR et al. 1986). Considerable variation in the normal thickness of the JZ has been reported, with a mean thickness ranging from 2 to 8 mm (BROWN et al. 1991; WICZYK et al. 1988; MITCHELL et al. 1990). In addition to an increase in thickness, the endometrium and myometrium both demonstrate a gradual increase in signal intensity from the follicular to the secretory phase (DEMAS et al. 1986; MCCARTHY et al. 1986).

On T1-weighted images, the zonal anatomy of the uterine corpus is usually inapparent (see Fig. 3.2). The uterus is of intermediate and homogeneous signal intensity, aside from the midsecretory phase, during which the endometrium may exhibit slightly greater signal intensity than the adjacent myometrium (HRICAK et al. 1983).

Considerable variation in the pattern of uterine enhancement may be observed, depending on the hormonal status of the patient and the imaging delay after injection (HIRANO et al. 1992; YAMASHITA et al. 1993a; ITO et al. 1994). Although the endometrium shows little enhancement during the dynamic phase of gadolinium administration, it shows marked enhancement on the delayed T1-weighted images. Peak myometrial enhancement has been reported to occur 120 s following gadolinium administration (YAMASHITA et al. 1993a). During the menstrual phase, intense early enhancement of the JZ may be observed at dynamic imaging (YAMASHITA et al. 1993a). Enhancement of a thin subendometrial layer followed by enhancement of the myometrium has been reported in postmenopausal women and in women during the proliferative phase of their menstrual cycle (YAMASHITA et al. 1993a). During the secretory phase, enhancement of the entire myometrium, predominantly in the outer muscle layer, may be seen on early dynamic images (YAMASHITA et al. 1993a). This pattern of enhancement may also be seen during the menstrual phase and in postmenopausal women (YAMASHITA et al. 1993a; ITO et al. 1994). On postcontrast delayed images, the signal intensity of the uterine corpus may parallel that seen with T2-weighted sequences: endometrium – high signal intensity, JZ – low signal intensity, and outer myometrium – intermediate signal intensity. However, the difference in contrast between the various layers is considerably diminished compared to T2-weighted sequences, and not infrequently the uterine zonal anatomy is completely obscured (HRICAK and KIM 1993).

## 3.5 Transvaginal Ultrasound Technique

### 3.5.1 General Guidelines

#### *3.5.1.1 Patient Preparation*

Ideally, the patient should be examined on a gynecologic examination table in which there is adequate leg support allowing the patient to elevate her pelvis. However, virtually any examination table or bed can be used. It is counterproductive to place the patient in a Trendelenburg position, but a slight anti-Trendelenburg may be beneficial because any fluid draining dependently will result in enhanced tissue interfaces during the examination.

The bladder should be empty in most cases in order to obtain the best results. Partially filled bladders become important in cases which the anterior cervical lip has to be emphasized on a sagittal scan, in cases of suspected placenta previa, or when cervical anatomy needs to be delineated. A distended urinary bladder may distort pelvic anatomy.

In many cases requiring pelvic ultrasonography it will be necessary to do a transabdominal examination as well as a transvaginal one. In such cases, if the patient presents with a distended urinary bladder, she should first be examined transabdominally then, after voiding, transvaginally.

Most examiners believe that an informed consent is not necessary; however, the procedure should first be explained to the patient. One should mention the similarity between the transvaginal examination and the routinely performed speculum examination. If there are any questions regarding the safety of the examination (e.g., ruptured membranes, placenta previa), the referring obstetrician should be contacted before the examination. There have been no documented reports of untoward effects of transvaginal ultrasonography. If a male examiner is to perform the examination, it is advisable to have a female aide, nurse, or sonographer present (Timor-Tristch et al. 1994).

#### *3.5.1.2 Equipment Preparation*

The tip to the transducer is covered with coupling gel and introduced into a condom or protective rubber sheath. A small amount of coupling gel is then applied on top of the probe, easing its vaginal insertion. Infertility patients close to midcycle should be scanned using saline or water to avoid exposure of the sperm to possible noxious effects of the coupling gels.

After completion of the examination and removal of the probe, the probe is gently cleaned with a paper towel and a disinfectant. A variety of disinfectant solutions are available in spray or other forms, and some work within as little as 10 min. It is wise to contact the manufacturer to find out its choices to keep the probes clean. As in all ultrasound examinations the examiner should wear gloves during the examination (Timor-Tristch et al. 1994).

### 3.5.2 Scanning Technique

A rigid and relatively strict scanning routine should be followed. The cervix should be scanned as the probe is introduced into the bladder. A quick examination of the bladder can be performed at this time. The uterus should then be localized and evaluated in longitudinal and transverse planes (Fig. 3.4). The cervix should be included in the sagittal scans of the uterus. This is accomplished by gently pulling out the probe and directing it toward the cervix. The adnexa should next be evaluated, including ovaries, fallopian tubes, and any pathologic process related to these structures. The cul-de-sac is evaluated by tilting the probe posteriorly. The probe should be extracted under continuous ultrasound observation and by tilting the probe upward upon complete re-

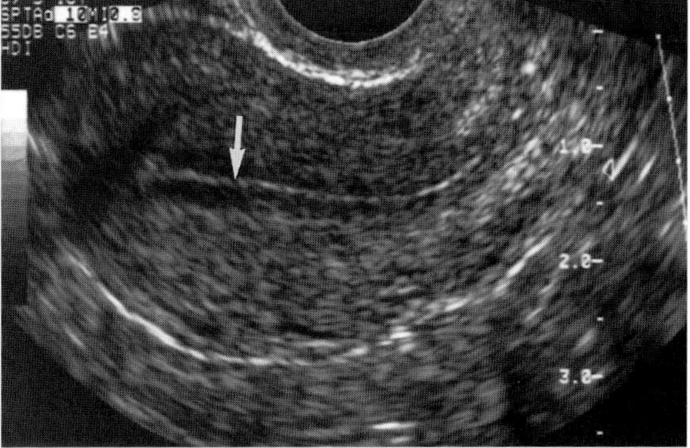

**Fig. 3.4.** Normal uterus. Sagittal transvaginal sonography of the uterus images the normal endometrium as an echogenic stripe (*arrow*), the result of opposing endometrial surfaces. (From Ascher et al. 1997)

moval. The insertion of the ureters into the bladder as well as the urethra can be evaluated. Transverse and sagittal planes of the urinary bladder, as well as the posterior bladder neck and its angle, can also be observed. If a complementary transabdominal examination is required after completion of the transvaginal examination, the formerly empty bladder should be sufficiently filled prior to imaging (Timor-Tristch et al. 1994).

## 3.6 Normal Sonographic Anatomy

The adult uterus is a thick-walled muscular structure which is usually anteverted, forming nearly a right angle with the vagina. The vagina is identified as a thin hyperechoic line on midline sagittal scans. The uterus can be identified by its usual central location, by its continuity with the vagina, and by the endometrial stripe or echo. The endometrial stripe is composed of the endometrial canal surrounded by two layers of endometrium. The brightness and thickness of this stripe vary with the patient's menstrual cycle, ranging from 2–3 mm (at the end of menses) to as much as 15 mm (at the start of menses). Occasionally, a striated appearance may be detected which seems to signify a time when the endometrium is more receptive to implantation. Although not always detected by ultrasound, a discrete hypoechoic inner myometrial zone may be identified deep to the endometrium, a possible US correlate of the JZ. The bulk of the myometrium, which is the largest component of the uterus, is identified beyond the JZ (if present) and has a uniform low-level echogenicity compared with the endometrium. The serosal surface is usually not appreciated, but occasionally subserosal veins may appear as prominent anechoic spaces (Kurtz and Middleton 1996).

## 3.7 Age-Related Physiologic Alterations

### 3.7.1 Premenarchal Uterus

In the premenarchal female the uterine corpus is small and the cervix accounts for more than half of the total length of the uterus (Demas et al. 1986). On T2-weighted sequences, the endometrium may be identified as a thin line. The JZ, although visible, appears indistinct. The overall signal intensity of the myometrium is lower than in women of reproductive age (Demas et al. 1986; Hricak et al. 1983). On ultrasound, the neonatal uterus has the shape of a fertile uterus with the body and fundus larger than the cervix. This is due to circulating maternal hormones. After the hormone effects dissipate, the fundus involutes, leaving a prominent cervix. The endometrial stripe is typically not identified but can infrequently be seen as a very thin hyperechoic line (Kurtz and Middleton 1986).

### 3.7.2 Postmenopausal Uterus

In postmenopausal women the uterus is small, with a 1:1 ratio of the corpus to the cervix. On T2-weighted sequences the endometrial stripe can be identified as a thin hyperintense structure. A few small series using MRI have reported a maximal endometrial thickness of 3 mm in women not receiving exogenous hormones and a thickness of 4–6 mm in women receiving hormonal replacement therapy (Demas et al. 1986; Hricak et al. 1983, 1987). The signal intensity of the myometrium on T2-weighted sequences is decreased and the JZ is not consistently visualized (Demas et al. 1986).

On ultrasound the postmenopausal uterus progressively atrophies, decreasing to its prepubertal size after 15–20 years. The body and fundus remain more prominent than the cervix, however. The endometrial stripe also atrophies and is either thin and hyperechoic or not visualized. Several sonographic studies of endometrial thickness in postmenopausal women have suggested an upper limit of 5 mm in patients not on hormone replacement (Sheth et al. 1993; Varner et al. 1991; Lin et al. 1991) (Fig. 3.5). With hormone replacement therapy, these changes are usually not as prominent and an upper limit of 8 mm for endometrial width is allowed (Kurtz and Middleton 1996).

The discrepancy between endometrial thickness on MRI and transvaginal sonography (TVS) is not unexpected; MRI measurements of endometrial width are usually less than the corresponding measurements obtained with ultrasound (Demas et al. 1986).

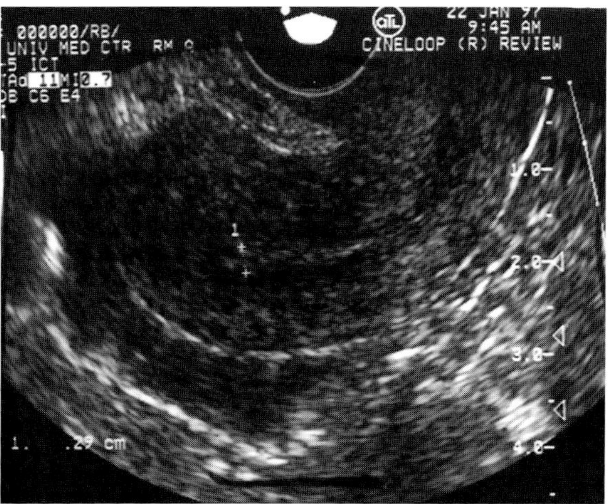


**Fig. 3.5.** Normal postmenopausal uterus. Sagittal transvaginal image of the uterus with an endometrial thickness of 3 mm

### 3.7.3 Myometrial Contractions

Uterine contractions occurring during pregnancy have been well described on ultrasound. At times, they demonstrate decreased echogenicity and may therefore closely mimic the appearance of leiomyomas (Lyons and Levi CS 1982; Fleischer et al, 1990). Although myometrial contractions are known to occur in the nongravid uterus, their role in menstrual discharge and implantation is currently not well understood. On T2-weighted images, myometrial contractions appear as areas of low signal intensity within the myometrium that result in distortion of the endometrial complex but typically do not deform the outer uterine contour (Togashi et al. 1993a,b). Myometrial contractions may closely resemble the appearance of focal adenomyosis or leiomyomas on MRI, depending on the shape and border definition of the resultant myometrial abnormality. Contractions are differentiated from true myometrial pathology on sequential imaging acquisitions by their transient nature and changing appearance over time. Myometrial contractions usually resolve within 30–45 min of onset (Lyons and Levi 1992; Fleischer et al. 1990). The cause of the low signal intensity on T2-weighted sequences observed with myometrial contractions is unknown but may be related to a regional decrease in vascularity (Togashi et al. 1993a).

## 3.8 Treatment-Induced Alterations and Postsurgical Change

### 3.8.1 Oral Contraceptives

With prolonged use of oral contraceptives the uterine corpus may decrease in size (Moghissi 1980). The endometrial thickness averages 2 mm and does not vary during the course of the menstrual cycle (Demas et al. 1986; McCarthy et al. 1986). Similarly, the JZ shows a decrease in maximal thickness compared with those who do not use oral contraceptives (McCarthy et al. 1986). The signal intensity of the myometrium is increased, consistent with the known myometrial edema that occurs with oral contraceptive intake (Moghissi 1980).

### 3.8.2 Exogenous Hormones

Changes induced by exogenous hormones will vary depending on the type of regimen used. The uterus of a postmenopausal woman on hormonal replacement therapy is similar in appearance to the premenopausal uterus. Exogenous hormones such as gonadotropin-releasing hormone (GnRH) used to treat leiomyomas, for example, will induce changes that parallel those of a postmenopausal uterus (Demas et al. 1986; Zawin et al. 1990a). These changes will revert to normal once the treatment is stopped. Hormonal therapy for the treatment of endometrial hyperplasia induces changes similar to those seen with oral contraceptive use (Togashi 1993).

### 3.8.3 Radiation Therapy

Irradiation of the uterus in the premenopausal woman results in a decrease in the size of the uterus, thinning of the endometrium, decreased signal intensity of the myometrium, and loss of uterine zonal anatomy on T2-weighted sequences (Arrive et al. 1989). The MRI appearance resembles that of a nonirradiated postmenopausal uterus. These changes likely reflect a combination of direct radiation effects on the uterus and loss of hormonal stimulation from ovarian function suppression. The appearance of the uterus in postmenopausal women does not significantly change following radiation therapy (Arrive et al. 1989).

### 3.8.4 Tamoxifen

Tamoxifen is a nonsteroidal antiestrogen that binds to estrogen receptors and is used as an adjuvant therapy in women with breast carcinoma. In addition to its antiestrogen effects on breast cancer tissue, tamoxifen acts as a weak estrogen agonist on the postmenopausal uterus. A spectrum of endometrial abnormalities has been reported in patients receiving tamoxifen therapy, including proliferative changes, hyperplasia, polyps, and carcinoma (De Muylder et al. 1991; Neven et al. 1990; Fornander et al. 1989) (Fig. 3.6). Currently, no definitive screening guidelines for monitoring patients on tamoxifen therapy have been established; however, a combination of TVS and endometrial sampling is most frequently used (Cohen et al. 1993). TVS findings include a thickened endometrium with multiple cystic spaces. Hann et al. (1997) suggested using 8 mm as the threshold for abnormal endometrial thickness in asymptomatic patients on tamoxifen therapy. In

a

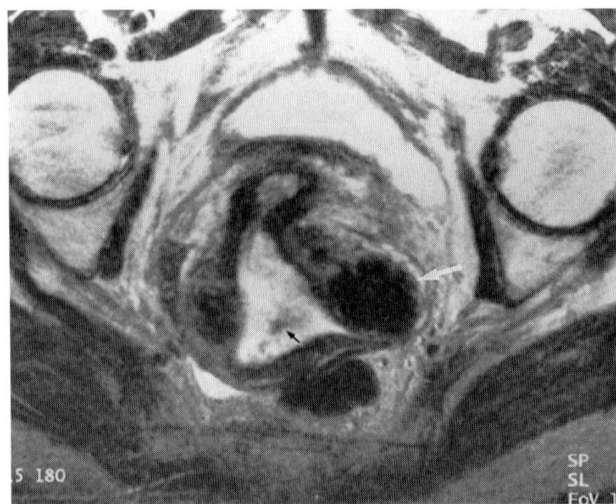

b

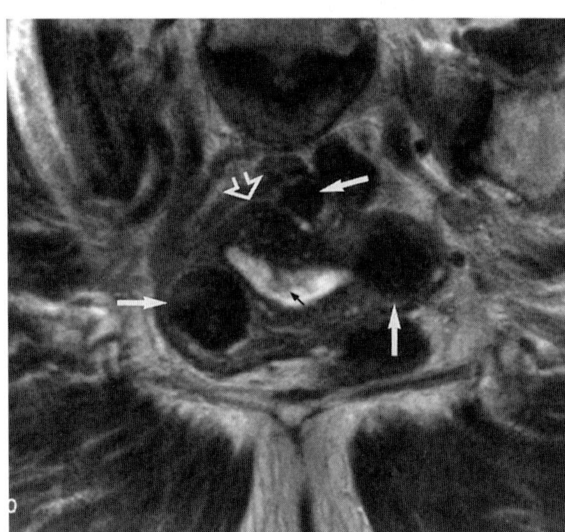

c

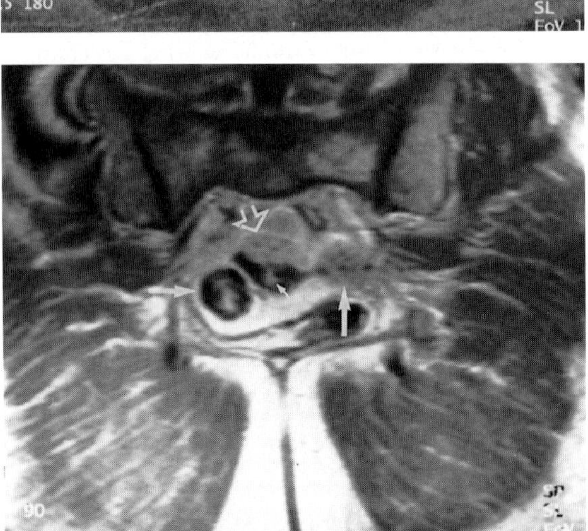

**Fig. 3.6 a–c.** Adenomyoma vs leiomyoma. An 81-year-old woman with breast carcinoma who was treated with tamoxifen for 24 months. T2-weighted TSE true coronal (**a**), true axial (**b**), and T1-weighted postcontrast uterus (**c**). This retropositioned uterus highlights many findings associated with tamoxifen therapy: widened endometrium with heterogeneous signal intensity, adenomyoma, and leiomyomas. The adenomyoma (*open white arrow*) demonstrates focal widening of the junctional zone with multiple punctate high-signal foci (**b**). These foci, which do not enhance postgadolinium administration (*open white arrow*, **c**), represent ectopic endometrium, dilated glands, and/or punctate hemorrhage. Several fibroids (*solid large white arrows*) demonstrate characteristic low signal with heterogeneous enhancement. A pedunculated polyp within the endometrial canal (*small black arrows*, **a**,**b**), is best visualized on the postcontrast image (*small white arrow*, **c**). Endometrial sampling showed a benign endometrial polyp and adenomyosis

symptomatic patients with vaginal bleeding, the authors relate that ultrasound has a limited role and that endometrial sampling is required. The use of saline sonohysterography may increase the detection of endometrial polyps or areas of asymmetric thickening that may appropriately be sampled. (Dubinsky et al. 1995; Cullinan et al. 1995).

There is a paucity of literature on the MRI appearance of uteri in women receiving tamoxifen therapy (Ascher et al. 1996). Consequently, the role of MRI in evaluating this group of patients is not yet known. However, in patients with technically inadequate or indeterminate TVS examinations, MRI may be helpful in determining which patients could benefit from further investigation. Ascher et al. (1996) described two distinct MRI patterns in women receiving tamoxifen therapy and correlated these results with findings at histopathology. In patients with atrophy or proliferative changes at histopathology, the endometrium was homogeneously hyperintense on T2-weighted images. After contrast administration, there was enhancement of the endometrial–myometrial interface with a persistent signal void in the lumen. In patients with polyps the endometrium was of heterogeneous signal intensity on T2-weighted images (Figs. 3.7, 3.8). On images obtained following gadolinium administration, a lattice-like pattern of enhancement was seen traversing the endometrial canal (Figs. 3.7, 3.8). Concomitant cystic atrophy was present in both groups at histopathology. The endometrial thickness was significantly greater in patients with polyps (mean, 1.8 cm) than in patients with atrophic or proliferative changes (mean, 0.5 cm). Additional findings included subendometrial cysts, adenomyosis, leiomyomas, and a small amount of intraperitoneal fluid (Ascher et al. 1996).

## 3.9 Benign Diseases of the Uterine Corpus

### 3.9.1 Endometrial Polyps and Hyperplasia

#### *3.9.1.1 General Considerations*

Transvaginal sonography is currently the standard imaging modality for assessing the endometrium in symptomatic patients (Sheth et al. 1993; Varner et al. 1991; Lin et al. 1991; Atri et al. 1994). A major indication for TVS evaluation of the endometrium is abnormal postmenopausal bleeding. Sonographic studies of endometrial thickness in postmenopausal women have suggested an upper limit of 5 mm in patients not on hormone replacement and 8 mm for patients receiving hormonal therapy (Sheth et al. 1993; Varner et al. 1991; Lin et al. 1991; Atri et al. 1994) (see Fig. 3.5). When these cut-off values are used as guidelines to determine which patients would benefit from endometrial sampling, TVS is highly sensitive for detecting endometrial pathology. Unfortunately, the presence of endometrial thickening on TVS is nonspecific and may be due to endometrial hyperplasia, polyps, or carcinoma (Atri et al. 1994; Hulka 1994) (Fig. 3.9). Endometrial sampling, however, is indicated in all cases of endometrial thickening in postmenopausal women because both endometrial hyperplasia and polyps may be seen in association with endometrial carcinoma (Jones and Jones 1982c). Although submucosal leiomyomas are usually differentiated from endometrial pathology by their location and typical sonographic appearance, distinction may not always be possible (Fig. 3.10). Improved differentiation between endometrial abnormalities and submucosal leiomyomas may be achieved with hysterosonography (Parsons and Lense 1993).

Nevertheless, TVS is a highly effective screening tool when the endometrium can be adequately visualized (Fig. 3.11). In some patients, however, accurate measurements of endometrial thickness may not be possible due to a vertical orientation of the uterus, the presence of multiple leiomyomas, or extensive adenomyosis. Under these circumstances, MRI may be able to provide additional information on the appearance of the endometrium, particularly in patients for whom endometrial sampling would be difficult, e.g., patients with cervical stenosis. However, it must be emphasized that MRI is not a first-line screening modality for endometrial pathology, and the accuracy of MRI in evaluating this subgroup of patients is not known.

#### *3.9.1.2 MR Imaging Considerations*

A combination of T2-weighted and contrast-enhanced T1-weighted sequences is used to evaluate benign endometrial pathology. Contrast-enhanced T1-weighted sequences considerably improve the detection rate of endometrial polyps. T2-weighted sagittal and transverse images are initially obtained through the pelvis. Short-axis views through the

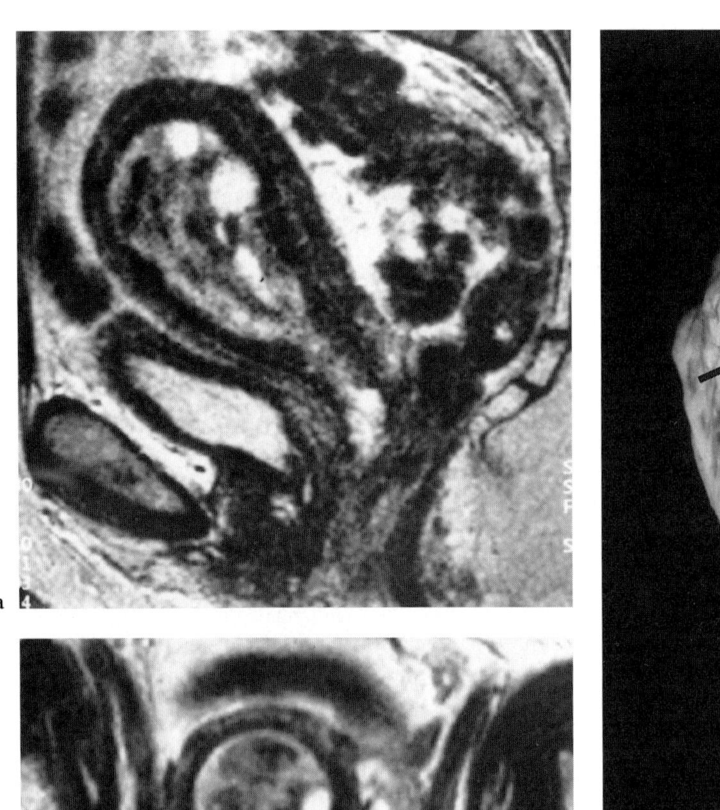

a

b

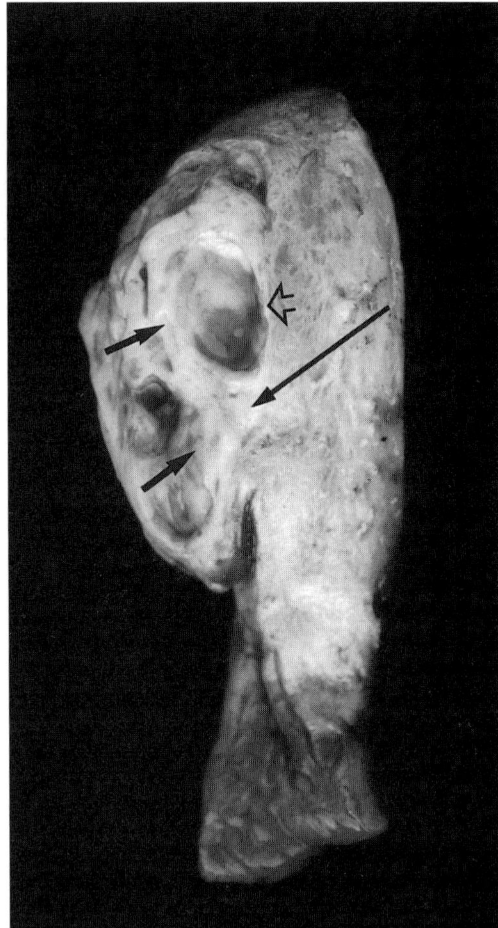

d

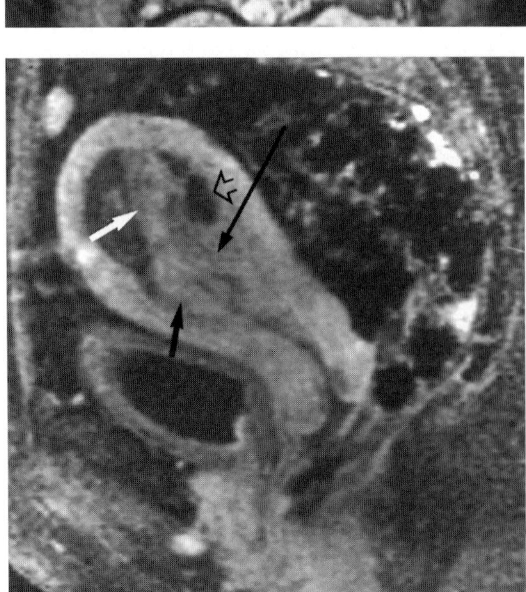

c

**Fig. 3.7 a–d.** Tamoxifen therapy. A 71-year-old woman with breast carcinoma who received tamoxifen for 42 months. **a,b** Orthogonal T2-weighted images of the uterus show a widened endometrium with heterogeneous signal intensity. **c** Contrast-enhanced sagittal T1-weighted fat-suppressed SGE image shows enhancing tissue traversing the endometrial canal. An enhancing stalk attaching to the posterior endometrium is well demonstrated (*long solid arrow*), as are superior and inferior branches of this polyp (*short solid arrows*). Signal voids represent cystic spaces between the enhancing interstices of the polyp (*open arrow*). **d** Hysterectomy specimen. The gross appearance correlates well with the imaging findings. A posteriorly attached benign endometrial polyp (*long solid arrow*) has superior and inferior components (*short solid arrows*) that circumscribe cystic spaces (*open arrow*)

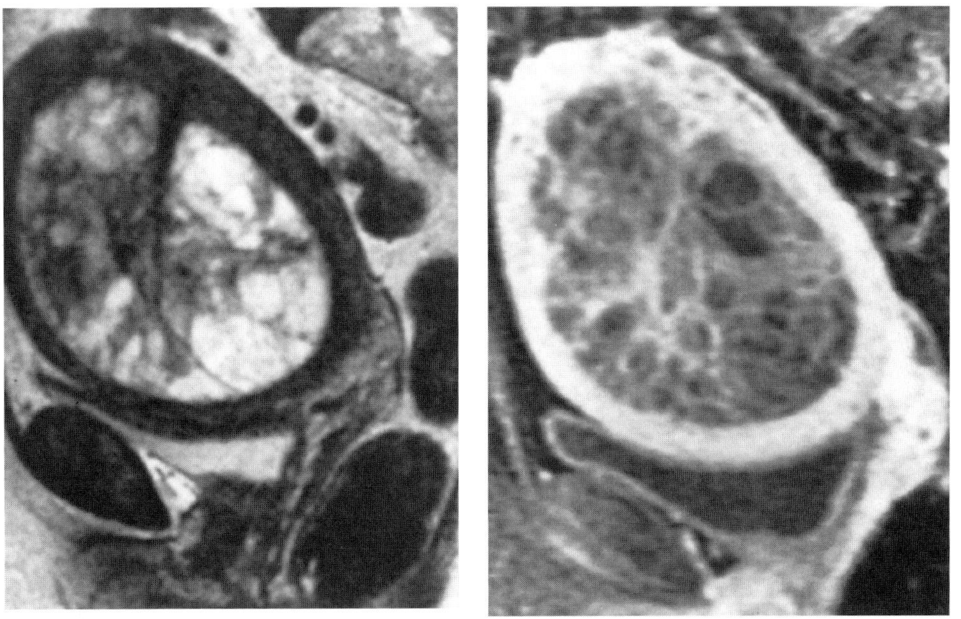

**Fig. 3.8 a,b.** Benign polyp. Sagittal T2-weighted TSE (**a**) and post-contrast T1-weighted fat-suppressed SGE (**b**) demonstrate a large, heterogeneous polyp expanding the entire endometrial canal

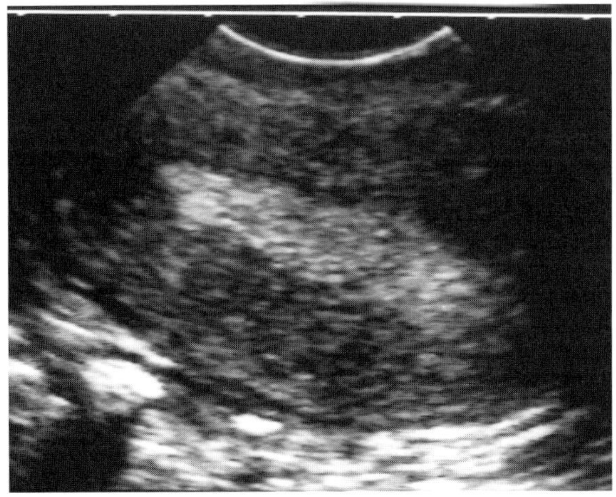

**Fig. 3.9.** Adenomatous hyperplasia. A 52-year-old patient with postmenopausal bleeding. The transvaginal ultrasound image shows an irregular, well-defined, and densely echogenic endometrium. (From ATRI et al. 1994)

uterus may be helpful in selected cases. Dynamic and delayed T1-weighted contrast-enhanced sequences are obtained following the T2-weighted sequences.

To date, the normal range of endometrial thickness in postmenopausal women with MRI has not been firmly established; however, a few small series using MRI have reported a maximal endometrial thickness of 3 mm in women not receiving exogenous hormones, and 4–6 mm in women receiving hormonal replacement therapy (DEMAS et al. 1986; HRICAK et al. 1983, 1987).

Endometrial hyperplasia usually presents as diffuse thickening of the endometrial stripe on T2-weighted images (Fig. 3.12). The signal intensity of the endometrial stripe is isointense or slightly hypointense relative to normal endometrium (HRICAK et al. 1987). These imaging characteristics, however, are nonspecific and are also seen with endometrial carcinoma.

On T2-weighted images, endometrial polyps most frequently present as masses of slightly lower signal intensity relative to normal endometrium. At times, however, they may be entirely isointense and present as diffuse or focal thickening of the endometrial stripe (JONES and JONES 1982b). Particularly when large, endometrial polyps may be markedly heterogeneous with areas of high and low signal intensity (see Fig. 3.8). A linear area of low signal corresponding to a stalk may be identified at the periphery of pedunculated polyps. After gadolinium administration, polyps show variable degrees of enhancement. Typically, polyps enhance less than the endometrium but similarly to or greater than the adjacent myometrium. Although contrast-enhanced images improve detection of endometrial polyps, the pattern of contrast enhancement is nonspecific and differentiation from early endometrial carcinoma is not possible (HRICAK and KIM 1993) (see Fig. 3.6).

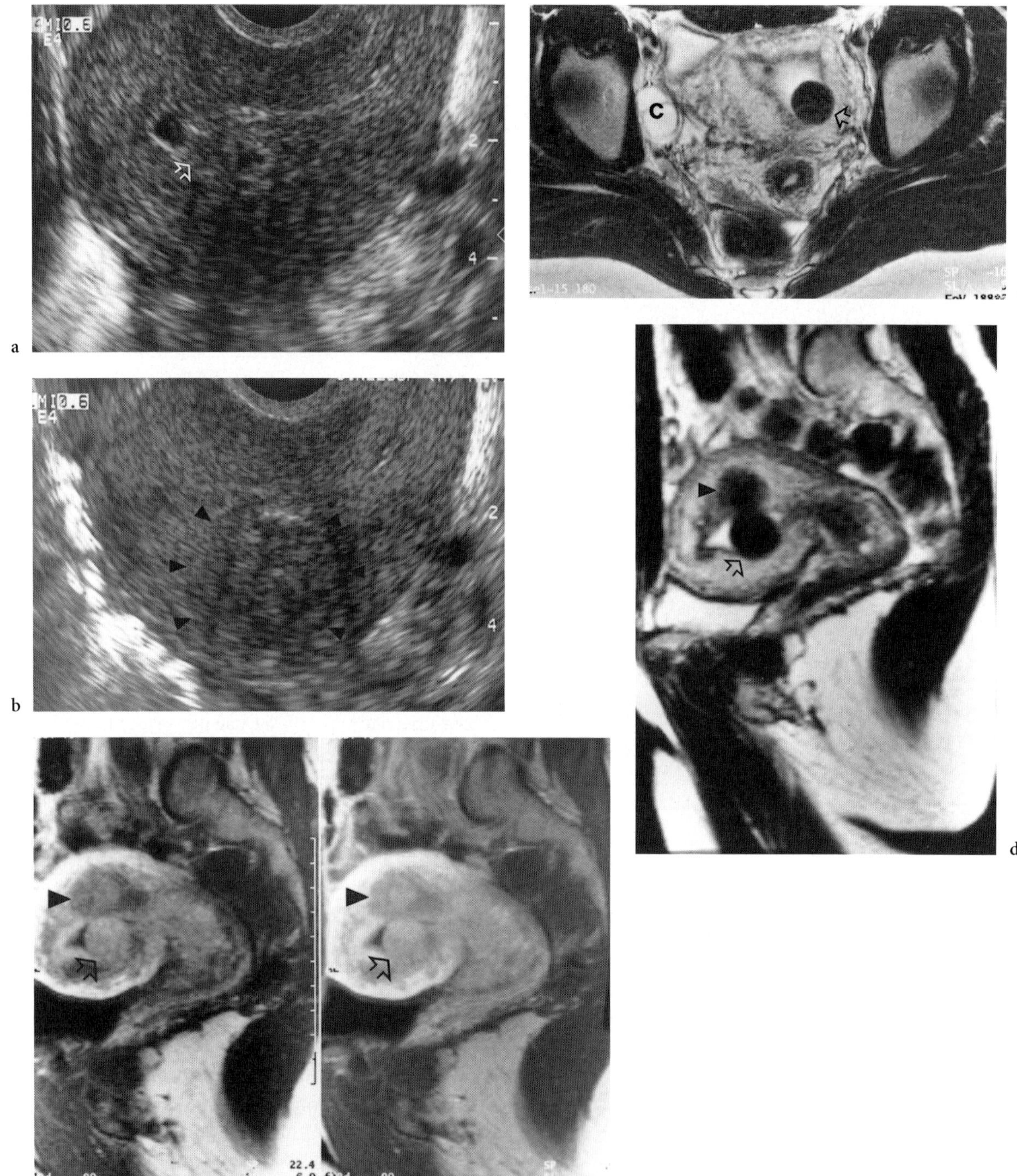

**Fig. 3.10 a–e.** Uterine leiomyomas. Sagittal (**a**) and transverse (**b**) transvaginal ultrasound images; MR coronal (**c**) and sagittal (**d**) T2-weighted TSE, and T1-weighted postcontrast (**e**) images of the uterus. There is soft tissue within the endometrial canal that mimics a polyp on TVS (*open arrow*, **a**). This correlates with a well-defined, low-signal mass which protrudes into the endometrium (*open arrows*, **c**,**d**) and enhances similar to myometrium on MRI (*open arrow*, **e**). The mass location and signal are characteristic for a submucosal fibroid. MRI also better defines the intramural fibroid (*arrowheads*, **d**,**e**) that is only vaguely seen on TVS (*arrowheads*, **b**). The exact relationship of a fibroid to the remainder of the uterus is important if uterine-sparing therapy is to be performed. Right ovarian cysts are seen on the coronal image (*c*,**c**)

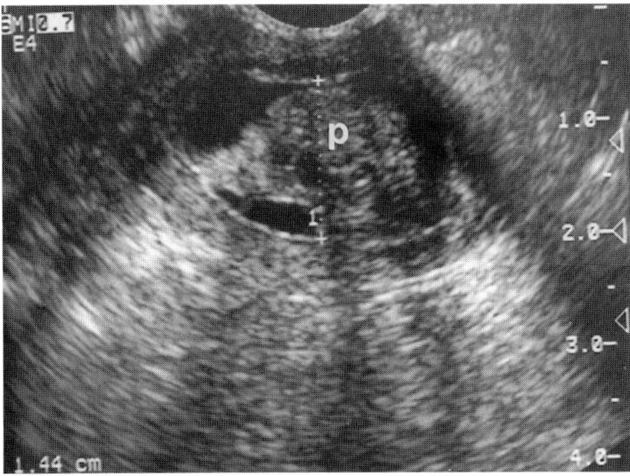

Fig. 3.11. Benign polyp. TVS in an asymptomatic postmenopausal patient with a benign polyp (*p*)

Submucosal leiomyomas may be differentiated from endometrial polyps on T2-weighted images by confirming their myometrial origin (see Fig. 3.10). In addition, leiomyomas are typically of low signal intensity on T2-weighted images. However, leiomyomas may exhibit variable signal intensities, and overlap in signal characteristics between degenerative leiomyomas and endometrial polyps is frequently noted (HRICAK et al. 1987).

## 3.9.2 Leiomyomas

### *3.9.2.1 General Considerations*

Leiomyoma is the most common type of uterine tumor and is estimated to be present in 20% of women over 35 years of age (JONES and JONES 1982d). Leiomyomas are estrogen-dependent, and therefore usually regress after the onset of menopause.

Leiomyomas are benign neoplasms of smooth muscle cell origin. They are sharply demarcated from the surrounding myometrium by a pseudocapsule of light areolar tissue (JONES and JONES 1982d). The smooth muscle cells are arranged in a whorl-like interlacing pattern, giving leiomyomas their characteristic gross appearance. Cellular leiomyomas are a specific subtype and are composed of densely packed smooth muscle tissue with little intervening collagen. Most leiomyomas undergo some degree of degeneration, which contributes to the variable appearance of these tumors on imaging (JONES and JONES 1982d; KLIEWER et al. 1995). Hyaline degeneration occurs to some extent in all leiomyomas, except the very small. Leiomyomas may also undergo myxomatous, cystic, fatty, or hemorrhagic (carneous) degeneration. In addition, leiomyomas frequently calcify, particularly in older women. Torsion, infection, and sarcomatous degeneration are rare complications.

Leiomyomas are usually classified according to location: submucosal, intramural, subserosal, or cervical. Uncommonly, a leiomyoma may be situated in the broad ligament or be entirely detached from the uterus, parasitizing the blood supply from other vascular beds, usually the omentum (RADER et al. 1990). Although leiomyomas may be entirely asymptomatic and present as incidental findings, they may be associated with a variety of symptoms, including menorrhagia, dysmenorrhea, pressure effects, infertility, second trimester abortions, and dystocia (JONES and JONES 1982d).

The role of imaging in evaluating patients with suspected leiomyomas is directed towards lesion detection, characterization, and localization. Ultrasound remains the initial imaging modality of choice for patients with suspected leiomyomas, and in the vast majority of routine clinical presentations no additional investigation is needed (GROSS et al. 1983; KARASICK et al. 1992). However, a number of limitations may be encountered with ultrasound when evaluating patients with suspected leiomyomas. Small leiomyomas (<2 cm) may not be consistently depicted with ultrasound, and although large leiomyomas are more likely to be symptomatic, small tumors may also produce symptoms depending on their location (GROSS et al. 1983) (see Fig. 3.10). The presence of multiple lesions and/or marked distortion of the uterus can adversely affect the ability of ultrasound to precisely locate leiomyomas (DUDIAK et al. 1988; ZAWIN et al. 1990b). In patients electing to undergo uterine-sparing surgery, accurate preoperative localization of leiomyomas is of paramount importance in planning myomectomy. Submucosal leiomyomas may be resected hysteroscopically, while laparoscopic or transabdominal myomectomy is required for intramural or subserosal leiomyomas. Similarly, visualization of the endometrium or ovaries may be obscured in patients with large or multiple leiomyomas (ZAWIN et al. 1990b). Therefore, distinction between a pedunculated leiomyoma and a solid ovarian mass may not always be possible (WEINREB et al. 1990). Although leiomyomas are usually easily recognized at ultrasound as localized hypoechoic masses with or without attenuation, the appearance

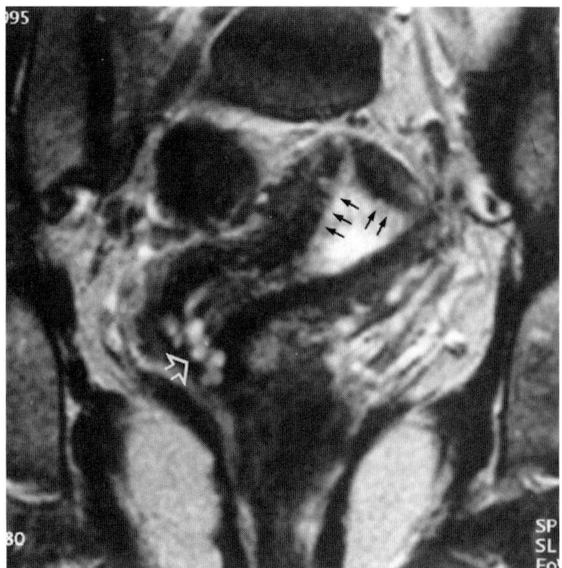


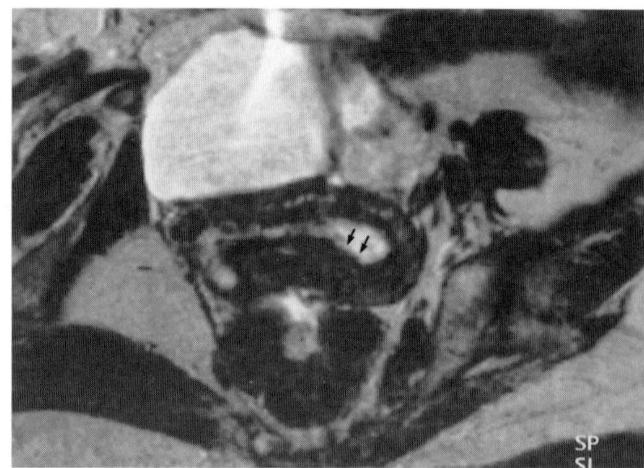


**Fig. 3.12 a,b.** Postmenopausal dysfunctional uterine bleeding. Paracoronal (**a**) and para-axial (**b**) T2-weighted TSE of the uterus. There is indistinct "feathering" along the endometrial/junctional zone interface in this patient with endometrial hyperplasia (*black arrows*). Thre are incidental nabothian cysts (*open white arrow*)

is nonspecific and overlap with other disease entities (for example, adenomyosis) may be present.

Under these circumstances, further evaluation with MRI is indicated. Several studies have demonstrated MRI to be superior to ultrasound for the detection and localization of uterine leiomyomas (Dudiak et al. 1988; Weinreb et al. 1990; Panageas et al. 1992; Hricak et al. 1986) (see Fig. 3.10). Furthermore, MRI is a useful adjunct for differentiating leiomyomas from other pathologic conditions (Weinreb et al. 1990; Mark et al. 1987) (Fig. 3.13).

### 3.9.2.2 MR Imaging Considerations

T2-weighted sequences provide optimal contrast between leiomyomas and the adjacent myometrium or endometrium (Hricak et al. 1986). In addition to standard sagittal and transverse views, coronal or oblique views may be indicated for accurate localization and for establishing the myometrial origin of a lesion (Panageas et al. 1992). T1-weighted sequences may be obtained if areas of degeneration are suspected. In addition, the presence of a fat plane on T1-weighted sequences may aid in the differentiation of a pedunculated leiomyoma and a solid ovarian mass. Contrast-enhanced T1-weighted images are not usually helpful in the detection or characterization of uterine leiomyomas. However, in cases where the myometrial origin of a mass has not been established with T2-weighted sequences, contrast-enhanced images with fat saturation may provide additional information by demonstrating the splaying of the myometrium around a portion of the lesion.

Leiomyomas typically appear as sharply marginated masses of low signal intensity relative to myometrium on T2-weighted sequences (see Figs. 3.10, 3.13). Lesions less than 0.5 cm in size are frequently identified. A rim of high signal intensity, representing a combination of dilated lymphatics, veins, and/or edema, may at times be seen surrounding intramural or subserosal leiomyomas (Mittl et al. 1991). Care must be taken not to mistake this high signal intensity rim for a displaced endometrial stripe. Leiomyomas greater than 3–5 cm in diameter may demonstrate heterogeneous areas of increased signal representing degeneration (see Fig. 3.13) (Hricak et al. 1986; Yamashita et al. 1993b). Accurate differentiation among the various types of degeneration is not possible with MRI, except for hemorrhagic degeneration, which typically demonstrates hyperintense areas on T1-weighted images (Hricak et al. 1986). Fatty degeneration in leiomyomas is rare, but may occur with advanced hyaline degeneration. However, when macroscopic areas of fat are present within a leiomyoma, the diagnosis of a benign mixed müllerian tumor or

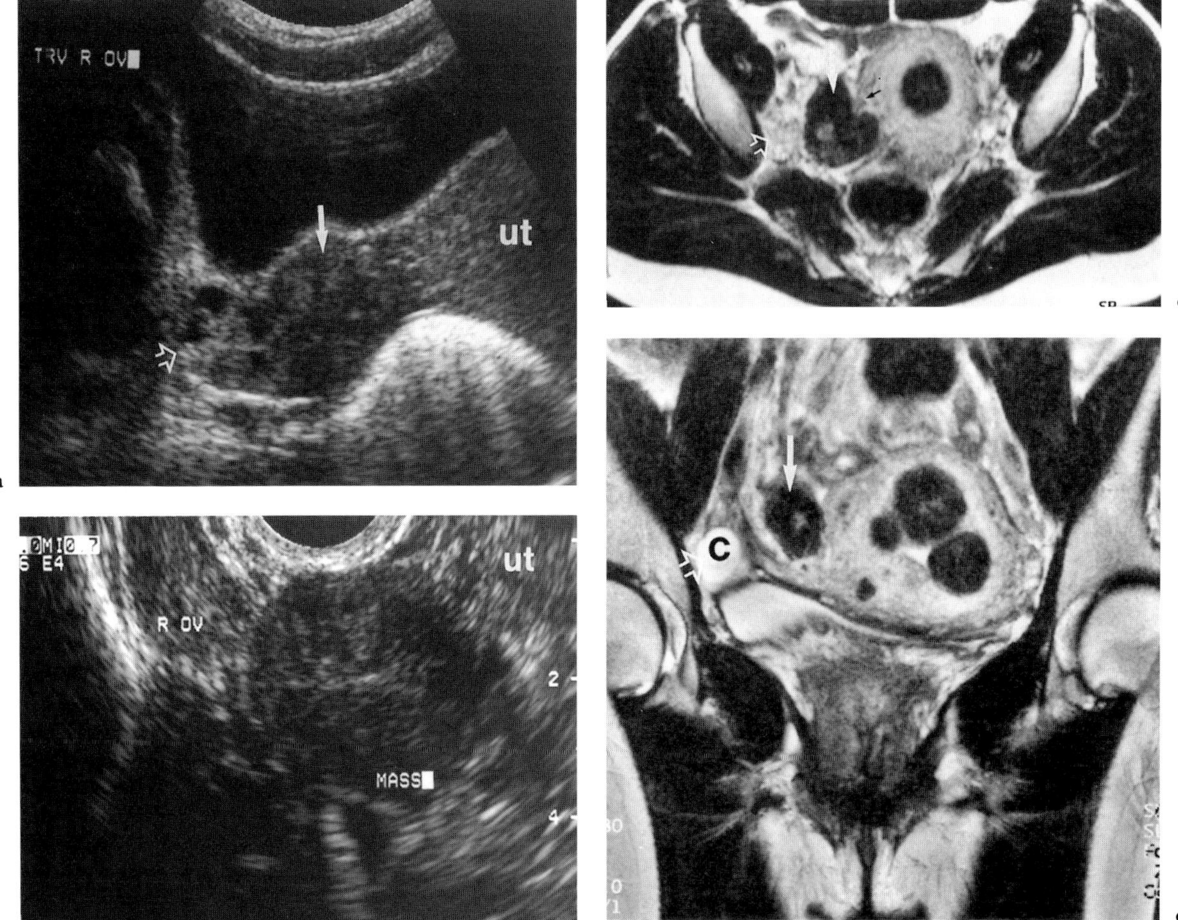


**Fig. 3.13 a–d.** MRI as a problem-solving tool. Transverse transabdominal (**a**) and transvaginal (**b**) ultrasonograms demonstrate a right adnexal mass (*solid white arrow*), contiguous with and medial to the right ovary (*open white arrow*) and lateral to the uterus (*ut*). High-resolution axial (**c**) and short-axis (**d**) T2-weighted TSE images illustrate the predominately low-signal characteristics of a subserosal fibroid (*solid white arrow*). Note the "claw" of uterine tissue at the posteriomedial aspect of the fibroid (*small black arrow*). Several other low-signal fibroids of varying size are also demonstrated. High signal within the fibroids is consistent with degeneration. A separate right ovary (*open arrow*, **c**,**d**) is seen with an incidental cyst (*c*)

lipoadenofibroma is probable (Jones and Jones 1982d). Extensive peripheral cystic degeneration in large leiomyomas may occasionally be seen. Cellular leiomyomas have been reported to be homogeneously hyperintense on T2-weighted sequences (Yamashita et al. 1993b). However, considerable overlap in the signal characteristics of cellular and degenerated leiomyomas is known to occur. Diagnosing cellular leiomyomas with MRI may be of interest, since this subtype has been reported to be more responsive to treatment with GnRH analogs (Yamashita et al. 1993b).

The appearance of leiomyomas following the administration of a gadolinium chelate is variable (Jones and Jones 1982b). On dynamic and delayed contrast-enhanced images, the majority of leiomyomas enhance to a lesser degree than the surrounding myometrium and remain well marginated (Fig. 3.14). However, intense early enhancement may also be seen and has been reported to occur most frequently with the cellular subtype (Yamashita et al. 1993b). The enhancement pattern is heterogeneous in the majority of leiomyomas (Jones and Jones 1982b) (see Fig. 3.10).

Leiomyomas can be accurately localized with MRI as submucosal, intramural, subserosal, or cervical. In patients with prolapsed submucosal leiomyomas, accurate localization of the stalk may

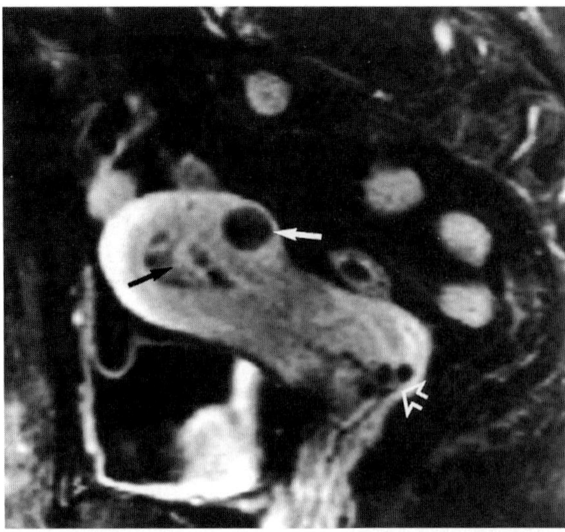

**Fig. 3.14.** Intramural fibroid. Sagittal postcontrast T1-weighted fat-suppressed SGE of the uterus. A well-defined, low-signal intramural fibroid (*solid white arrow*) enhances to a lesser degree than the surrounding myometrium. Note the enhancing pedunculated polyp within the endometrial canal (*black arrow*) and the multiple nabothian cysts (*open white arrow*)

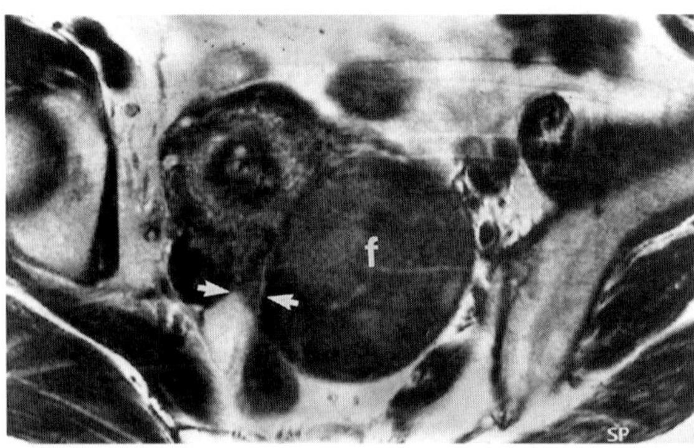


**Fig. 3.15.** Subserosal fibroid. True axial high-resolution T2-weighted TSE of the lower uterine segment. Note the "claw" of myometrium (*solid arrows*) extending around a portion of the fibroid (*f*)

facilitate hysteroscopic resection (Panageas et al. 1992).

Magnetic resonance imaging has proved useful in differentiating leiomyomas from other solid pelvic masses when sonographic findings are indeterminate (Weinreb et al. 1990) (see Fig. 3.13). Establishing the myometrial origin of a mass by demonstrating splaying of the uterine serosa or myometrium usually allows a confident diagnosis of leiomyoma to be made (Fig. 3.15). In addition, the presence of tumor-feeding vessels arising from the myometrium lends further support to the myometrial origin of a pelvic mass. Signal characteristics of a pelvic mass can also be used to suggest the diagnosis of a leiomyoma. If a mass is predominantly of low signal intensity relative to myometrium on T2-weighted images, the diagnosis of leiomyoma is probable. While the signal characteristics of leiomyomas may be indistinguishable from those of fibrothecomas of the ovary, the consequence of a misdiagnosis is probably not significant since these tumors are rarely malignant (Weinreb et al. 1990; Jones and Jones 1982e; Hamlin et al. 1985). However, if a mass adjacent to the uterus is of intermediate or increased signal intensity, the differential diagnosis includes a degenerated leiomyoma as well as benign or malignant extrauterine tumors. Under these circumstances, a specific diagnosis of leiomyoma should not be made unless the myometrial origin of a mass can be unequivocally demonstrated (Weinreb et al. 1990). Submucosal leiomyomas may be differentiated from endometrial polyps by confirming their myometrial origin and by their typical low signal intensity on T2-weighted images (see Fig. 3.10). Unfortunately, leiomyomas may exhibit variable signal intensities, and overlap in signal characteristics between leiomyomas and endometrial polyps is frequently noted (Hricak et al. 1987). Leiomyomas must also be differentiated from adenomyosis on MRI (see Fig. 3.6). For a discussion on the features distinguishing leiomyomas and adenomyosis see Sect. 3.9.3.2. Myometrial contractions may mimic the appearance of leiomyomas on MRI. Contractions can be differentiated from true myometrial pathology on sequential imaging acquisitions by their transient nature and changing appearance over time.

Malignant degeneration of a leiomyoma occurs rarely, but is suspected if a leiomyoma enlarges suddenly, especially following menopause, or if an indistinct border or irregular contour is noted. MR signal characteristics are not reliable in differentiating leiomyomas from leiomyosarcomas.

Benign metastasizing leiomyoma is one of several unusual variants that include intravenous leiomyomatosis and leiomyomatosis peritonealis disseminata. In benign metastasizing leiomyoma, histologically benign-appearing smooth muscle tumors are located in the parenchyma of distant organs, such as the lung. Although histologically benign, it is generally believed that this form of leiomyoma is a variant of low-grade leiomyosarcoma (Jones and Jones 1982d).

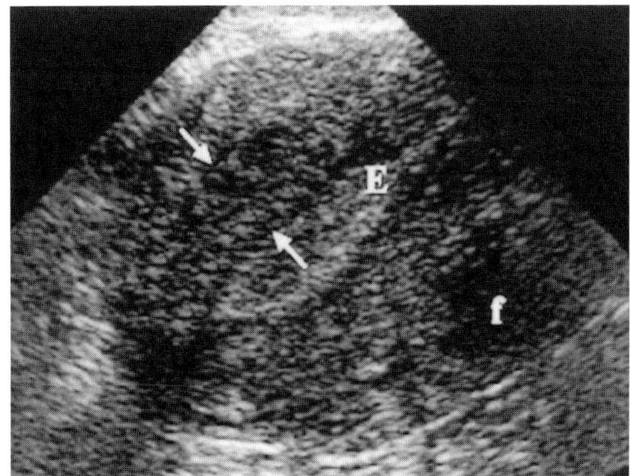


a

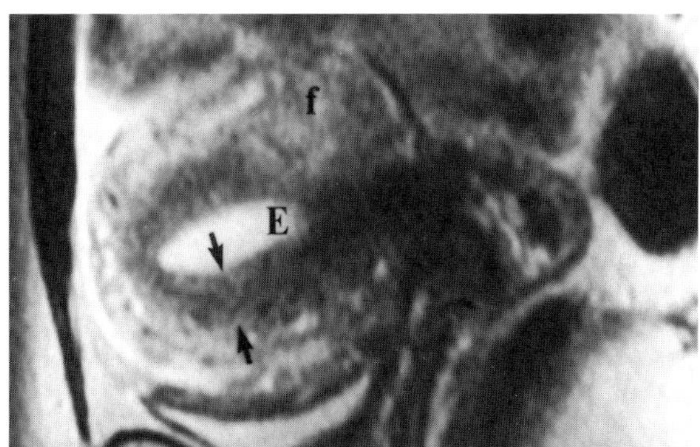


b

**Fig. 3.16a,b.** Adenomyosis. True-positive findings at transvaginal ultrasound and MRI in a patient with histopathologically proved diffuse adenomyosis extending to involve the middle third of the myometrium. *E*, Endometrium; *f*, fibroid. **a** Sagittal TVS through the uterus demonstrates the inner half of the ventral myometrium to be heterogeneous and of decreased echogenicity consistent with the presence of adenomyosis (*arrows*). The same findings were present dorsally at real-time imaging but are not as well depicted on this static image. **b** Sagittal T2-weighted conventional SE MR image in the same patient demonstrates diffuse thickening of the JZ (*arrows*) consistent with adenomyosis. The $JZ_{max}$ was 21 mm. (From REINHOLD et al. 1995)

## 3.9.3 Adenomyosis

### *3.9.3.1 General Considerations*

Uterine adenomyosis is a common disease that results from the presence of heterotopic endometrial glands and stroma in the myometrium with adjacent myometrial hyperplasia. Cyclic hemorrhage is infrequently observed with adenomyosis, since the ectopic endometrial tissue originates from the stratum basale and is typically unresponsive to hormonal stimuli. The associated myometrial hyperplasia interdigitates with the normal myometrium, resulting in poorly marginated borders that are not encapsulated. Adenomyosis may be microscopic, focal, or diffuse. The term adenomyoma is reserved for the nodular form of adenomyosis (AZZIZ 1989). The incidence of adenomyosis in unselected hysterectomy specimens ranges from 8.8% to 31% (OWOLABI and STRICKLER 1977; BENSON and SNEEDEN 1958; MOLITOR 1971; BIRD et al. 1972).

While adenomyosis is most frequently diagnosed in multiparous, premenopausal women, it is not uncommon in postmenopausal women (REINHOLD et al. 1995). Although adenomyosis may be entirely asymptomatic, it frequently presents with symptoms of pelvic pain, hypermenorrhea, and uterine enlargement. These symptoms and signs, however, are nonspecific and can be seen in other common gynecologic disorders such as dysfunctional uterine bleeding, leiomyomas, and endometriosis (JONES and JONES 1982e; MUSE 1990). It is hardly surprising, therefore, that the clinical diagnosis of adenomyosis is fraught with error, and until recently the diagnosis of adenomyosis was rarely established prior to surgical exploration (OWOLABI and STRICKLER 1977; BENSON and SNEEDEN 1958; MOLITOR 1971; ISRAEL and ARNOLD 1995). Establishing the correct diagnosis preoperatively is essential, since uterine-conserving therapy is possible with leiomyomas, whereas hysterectomy is the definitive treatment for debilitating adenomyosis.

Studies published on the accuracy of ultrasound in diagnosing adenomyosis report a wide range of results. Early reports on transabdominal sonography concluded that ultrasound is able neither to reliably diagnose adenomyosis nor to consistently differentiate it from leiomyomas (BOHLMAN et al. 1987; BULIC et al. 1986). However, the advent of TVS with its improved resolution has renewed interest in diagnosing this disease. Several series have reported the sensitivity of TVS for diagnosing adenomyosis as ranging from 53% to 89% with a specificity of 50%–98% (REINHOLD et al. 1996, 1995; FEDELE et al. 1992a,b; ASCHER et al. 1994; BROSENS et al. 1995). The wide range of reported accuracies reflects, in part, the high degree of operator dependence of TVS. The findings of adenomyosis on TVS are subtle and can only be diagnosed if the examination is performed meticulously and in real time (Figs. 3.16, 3.17). In one study of 100 patients undergoing hysterectomy, TVS depicted 25 of 29 pathologically

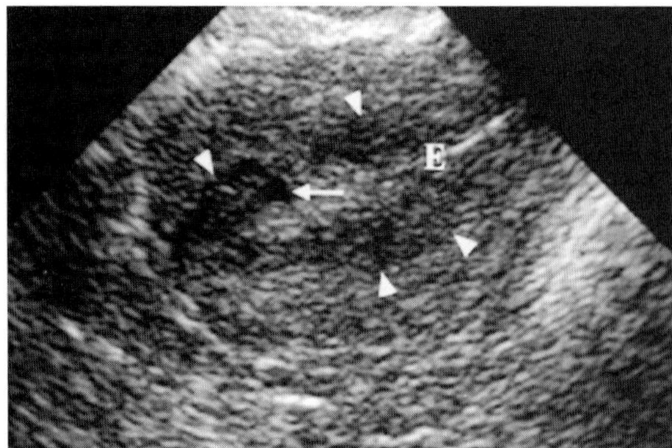


a

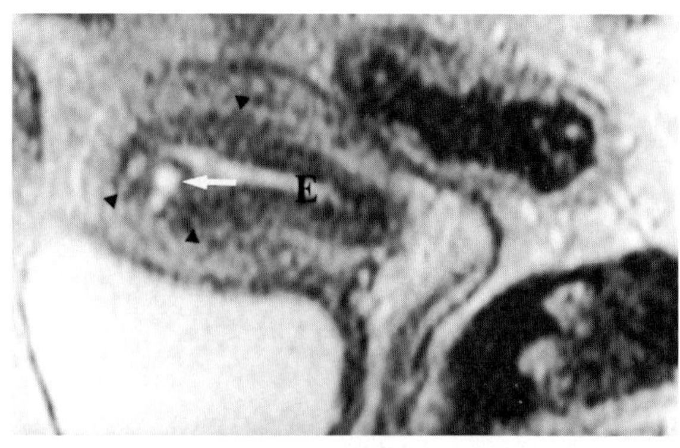


b

**Fig. 3.17 a,b.** Adenomyosis. True-positive findings at TVS and MRI in a patient with histopathologically proved adenomyosis and hemorrhagic foci in the ventral myometrium. **a** Sagittal TVS through the uterus demonstrates decreased echogenicity and heterogeneity of the inner myometrium (*arrows*), consistent with adenomyosis. In addition a small myometrial cyst (*arrowhead*) is present ventrally. *E*, Endometrium. **b** Sagittal T2-weighted conventional SE MR image demonstrates uneven thickening of the JZ (*arrowheads*), consistent with adenomyosis. This corresponds well to the findings at TVS. Two myometrial cysts are present; only the larger of the two (*arrowhead*) could be resolved with use of TVS. (From Reinhold et al. 1995)

proven cases of adenomyosis. Myometrial findings suggestive of adenomyosis included: (1) heterogeneous and hypoechoic areas with or without the presence of cysts (84% of patients); (2) hypoechoic areas with cysts (12% of patients); and (3) heterogeneous areas (4% of patients) (Reinhold et al. 1995).

Magnetic resonance imaging offers several advantages over TVS in the diagnosis of adenomyosis. The presence of mural leiomyomas can limit the assessment of the adjacent myometrium with TVS. MRI is considerably less operator-dependent and provides images that are standard and reproducible from one examination to another. TVS may not be suitable for monitoring the evolution of adenomyosis, since identical views from one examination to the next may be difficult to reproduce. Several studies have demonstrated MRI to be highly accurate in diagnosing adenomyosis, with sensitivities and specificities ranging from 86% to 100% (Jones and Jones 1982b; Reinhold et al. 1996; Mark et al. 1987; Ascher et al. 1994; Togashi et al. 1988, 1989) (see Figs. 3.16, 3.17).

### 3.9.3.2 MR Imaging Considerations

T2-weighted sequences are used to diagnose adenomyosis because they provide optimal depiction of the uterine zonal anatomy. In addition to standard sagittal and transverse imaging planes, short-axis views of the uterine corpus may be indicated for accurate measurements of junctional zone (JZ) thickness. On T1-weighted sequences, small hyperintense foci representing hemorrhage within the ectopic endometrial tissue may be seen in approximately 20% of patients (Jones and Jones 1982b; Reinhold et al. 1996). The addition of contrast-enhanced images does not improve the detection or characterization of adenomyosis (Jones and Jones 1982b).

Diagnostic criteria used for diagnosing adenomyosis on T2-weighted sequences include: (1) a low-signal-intensity lesion adjacent to the endometrium presenting as focal or diffuse thickening of the JZ, or (2) the presence of a low-signal-intensity myometrial mass with ill-defined borders (adenomyoma) (Fig. 3.18). Cutoff values for JZ thickness used to differentiate patients with adenomyosis from those without adenomyosis have been reported as greater than 5 mm by some investigators and greater than or equal to 12 mm by others (Reinhold et al. 1996; Mark et al. 1987; Ascher et al. 1994). In practice, we have found that a maximal JZ thickness greater than or equal to 12 mm is highly predictive of the presence of adenomyosis, while a JZ thickness less than or equal to 8 mm usually excludes the disease. In patients with a JZ thickness measuring between 8 and 12 mm, ancillary findings such as relative thickening of the JZ in a localized area, poor definition of borders, or the presence of high-signal foci on T2- or T1-weighted sequences can be used to diagnose adenomyosis. High-signal foci within the lesion on T2-weighted sequences have been reported in 50%–88% of cases

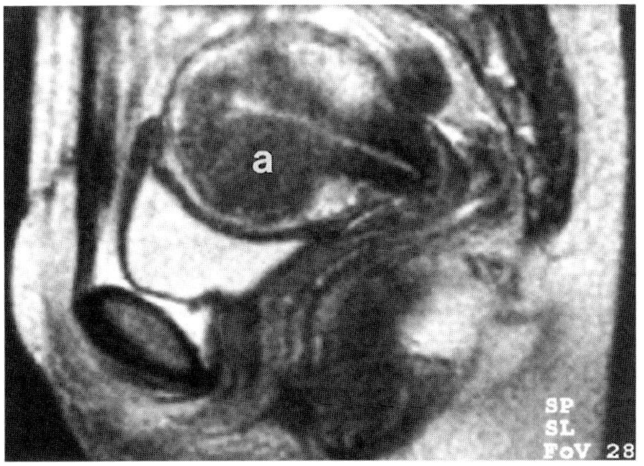


**Fig. 3.18.** Adenomyoma. Sagittal T2-weighted TSE. Note the focal widening of the inferior JZ consistent with an adenomyoma (*a*). Less pronounced changes are noted along the superior fundus

and may represent islands of ectopic endometrium, cystically dilated endometrial glands, and/or hemorrhagic fluid (Reinhold et al. 1996; Jones and Jones 1982a; Togashi et al. 1988) (see Fig. 3.6). In some patients, linear striations of increased signal can be seen radiating out from the endometrium into the myometrium on T2-weighted sequences. These striations likely represent direct invasion of the basal endometrium into the myometrium. On T1-weighted sequences, adenomyosis is isointense to the surrounding myometrium, except for the presence of bright foci, which have been shown to correspond to small areas of hemorrhage at histopathology (Togashi et al. 1989).

Practically, the most important differential diagnosis of adenomyosis is leiomyoma (see Fig. 3.6). Differentiating the two conditions is essential, since uterine-conserving therapy is possible with leiomyomas, whereas hysterectomy is the traditional definitive treatment for debilitating adenomyosis. Although MRI has been shown to be highly accurate in differentiating adenomyosis from leiomyomas, the imaging characteristics may overlap, particularly in the case of adenomyomas (Mark et al. 1987; Togashi et al. 1989). Features that favor the diagnosis of adenomyosis include: (1) a lesion with poorly defined borders, (2) a lesion that extends along endometrium and usually has an elliptical shape, (3) minimal mass effect on the endometrium relative to the size of the lesion, and (4) linear striations radiating out from endometrium into the myometrium.

Myometrial contractions may closely resemble the appearance of focal adenomyosis on MRI. Contractions can be differentiated from true myometrial pathology on sequential imaging acquisitions by their transient nature and changing appearance over time. In addition, the presence of muscular hypertrophy of the uterus at histopathology may result in thickening of the JZ at MRI, mimicking the appearance of diffuse adenomyosis (Reinhold et al. 1996).

## 3.10 Benign Diseases of the Cervix

### 3.10.1 Nabothian Cysts

#### *3.10.1.1 General Considerations*

Nabothian cysts result from mucous distention of endocervical glands or clefts, either as a result of an inflammatory process or due to squamous metaplasia (Hill and Pernoll 1994). Although nabothian cysts are common, they are rarely symptomatic and require no treatment. Occasionally, nabothian cysts reach 2–4 cm in diameter and, when multiple, result in marked enlargement of the cervix. Their ultrasound appearance, as with other cysts, will typically be that of a round, anechoic structure with a thin, imperceptible wall and enhanced through-transmission.

#### *3.10.1.2 MR Imaging Considerations*

Nabothian cysts are well depicted on T2-weighted sagittal and transverse images (see Fig. 3.12). Nabothian cysts demonstrate medium-to-high signal intensity on T1-weighted images and are hyperintense on T2-weighted images. They show no enhancement after gadolinium chelate administration (see Fig. 3.14). Nabothian cysts are differentiated from most cervical neoplasms by their small size and well-defined margins.

Adenoma malignum of the cervix has been reported to mimic nabothian cysts at MRI (Yamashita et al. 1994). Adenoma malignum is a rare tumor that accounts for approximately 3% of adenocarcinomas of the cervix and forms nodular masses with mucin-rich cystic spaces. Therefore, if cystic lesions are observed in a patient with adenocarcinoma of the cervix at histopathology, adenoma malignum may be considered in the differential diagnosis.

In addition, hemorrhagic foci associated with cervical endometriosis may mimic the MRI appearance of nabothian cysts.

## 3.10.2 Cervical Stenosis

### 3.10.2.1 *General Considerations*

Cervical stenosis may be congenital, inflammatory, neoplastic, or iatrogenic in origin (Hill and Pernoll 1994). Most cases of cervical stenosis involve the external os and are associated with extensive surgical manipulation (e.g., conization, electocoagulation, cyotherapy) or are radiation induced (Hill and Pernoll 1994). Senile atrophy may also result in cervical stenosis. The role of imaging is to exclude mechanical obstruction, most commonly due to the presence of endometrial or cervical carcinoma. When the obstruction of the cervix is complete, hematometra or pyometra may result with a fluid-filled uterus seen on ultrasound. Depending on the fluid contents, it will either be anechoic or contain internal echoes.

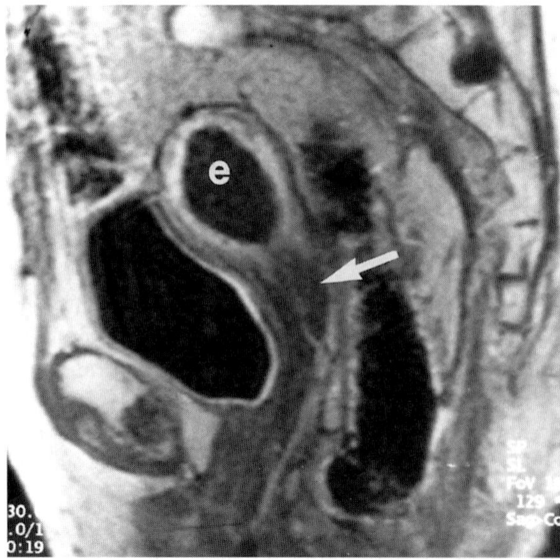


Fig. 3.19. Cervical stenosis. Sagittal T2-weighted TSE (**A**) and post-contrast T1-weighted fat-suppressed SGE (**B**) of the uterus in this patient with a history of radiation therapy. The endometrial canal is distended with fluid (*e*). The persistent low signal of the cervix (*arrow*), which does not enhance, is consistent with radiation-induced fibrosis

### 3.10.2.2 *MR Imaging Considerations*

T2- and T1-weighted sagittal images through the uterus are best to demonstrate the relationship of the distended uterine cavity to the cervical stenosis (Fig. 3.19). Unenhanced and contrast-enhanced sequences are necessary to differentiate tumor from debris or blood within the uterine cavity.

Magnetic resonance imaging can identify the presence and location of the cervical stenosis. In cases of complete obstruction, the uterine cavity is distended by material of variable signal intensity, depending on its composition (e.g., retained secretions, pus, blood, or tumor).

## 3.10.3 Cervical Incompetence

### 3.10.3.1 *General Considerations*

Cervical incompetence occurs in less than 1% of all pregnancies but may account for up to 16% of second- or third-trimester abortions (Stromme and Haywa 1963). The etiology of cervical incompetence is as follows: (1) congenital – including congenital uterine malformation, in utero exposure to diethylstilbestrol (DES), and decreased collagen content, or (2) acquired – including obstetric or gynecologic trauma, multiple gestations, and hormonal disorders (Stromme and Haywa 1963; Ansari and Reynolds 1987). The MR findings of the cervix in the nonpregnant woman with a history of cervical incompetence have been described and will be addressed in the ensuing section (Hricak et al. 1990).

### 3.10.3.2 *MR Imaging Considerations*

One or more of the following findings at MRI or ultrasound can suggest the presence of cervical incompetence in the nonpregnant woman: (1) cervical length less than or equal to 3.0 cm (measured from the internal os to the external os); (2) internal cervical os greater than or equal to 4.3 mm (distance between inner margins of the fibrous stroma); (3) thinning or increased signal intensity of the cervical fibrous stroma; and (4) irregular asymmetric widening of the endocervical canal (Hricak et al. 1990).

All measurements are obtained on T2-weighted sagittal images (Fig. 3.20).

In patients with cervical incompetence related to DES exposure, the endocervical canal usually measures less than 2.5 cm. The width of the internal os and the signal intensity of the cervical stroma, however, remain normal. (Hricak et al. 1990; van Gils et al. 1989).

## 3.11 Conclusion

The role of MRI in the evaluation of the female pelvis has increased in significance due to recent developments which have improved soft tissue differentiation as well as decreased scan time. In patients with suspected adenomyosis or for preoperative planning in patients with leiomyomas, MRI has distinct advantages over ultrasound. Similarly, if the origin of a pelvic mass cannot be discerned on ultrasound, MRI can provide valuable complementary information. Ultrasound does remain an important screening modality for endometrial conditions, but if technically suboptimal or nondiagnostic, MRI should be the next step in imaging assessment.

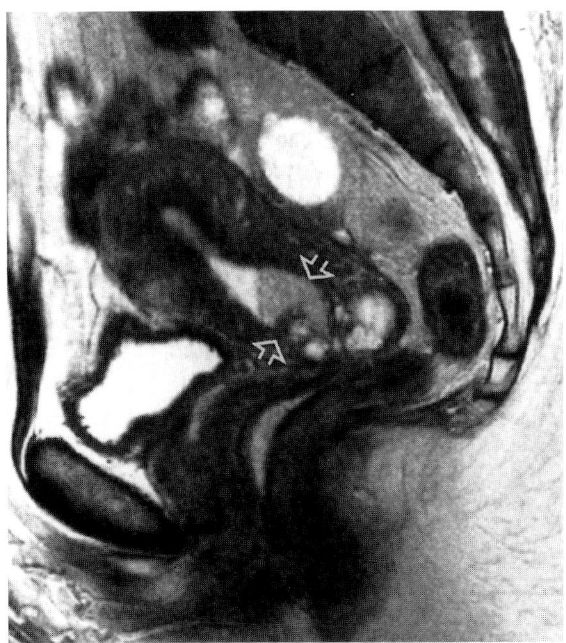

**Fig. 3.20.** Cervical incompetence. Sagittal T2-weighted TSE. Note increased endocervical width (*open arrows*)

## References


Ansari AH, Reynolds RA (1987) Cervical incompetence. A review. J. Reprod Med 32:161–171

Arnold LL, Ascher SM, Schruefer JJ, Simon JA (1995) The nonsurgical diagnosis of adenomyosis. Obstet Gynecol 86:461–465

Arrive L, Chang YC, Hricak H, Brescia RJ, Aufferman W, Quivey JM (1989) Radiation-induced uterine changes: MR imaging. Radiology 170:55–58

Ascher SM, Arnold LL, Patt RH, et al. (1994) Adenomyosis: prospective comparison of MR imaging and transvaginal sonography. Radiology 190:803–806

Ascher SM, Johnson JC, Barnes WA, Bae CJ, Patt RH, Zeman RK (1996) MR imaging appearance of the uterus in postmenopausal women receiving tamoxifen therapy for breast cancer: Histopathologic correlation. Radiology 200:105–110

Ascher SM, Brown JJ, Walsh JW (1997) In: Hoskins WJ, Perez CA, Young RC (eds) Principles and practice of gynecologic oncology, 2nd edn. Lippincott-Raven, Philadelphia, pp 593–597

Atri M, Nazarnia S, Aldis AE, Reinhold C, Bret PM, Kintzen G (1994) Transvaginal US appearance of endometrial abnormalities. Radiographics 14:483–492

Azziz R (1989) Adenomyosis: current perspectives. Obstet Gynecol Clin North Am 16:221–235

Benson RC, Sneeden VD (1958) Adenomyosis: a reappraisal of symptomatology. Am J Obstet Gynecol 76:1044–1061

Bird CC, McElin TW, Manalo-Estrella P (1972) The elusive adenomyosis of the uterus – revisited. Am J Obstet Gynecol 112:583–593

Bloom W, Fawcett DW (1975) A textbook of histology. Saunders, Philadelphia, p 894

Bohlman ME, Ensor RE, Sanders RC (1987) Sonographic findings in adenomyosis of the uterus. Am J Roentgenol 148:765–766

Brosens JJ, DeSouza NM, Barker FG, Paraschos T, Winston RML (1995) Endovaginal ultrasonography in the diagnosis of adenomyosis uteri: identifying the predictive characteristics. Br J Obstet Gynaecol 102:471–474

Brown HK, Stoll BS, Nicosia SV, et al. (1991) Uterine junctional zone: correlation between histologic findings and MR imaging. Radiology 179:409–413

Bulic M, Kasnar V, Dukovic I (1986) Use of ultrasound in the diagnosis of genital endometriosis. Jugosl Ginekol Perinatol 26:33–34

Chang YC, Hricak H (1989) Current status of MR imaging of the female pelvis. Crit Rev Diagn Imaging 29:337–356

Cohen I, Rosen DJ, Tepper R, et al. (1993) Ultrasonographic evaluation of the endometrium and correlation with endometrial sampling in postmenopausal patients treated with tamoxifen. J Ultrasound Med 12:275–280

Constable RT, Anderson AW, Zhong J, Gore JC (1992) Factors influencing contrast in fast spin-echo MR imaging. Magn Reson Imaging 10:497–511

Constable RT, Gore JC (1992) The loss of small objects in variable TE imaginng: implications for FSE, RARE, and EPI. Magn Reson Med 28:9–24

Cullinan JA, Fleischer AC, Kepple DM, Arnold AL (1995) Sonohysterography: technique for endometrial evaluation. Radiographics 15:501–514

De Muylder X, Neven P, De Somer M, Van Belle Y, Vanderick G, De Muylder E (1991) Endometrial lesions in patients undergoing tamoxifen therapy. Int J Gynecol Obstet 36:127–130

Demas BE, Hricak H, Jaffe RB (1986) Uterine MR imaging: effects of hormonal stimulation. Radiology 159:123–126

deSouza NM, Hawley IC, Schwieso JE, Gilderdale DJ, Soutter WP (1994) The uterine cervix on in vitro and in vivo MR images: a study of zonal anatomy and vascularity using an enveloping cervical coil. Am J Roentgenol 163:607–612

Dubinsky TJ, Parvey R, Gormaz G, Curtis M, Maklud N (1995) Transvaginal hysterosonography: comparison with biopsy in the evaluation of postmenopausal bleeding. J Ultrasound Med 14:887–893

Dudiak CM, Turner DA, Patel SK, Archie JT, Silver B, Norusis M (1988) Uterine leiomyomas in the infertile patient: preoperative localization with MR imaging versus US and hysterosalpingography. Radiology 167:627–630

Fedele L, Bianchi S, Dorta M, Arcaini L, Zanotti F, Carinelli S (1992a) Transvaginal ultrasonography in the diagnosis of diffuse adenomyosis. Fertil Steril 58:94–97

Fedele L, Bianchi S, Dorta M, Zanotti F, Brioschi D, Carinelli S (1992b) Transvaginal ultrasonography in the differential diagnosis of adenomyoma versus leiomyoma. Am J Obstet Gynecol 167:603–606

Fleischer AC, Shah DM, Entman SS (1990) Sonographic evaluation of maternal disorders during pregnancy. Radiol Clin North Am 28:51–58

Fornander T, Rutqvist LE, Cedermark B, et al. (1989) Adjuvant tamoxifen in early breast cancer: occurrence of new primary cancers. Lancet 1:117–120

Gross BH, Silver TM, Jaffe MH (1983) Sonographic features of uterine leiomyomas: analysis of 41 proven cases. J Ultrasound Med 2:401–406

Hamlin DJ, Fitzsimmons JR, Pettersson H, et al. (1985) Magnetic resonance imaging of the pelvis: evaluation of ovarian masses at 0.15 T. AJR 145:585–590

Hann LE, Giess CS, Bach AM, et al. (1997) Endometrial thickness in tamoxifen-treated patients: correlation with clinical and pathologic findings. AJR 168:657–661

Haramati N, Penrod B, Staron RB, Barax CN (1994) Surgical sutures: MR artifacts and sequence dependence. J Magn Reson Imaging 4:209–211

Haynor DR, Mack LA, Soules MR, Shuman WP, Montana MA, Moss AA (1986) Changing appearance of the normal uterus during the menstrual cycle: MR studies. Radiology 161:459–462

Hill EC, Pernoll ML (1994) Benign disorders of the uterine cervix. In: DeCherney AH, Pernoll ML (eds) Current obstetric & gynecologic diagnosis & treatment, 8th edn. Appleton & Lange, Norwalk, CT, pp 713–730

Hirano Y, Kubo K, Hirai Y, et al. (1992) Preliminary experience with gadolinium-enhanced dynamic MR imaging for uterine neoplasms. Radiographics 12:243–256

Horie Y, Ikawa S, Kadowaki K, Minagawa Y, Kigawa J, Terekawa N (1995) Lipoadenofibroma of the uterine corpus. Report of a new variant of adenofibroma (benign mullerian mixed tumor). Arch Pathol Lab Med 119:274–276

Hricak H (1986) MRI of the female pelvis: a review. AJR 146:1115–1122

Hricak H (1993) Current trends in MR imaging of the female pelvis. Radiographics 13:913–919

Hricak H, Kim B (1993) Contrast-enhanced MR imaging of the female pelvis. J Magn Reson Imaging 3:297–306

Hricak H, Alpers C, Crooks LE, Sheldon PE (1983) Magnetic resonance imaging of the female pelvis: initial experience. AJR 141:1119–1128

Hricak H, Tscholakoff D, Heinrichs L, et al. (1986) Uterine leiomyomas: correlation of MR histopathologic findings, and symptoms. Radiology 158:385–391

Hricak H, Stern JL, Fischer MR, Shapeero LG, Winkler ML, Conley GL (1987) Endometrial carcinoma staging by MR imaging. Radiology 162:297–305

Hricak H, Chang YC, Cann CE, Parer JT (1990) Cervical incompetence: preliminary evaluation with MR imaging. Radiology 174:821–826

Hricak H, Finck S, Honda G, Goeranson H (1992) MR imaging in the evaluation of benign uterine masses: value of gadopentetate dimeglumin-enhanced T1-weighted images. Am J Roentgenol 158:1043–1050

Hulka CA, Hall DA, McCarthy K, Simeone JF (1994) Endometrial polyps, hyperplasia and carcinoma in postmenopausal women: differentiation with endovaginal sonography. Radiology 191:755–758

Israel SL, Woutersz TB (1959) Adenomyosis: a neglected diagnosis. Obstet Gynecol 14:168–173

Ito K, Fujita T, Uchisako H, et al. (1994) MR imaging of the uterus: findings from high-resolution multisection dynamic imaging with a surface coil. Am J Roentgenol 163:873–879

Jolesz FA, Jones KM (1993) Fast spin-echo imaging of the brain. Top Magn Reson Imaging 5:1–13

Jones HW, Jones GS (1982a) Gynecology, 3rd edn. Williams & Wilkins, Baltimore, MD, pp 1–8

Jones HW, Jones GS (1982b) Gynecology, 3rd edn. Williams & Wilkins, Baltimore, MD, pp 46–68

Jones HW, Jones GS (1982c) Gynecology, 3rd edn. Williams & Wilkins, Baltimore, MD, pp 222–229

Jones HW, Jones GS (1982d) Gynecology, 3rd edn. Williams & Wilkins, Baltimore, MD, pp 245–253

Jones HW, Jones GS (1982e) Gynecology, 3rd edn. Williams & Wilkins, Baltimore, MD, pp 334–345

Karasick S, Lev-Toaff AS, Toaff ME (1992) Imaging of uterine leiomyomas. Am J Roentgenol 158:799–805

Kasai M (1990) Clinical application of magnetic resonance imaging (MRI) in uterine disease. Acta Obstet Gynaecol Jpn 42:711–718

Kliewer MA, Hertzberg BS, George PY, McDonald JW, Bowie JD, Carroll BA (1995) Acoustic shadowing from uterine leiomyomas: sonographic-pathologic correlation. Radiology 196:99–102

Kurtz AB, Middleton WD (1996) Ultrasound: the requisites. Mosby, St. Louis, MO, pp 359–368

Lange RC, Duberg AC, McCarthy SM (1991) An evaluation of MRI contrast in the uterus using synthetic imaging. Magn Reson Med 17:279–284

Langlois LP (1970) The size of the normal uterus. J Reprod Med 4:220–228

Lee JKT, Gersell DJ, Balfe DM, Worthington JL, Picus D, Gapp G (1985) The uterus: in vitro MR anatomic correlation of normal and abnormal specimens. Radiology 157:175–179

Lin MC, Gosink BB, Wolf SI, et al. (1991) Endometrial thickness after menopause: effect of hormone replacement. Radiology 180:427–432

Lyons EA, Levi CS (1982) Ultrasound in the first trimester of pregnancy. Radiol Clin North Am 20:259–270

Mark AS, Hricak H (1987) Intrauterine contraceptive devices: MR imaging. Radiology 162:311–314

Mark AS, Hricak H, Heinrichs LW, et al. (1987) Adenomyosis and leiomyoma: differential diagnosis with MR imaging. Radiology 163:527–529

McCarthy S, Tauber C, Gore J (1986) Female pelvic anatomy: MR assessment of variations during the menstrual cycle and with use of oral contraceptives. Radiology 160:119–123

McCarthy S, Scott G, Majumdar S, et al. (1989) Uterine junctional zone: MR study of water content and relaxation properties. Radiology 171:241–243

McCauley TR, McCarthy S, Lange R (1992) Pelvic phased array coil: image quality assessment for spin-echo MR imaging. Magn Reson Imaging 10:513–522

Mitchell DG, Schonholz L, Hilpert PL, Pennell RG, Blum L, Rifkin MD (1990) Zones of the uterus: discrepancy between US and MR images. Radiology 174:827–831

Mittl RL, Yeh I, Kressel HY (1991) High-signal-intensity rim surrounding uterine leiomyomas on MR images: pathologic correlation. Radiology 180:81–83

Moghissi K (1980) Effects of steroidal contraceptives on the reproductive system. In: Hafez E (ed) Human reproduction. Harper & Row, Hungerstown, pp 529–537

Molitor JJ (1971) Adenomyosis: a clinical and pathological appraisal. Am J Obstet Gynecol 110:275–284

Muse KN (1990) Cyclic pelvic pain. Obstet Gynecol Clin North Am 17:427–440

Neven P, De Muylder X, Van Belle Y, Vanderick G, De Muylder E (1990) Hysteroscopic follow-up during tamoxifen treatment. Eur J Obstet Gynecol Reprod Biol 35:235–238

Nghiem HV, Herfkens RJ, Francis IR, et al. (1992) The pelvis: T2-weighted fast spin-echo MR imaging. Radiology 185:213–217

Owolabi TO, Strickler RC (1977) Adenomyosis: a neglected diagnosis. Obstet Gynecol 50:424–427

Panageas E, Kier R, McCauley TR, McCarthy S (1992) Submucosal uterine leiomyomas: diagnosis of prolapse into the cervix and vagina based on MR imaging. Am J Roentgenol 159:555–558

Parsons AK, Lense JJ (1993) Sonohysterography for endometrial abnormalities. J Clin Ultrasound 21:87–95

Rader JS, Binette SP, Brandt TD, Sreekanth S, Chhablani A (1990) Ileal hemorrhage caused by a parasitic uterine leiomyoma. Obstet Gynecol 76:531–534

Reinhold C, Atri M, Mehio A, Zakarian R, Aldis AE, Bret PM (1995) Diffuse uterine adenomyosis: morphologic criteria and diagnostic accuracy of endovaginal sonography. Radiology 197:609–614

Reinhold C, McCarthy S, Bret PM, et al. (1996) Diffuse adenomyosis: comparison of endovaginal US and MR imaging with histopathologic correlation. Radiology 199:151–158

Schwalm H, Dubrauszky V (1966) The structure of the musculature of the human uterus: muscles and connective tissue. Am J Obstet Gynecol 94:391–404

Scoutt LM, Flynn SD, Luthringer DJ, McCauley TR, McCarthy SM (1991) Junctional zone of the uterus: correlation of MR imaging and histologic examination of hysterectomy specimens. Radiology 179:403–407

Sheth S, Hamper UM, Kurman RJ (1993) Thickened endometrium in the postmenopausal woman: sonographic-pathologic correlation. Radiology 187:135–139

Smith RC, Reinhold C, Lange RC, McCauley TR, Kier R, McCarthy S (1992a) Fast spin-echo MR imaging of the female pelvis. I. Use of a whole-volume coil. Radiology 184:665–669

Smith RC, Reinhold C, McCauley TR, et al. (1992b) Multicoil high-resolution fast spin-echo MR imaging of the female pelvis. Radiology 184:671–675

Stromme WB, Haywa EW (1963) Intrauterine fetal death in the second trimester. Am J Obstet Gynecol 85:223–233

Timor-Tristch IE, Monteagudo A, Brown GM (1994) In: Callen PW (ed) Ultrasonography in obstetrics and gynecology, 3[rd] edn. Saunders, Philadelphia, pp 52–57

Togashi K (1993) MRI of the female pelvis. Igaku-Shoin, Tokyo, p 33

Togashi K, Nishimura K, Itoh K, et al. (1988) Adenomyosis: diagnosis with MR imaging. Radiology 166:111–114

Togashi K, Ozasa H, Konishi I, et al. (1989) Enlarged uterus: differentiation between adenomyosis and leiomyoma with MR imaging. Radiology 171:531–534

Togashi K, Kawakami S, Kimura I, et al. (1993a) Sustained uterine contractions: a cause of hypointense myometrial bulging. Radiology 187:707–710

Togashi K, Kawakami S, Kimura I, et al. (1993b) Uterine contractions: possible diagnostic pitfall at MR imaging. J Magn Reson Imaging 3:889–893

van Gils APG, Tham RTOTA, Falke THM, Peters AAW (1989) Abnormalities of the uterus and cervix after Diethylstilbesterol exposure: correlation of findings on MR and hysterosalpingography. Am J Roentgenol 153:1235–1238

Varner RE, Sparks JM, Cameron CD, Roberts LL, Soong S (1991) Transvaginal sonography of the endometrium in postmenopausal women. Obstet Gynecol 78:195–199

Weinreb JC, Barkoff ND, Megibow A, Demopoulos R (1990) The value of MR imaging in distinguishing leiomyomas from other solid pelvic masses when sonography is indeterminate. Am J Roentgenol 154:295–299

Wiczyk HP, Janus CL, Richards CJ, et al. (1988) Comparison of magnetic resonance imaging and ultrasound in evaluating follicular and endometrial development throughout the normal cycle. Fertil Steril 49:969–972

Yamashita Y, Harada M, Sawada T, Takahashi M, Miyazaki K, Okamura H (1993a) Normal uterus and FIGO Stage I endometrial carcinoma: dynamic gadolinium-enhanced MR imaging. Radiology 186:495–501

Yamashita Y, Torashima M, Takahashi M (1993b) Hyperintense uterine leiomyoma at T2-weighted MR imaging: differentiation with dynamic enhanced MR imaging and clinical implications. Radiology 189:721–725

Yamashita Y, Takahashi M, Katabuchi H, Fukumatsu Y, Miyazaki K, Okamura H (1994) Adenoma malignum: MR appearances mimicking nabothian cysts. Am J Roentgenol 162:649–650

Zawin M, McCarthy S, Scoutt L, et al. (1990a) Monitoring therapy with a gonadotropin-releasing hormone analog: utility of MR imaging. Radiology 175:503–506

Zawin M, McCarthy S, Scoutt LM, Comite F (1990b) High-field MRI and US evaluation of the pelvis in women with leiomyomas. Magn Reson Imaging 8:371–376

# 4 Color Doppler Ultrasound in the Assessment of Benign and Malignant Neoplasms of the Female Pelvis

U.M. Hamper, S. Sheth, and C.I. Caskey

CONTENTS



## 4.1 Role of Color and Doppler Ultrasound in the Evaluation of Pelvic Neoplasms

### 4.1.1 Introduction

Ultrasound (US) is a well-established modality for evaluating the female pelvis. Advances in US technology such as the advent of endovaginal US (EVS) and, recently, EVS coupled with color flow and power color Doppler have increased the diagnostic accuracy of US in determining the nature and etiology of uterine, adnexal, and ovarian masses. Close proximity of the pelvic organs to the transducer and the use of higher frequency transducers (5–7.5 MHz) allow better image resolution.

This chapter will review endovaginal applications for the evaluation of a selected number of adnexal and uterine conditions and specifically address the current status and role of color Doppler US and power Doppler US for the evaluation of ovarian, endometrial, and selected pelvic lesions.

### 4.1.2 Instrumentation and Examination Technique

In most US laboratories the standard examination of the female pelvis consists in the traditional transabdominal/transvesical approach followed by EVS and in selected cases endovaginal color Doppler or power Doppler US. Transabdominal sonography (TAS) is performed through the full urinary bladder usually using 3.5-MHz transducers; however, in some patients it is possible to use 5-MHz or 7.5-MHz probes. TAS provides a wider field of view than the endovaginal approach and allows better visualization of superficial structures and structures remote from the vagina.

Endovaginal US demonstrates exquisite anatomic detail of the uterus, ovaries, and adnexa which cannot be achieved by TAS. Endovaginal scanning is performed with 5 to 7.5-MHz transducers. The uterus is examined in longitudinal and semiaxial/coronal planes. The ovaries are usually easily seen on an angled long-axis scan immediately medial to the pelvic vessels. The axial or semicoronal view is the best view to evaluate the ovaries and adnexae. State-of-the-art probes allow color Doppler and power Doppler imaging with frequencies ranging from 3 to 5 MHz. Color velocity settings (pulse repetition frequency), output power, color gain, filter settings and focal zone placement are optimized in each individual patient.

U.M. Hamper, MD, Division of Ultrasound, Department of Radiology and Radiological Sciences, The Johns Hopkins Medical Institutions, 600 North Wolfe Street, Baltimore, MD 21287, USA
S. Sheth, MD, Division of Ultrasound, Department of Radiology and Radiological Sciences, The Johns Hopkins Medical Institutions, 600 North Wolfe Street, Baltimore, MD 21287, USA
C.I. Caskey, MD, Division of Ultrasound, Department of Radiology and Radiological Sciences, The Johns Hopkins Medical Institutions, 600 North Wolfe Street, Baltimore, MD 21287, USA; current address: Department of Radiology University of Texas–Houston LBJ General Hospital 5656 Kelly Street Houston, TX 77026, USA

## 4.2 Evaluation of Ovarian Neoplasms

### 4.2.1 Ovarian Neoplasms: Background

Ovarian cancer is the most common cause of death due to gynecologic malignancy in the United States. One in 70 women will develop it during their lifetime. In 1998, 25400 women will be diagnosed with ovarian cancer and more than 50% (14500) will die of their disease (Cancer Facts and Figures 1998). Histologically, epithelial neoplasms account for 65%–75% of ovarian tumors and 90% of ovarian malignancies. Ovarian cancer is usually only detected in advanced stages (III and IV). The overall survival rate for patients with ovarian cancer is only 30%. Patients with early stage I cancers, however, have a much better survival rate, about 85%–90%. Until a new therapeutic regimen is developed, the only way to improve survival rates is to improve our ability to detect the disease at an early stage (Cancer Facts and Figures 1998).

### 4.2.2 Screening Techniques

Although many questions cannot be answered yet, exploration of possible methods of early detection of ovarian cancer have been sought. The clinical vaginal examination is of limited value. Several studies have shown that the pelvic examination detects less than 50% of pathology detected at laparoscopy (Averette and Donato 1990; Campbell et al. 1989; Sparks and Varner 1991). The CA-125 marker is an antigen identified by a murine monoclonal antibody to human ovarian cancer tissue. Levels greater than 35 U/ml are considered elevated. Eighty percent of women with nonmucinous epithelial ovarian cancers have elevated CA-125 levels, with 1% of the normal female population having a false-positive result. It can also be elevated in a variety of nonmalignant or malignant conditions. The tumor marker does seem to reflect the amount of tumor present; consequently, there is poor sensitivity in patients targeted for screening, i.e., those with stage I disease (Einhorn et al. 1992; Hata et al. 1992a; Mann et al. 1988; Patsner 1991).

### 4.2.3 Ultrasound and Ovarian Cancer Detection

Diagnostic US has played an increasingly important role in recent years in the evaluation of the gynecologic patient. With reference to the ovaries, a large amount of literature has been devoted to describing their morphology and size, especially in the postmenopausal woman (Andolf et al. 1986, 1987; Campbell et al. 1982; Goswamy et al. 1988; Jain and Jeffrey 1994; Levine and Gosink 1992; Timor-Tritsch et al. 1993; Sassone et al. 1991; Wolf et al. 1991). Ovarian volume measurements have been shown to be very accurate, when compared to surgery. Morphologic changes, although readily detected, have been shown to be disappointing in predicting the correct pathologic diagnosis due to the lack of tissue specificity.

Scoring systems to differentiate between benign and malignant adnexal masses have been reported to provide encouraging results in terms of sensitivity and negative predictive values (100%); however, significant limitations exist in terms of specificity (73%–83%) and positive predictive values (32%–46%) (Jain and Jeffrey 1994; Sassone 1991; Timor-Tritsch et al. 1993).

The likelihood of malignancy in an ovarian mass increases with size. There is an approximately 56% malignancy rate in masses >15 cm, 40% for the 5- to 15-cm range, and 4% with masses <5 cm. If a mass is a simple cyst, however, it is almost always benign. Simple cysts have been identified in about 14% of otherwise normal postmenopausal women (Wolf et al. 1991).

The development of endovaginal US techniques and the availability of color flow Doppler have been used in an attempt to diagnose early, i.e., stage I ovarian carcinoma. A recent flurry of reports have appeared in the literature in an effort to determine the role of US in ovarian cancer screening (Andolf et al. 1986; Bourne et al. 1989, 1991a,c; Brown et al. 1994; Fleischer et al. 1991a,b, 1992, 1993; Hamper et al. 1993; Hata et al. 1989; Jain and Jeffrey 1994; Kawai et al. 1992; Kurjak et al. 1991, 1993b; Stein et al. 1995; Timor-Tritsch et al. 1993; Weiner et al. 1992). The first study by Campbell et al. (1989) from Kings College Hospital in London described a large ovarian cancer screening program enrolling 5479 women undergoing 15977 transabdominal scans. A positive scan with abnormal ovarian morphology was found in 2.3%, and five patients were found to have stage I ovarian cancer. US in this study was unable to distinguish benign from malignant processes based on abnormal ovarian morphology (inhomogeneous texture, irregular borders, abnormal volume) with transabdominal scanning techniques. The advent of transvaginal sonography has enabled the production or more detailed images of ovarian morphology. The complementary use of pulsed, color, and power Doppler endovaginal sonography has been introduced to study blood flow in the arteries supplying the uterus and ovaries. A number of recent reports have advocated the use of this technique to characterize blood flow in ovarian and uterine lesions (ANDOLF et al. 1986; BOURNE et al. 1989, 1991b,c; BROWN et al. 1994; FLEISCHER et al. 1991a,b, 1992, 1993; HAMPER et al. 1993; HATA et al. 1989; JAIN 1994; KAWAI et al. 1992; KURJAK and ZALUD 1991; KURJAK et al. 1991, 1993a; STEIN et al. 1995; TIMOR-TRITSCH et al. 1993; WEINER et al. 1992). Quantitative results can be obtained by measuring the resistive index (RI):

$$\mathrm{RI} = \frac{\text{peak systolic velocity} - \text{end diastolic velocity}}{\text{peak systolic velocity}}$$

or the pulsatility index (PI):

$$\mathrm{PI} = \frac{\text{peak systolic velocity} - \text{end diastolic velocity}}{\text{mean velocity}}.$$

Flow patterns to the ovarian artery have been shown to vary depending on the phase of the menstrual cycle (DE ZIEGLER et al. 1991; BOURNE et al. 1991a; STEER et al. 1990; TAYLOR et al. 1985). Animal and human studies have shown increased ovarian blood flow near the time of ovulation, manifested by a lower PI or RI. In addition, preliminary data suggest that it may be possible to detect the vascular changes associated with early ovarian cancer using color Doppler US. In malignant lesions blood flow can be detected throughout diastole, reflecting a decrease in impedance to flow distal to the point of sampling. This may be explained by neovascularity associated with carcinoma, with the tumor vessels having limited vascular tone due to an absent or attenuated muscular coat or low-impedance shunts.

Previous papers by BOURNE et al. (1989) suggest that the specificity of EVS can be improved by measuring ovarian blood flow impedance with color Doppler techniques. The PI in his study of 50 women referred for suspicious pelvic masses was >1 in 41/42 normal scans or benign lesions and <1 in seven of eight malignancies. WEINER et al. (1992) showed similar findings in the preoperative evaluation of ovarian masses with PI >1 in 35/36 benign and PI <1 in 16/17 malignant lesions. KAWAI et al. (1992) evaluated 24 ovarian masses and used a PI of 1.25 to determine benign versus malignant masses. They had a correct diagnosis in 23/24 masses, eight of which were malignant. KURJAK et al. (1991, 1993a,b) wrote several papers using the RI cutoff of 0.4 to discriminate between malignant (RI <0.4) and benign (RI >0.4) lesions. HATA et al. (1989) studied eight malignant masses and found a mean RI of 0.503 ± 0.216 showing overlap between cancers and corpus luteum and endometrioid cysts. FLEISCHER et al. (1991a,b, 1993) studied 43 surgically proven ovarian masses; the PI of benign lesions ($n$ = 32) was 1.8 ± 0.8, while that of malignant masses ($n$ = 4) was 0.8 ± 0.6, again demonstrating overlap between benign and malignant lesions. Published data from our institution (HAMPER et al. 1993) demonstrate overlap of PIs and RIs in benign and malignant lesions (Figs. 4.1, 4.2) The mean PI and RI for benign lesions were 1.93 ± 1.02 (PI) and 0.77 ± 0.22 (RI), and for malignant lesions 0.77 ± 0.33 (PI) and 0.5 ± 0.17 (RI). BROWN et al. (1994) confirmed these findings in 44 ovarian masses: the PI of benign lesions ($n$ = 30) was 1.24 ± 0.71 and the RI, 0.62 ± 0.16; the PI of malignant lesions ($n$ = 8) was 0.56 ± 0.13 and the RI, 0.39 ± 0.09. However, despite the trend toward lower values in malignant masses, BROWN et al. did observe overlap between benign and malignant lesions. The most recent study by STEIN et al. (1995) evaluated 170 adnexal masses (123 benign and 47 malignant) and concluded that spectral Doppler analysis with PI and RI was not useful as no reliable discriminatory value with high sensitivity and specificity could be found because of an overlap in values for benign and malignant masses. A study by COLEMAN et al. (1994) showed that power Doppler US was more sensitive than color Doppler US in the depiction of longer vessel segments in the ovary (Fig. 4.3), though limitations were sensitivity to motion and the probe's decreased depth of penetration. The true potential of power Doppler US, however, has yet to be explored.

In summary, to date no adequate screening test exists for ovarian cancer. The multitude of recent reports describing experience with color Doppler endovaginal techniques support the general trend toward lower PI and RI values in malignant masses; however, the sensitivity and specificity of this technique are limited due to overlap of both indices in benign and malignant lesions. A prospective randomized trial is needed to evaluate the role of endovaginal color Doppler US for the evaluation of ovarian cancer and to answer the question of whether screening and thus earlier treatment will reduce the high mortality from this disease.

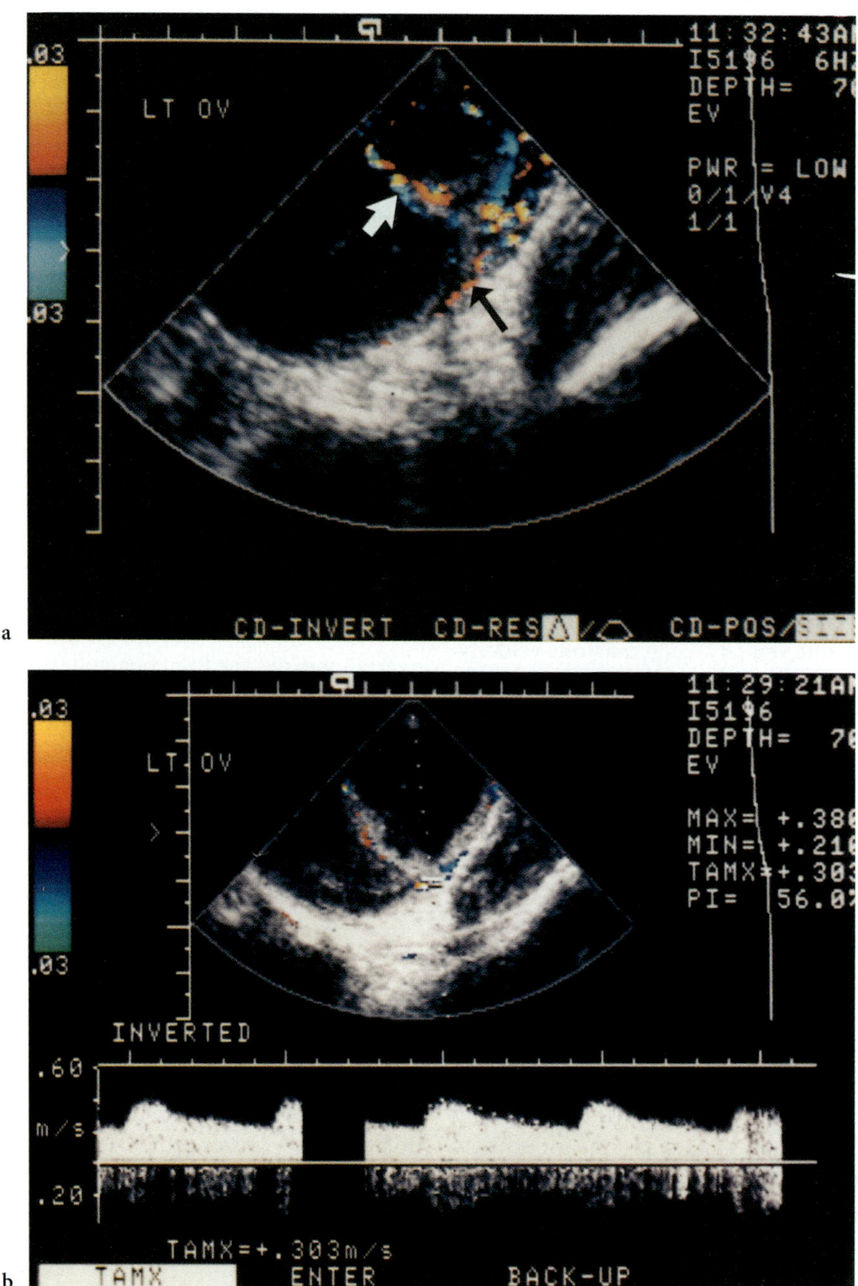


**Fig. 4.1.** **a** Color flow Doppler transvaginal sonogram of a septated, predominantly cystic, left-sided adnexal mass with peripheral (*black arrow*) and central (*white arrow*) vascularity within septa. **b** Pulsed Doppler sonogram shows low-resistance flow with a PI of 0.56 and an RI of 0.45. The patient had a family history of ovarian carcinoma and an elevated level of the tumor marker CA-125. **c** The pathologic specimen shows an endometrioma with multiple thin-walled vessels (*arrows*) lining endometriotic cystic wall. H&E; original magnification, ×40. (From Hamper et al. 1993)

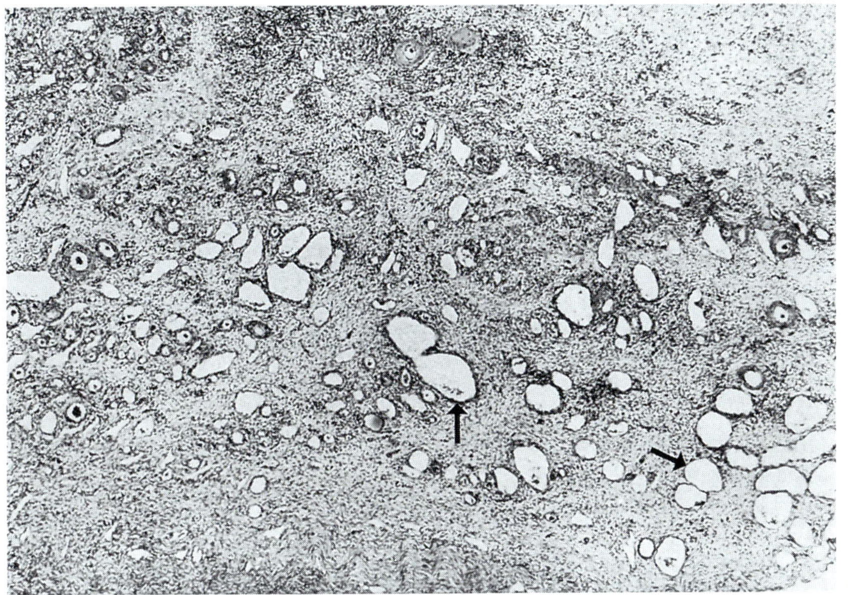

c

**Fig. 4.1.** *Continued*

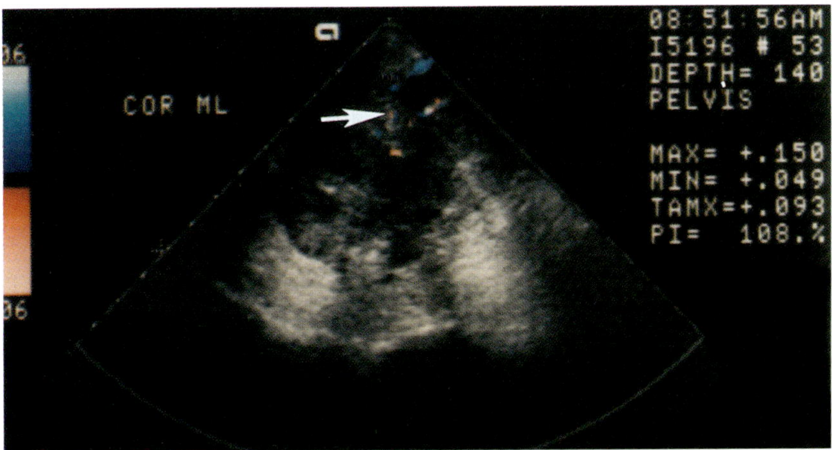


a

**Fig. 4.2.** **a** Color Doppler transvaginal sonogram of bilateral complex adnexal masses shows only minimal central vascularity (*arrow*). **b** Pulsed Doppler sonogram shows a relatively high PI of 0.98 and an RI of 0.62. **c** The pathologic specimen shows a poorly differentiated papillary serous cystadenocarcinoma of the ovary with multiple thin-walled vessels filled with tumor emboli (*arrows*), presumably accounting for the relatively high resistance to flow. H&E; original magnification, ×100. (From Hamper et al. 1993)

## 4.3 Evaluation of Endometrial Neoplasms

### 4.3.1 Endometrial Neoplasms: Background, Clinical Presentation, and Diagnosis

Endometrial cancer is the most common gynecologic malignancy in the United States, with 36 100 new cancers expected to occur in 1998. While it is among the six leading causes of cancer death in women, the cure rate for endometrial cancer is very high for well-differentiated and localized tumors. This underscores the importance of early detection and treatment (Cancer Facts and Figures 1998). Endometrial cancer predominantly affects peri- and postmenopausal women (75% of cases occur after age 50), with a peak incidence at age 58–60. Risk factors include age, obesity, diabetes, and prolonged estrogen unopposed stimulation of the endometrium.

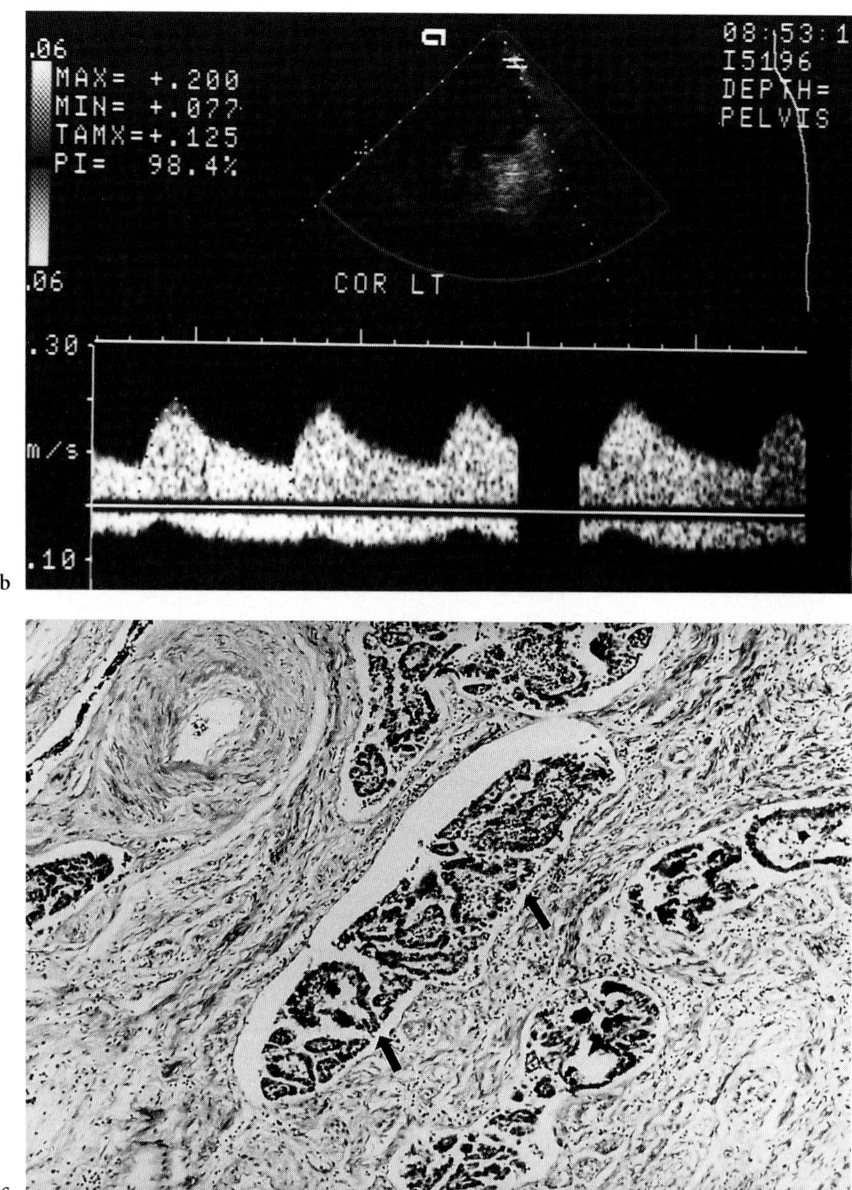


Fig. 4.2. *Continued*

The predominant histologic type is an adenocarcinoma arising from the glandular endometrial epithelium. Less common malignancies of the uterine corpus include endometrial sarcomas, mixed mesodermal cell tumors, and adenosquamous, clear cell, and papillary serous carcinomas. Endometrial hyperplasia, particularly if associated with atypia, is thought to be a precursor of endometrial cancer. Rarely, it may arise within an endometrial polyp.

The most common presenting symptom is postmenopausal vaginal bleeding. However, endometrial cancer is found in only 10% of women who present with postmenopausal bleeding. In fact, in the majority of these women, bleeding is caused by benign endometrial conditions such as endometrial atrophy, endometrial hyperplasia, or endometrial polyps (Ross 1988). Definitive diagnosis of endometrial cancer requires histologic sampling of the endometrium, either by endometrial biopsy or dilatation and curettage, preferably combined with hysteroscopy.

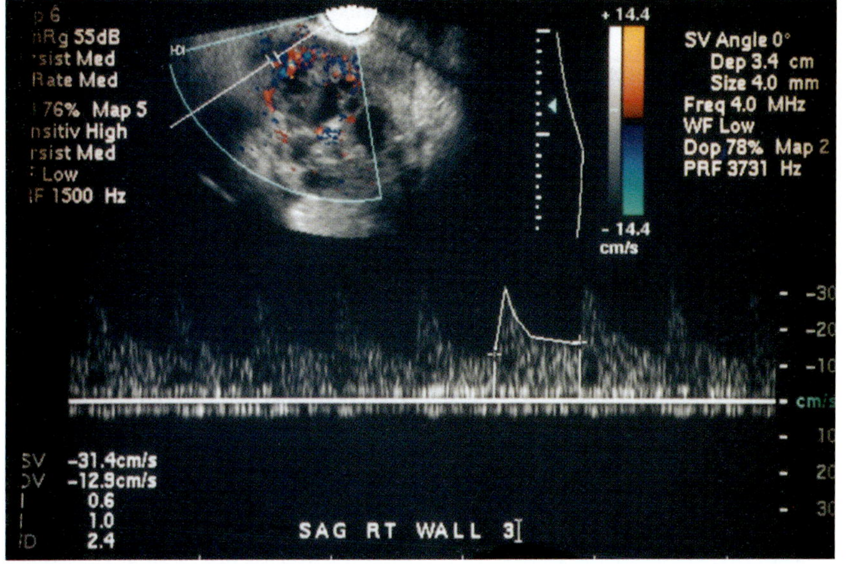


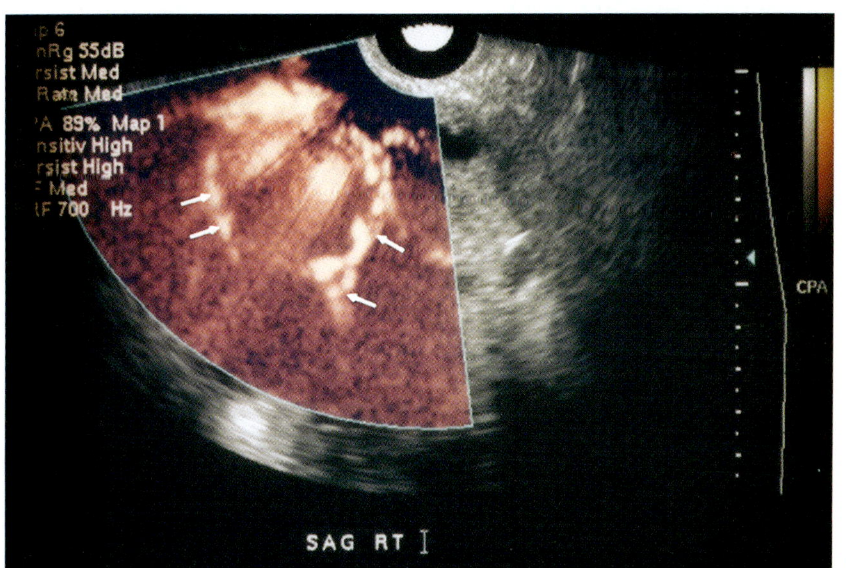


**Fig. 4.3.** **a** Color Doppler EV image of a mucinous cystadenocarcinoma of the ovary. **b** Power Doppler image nicely demonstrates the full length of the tumor vessels (*arrow*)

### 4.3.2
### Role of Color Doppler Endovaginal Sonography in the Detection and Diagnosis of Endometrial Cancer

Endovaginal sonography has been shown to be quite sensitive in depicting endometrial abnormalities, and is now widely used to evaluate the postmenopausal endometrium (Mendelson et al. 1988; Mogavero et al. 1993).

Common indications include postmenopausal bleeding, women on hormonal replacement regimens or taking long-term tamoxifen as adjuvant therapy for breast cancer, and screening of asymptomatic women at risk of developing endometrial cancer (Kurjak et al. 1994). The normal postmenopausal endometrium is thin (5 mm in thickness or less) and avascular on color Doppler EVS (CDEVS). However, endometrial thickness and possibly vascularity may be influenced by the presence of exogenous administration of estrogen (Bourne et al. 1991b; Zalud et al. 1993). Several authors have shown that if the endometrial stripe is clearly visible and is thin (less than 5 mm double layer measurement), it correlates with an atrophic endometrium at histology and virtually excludes the presence of endometrial cancer, with the consequence that biopsy may be avoided (NASRI and COAST 1989; NASRI et al. 1991; GOLDSTEIN et al. 1990; ROSS 1988).

The cardinal sonographic sign of endometrial carcinoma is an abnormally thick endometrium. However, this is a nonspecific finding as benign endometrial lesions such as hyperplasia, polyps, endometritis, or submucous myoma are more commonly found at pathology in women with a thickened endometrium (SHETH et al. 1993; NASRI and COAST 1989). Analysis of endometrial texture may be of some help. The presence of small cystic spaces within an otherwise echogenic endometrium is suggestive of cystic hyperplasia/atrophy or an endometrial polyp, while a heterogeneous echotexture favors endometrial cancer (SHETH et al. 1993; HULKA et al. 1994). However, there is an overlap between the various causes of endometrial thickening (HULKA et al. 1994). In an attempt to increase the specificity of EVS, and differentiate benign from malignant causes of endometrial thickening, several investigators have advocated color and duplex Doppler evaluation of the uterine arteries and endometrial blood flow.

Malignant tumors produce an angiogenesis factor that stimulates the formation and growth of tumor vessels. These vessels have an irregular pattern, lack intimal smooth muscle, and have numerous areas of arteriovenous shunting (FOLKMAN et al. 1989). Such abnormal tumor vessels are responsible for areas of increased vascularity and decreased impedance to blood flow demonstrated by color and duplex Doppler US in many solid malignant tumors (TAYLOR et al. 1988). In the uterus, various parameters have been investigated, i.e., measurements of RI and PI in the main uterine arteries (BOURNE et al. 1990, 1991b), visual evaluation of endometrial blood flow as depicted by color Doppler US, and measurement of intratumoral RI and PI (CARTER et al. 1993; KURJAK and ZALUD 1991; KURJAK et al. 1993b; SHETH et al. 1995a,b; ALEEM et al. 1995).

Early publications showed promising results. BOURNE and his colleagues (1990, 1991b) studied 34 women with postmenopausal bleeding and found that the uterine artery PI of 17 patients with endometrial cancer was significant lower (mean = 0.91) than that in women with normal endometrial histology (mean = 3.83). They recommended using a cutoff PI value of 2.0 to exclude endometrial cancer. et al. KURJAK and co-workers found increased endometrial vascularity in virtually all cases of endometrial cancer. By contrast, all cases of atrophic endometrium and 92% of hyperplastic endometria

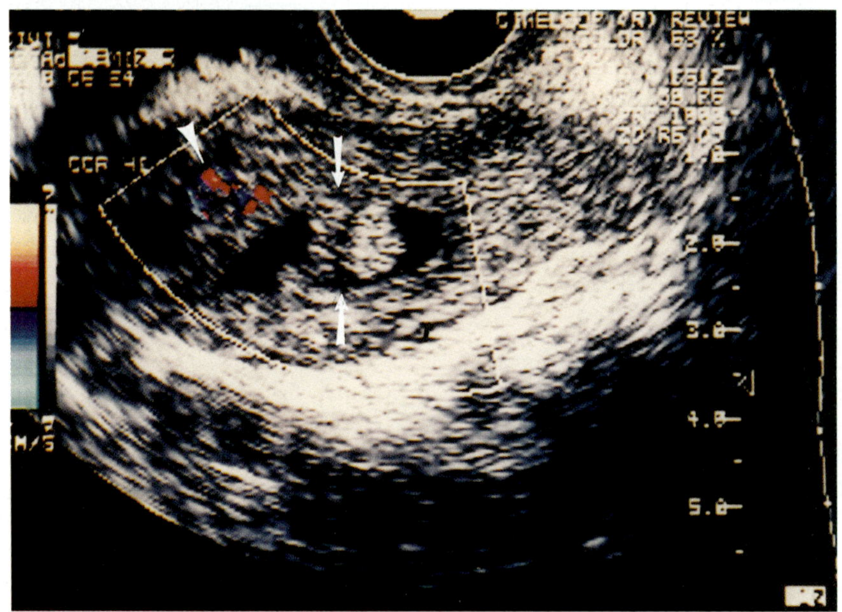

**Fig. 4.4. a** Coronal CDEVS of the uterus from a 74-year-old woman with endometrial cancer demonstrated on previous endometrial biopsy shows an irregular thickened endometrium (*arrows*) with several polypoid masses and a fluid component. A cluster of vessels is demonstrated at the edge of the lesion (*arrowhead*). **b** The Doppler spectrum shows low resistance, high diastolic flow with a PI of 0.44 and an RI of 0.34. **c** Photomicrograph demonstrates several thin-walled vessels (*v*) at the periphery of the tumor. H&E; original magnification ×40. (From SHETH et al. 1995a)

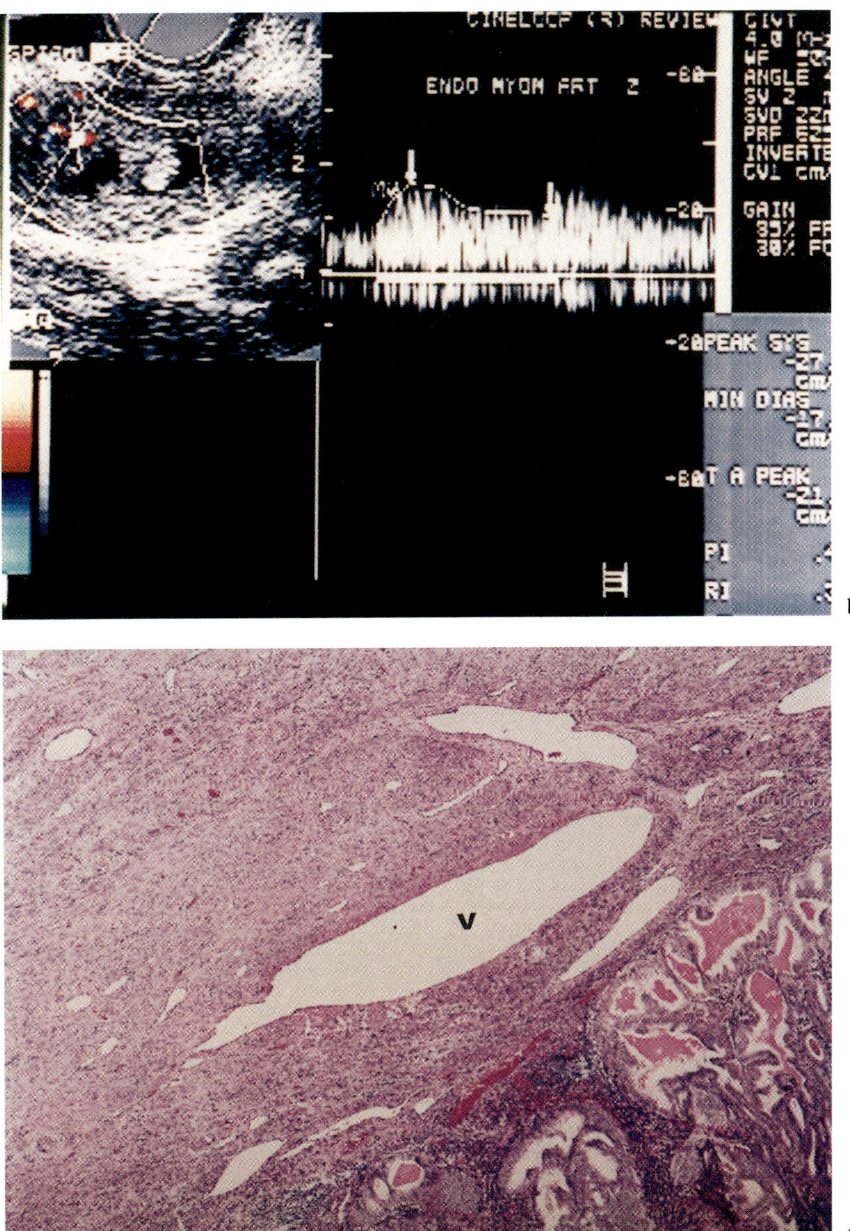


**Fig. 4.4.** *Continued*

were avascular. They concluded that an endometrial RI of 0.40 should be considered as a cutoff value in differentiating benign from malignant lesions of the endometrium (KURJAK and ZALUD 1991; KURJAK et al. 1993b). Similar results were reported by CARTER et al. (1993) and HATA and colleagues (1992b). ALEEM and co-workers (1995) were hopeful that CDEVS would allow improve differentiation between benign and malignant endometrial disease and help reduce the number of dilatation and curettage procedures performed in postmenopausal women.

Other investigators have not shared this optimism, however. FLAM et al. (1995) compared uterine artery PI in 27 women with endometrial cancer and in a control group and found no significant difference in PI values. We evaluated endometrial vascularity in 45 postmenopausal women with a thick endometrium (≥8 mm double layer) and observed increased endometrial vascularity and low impedance arterial

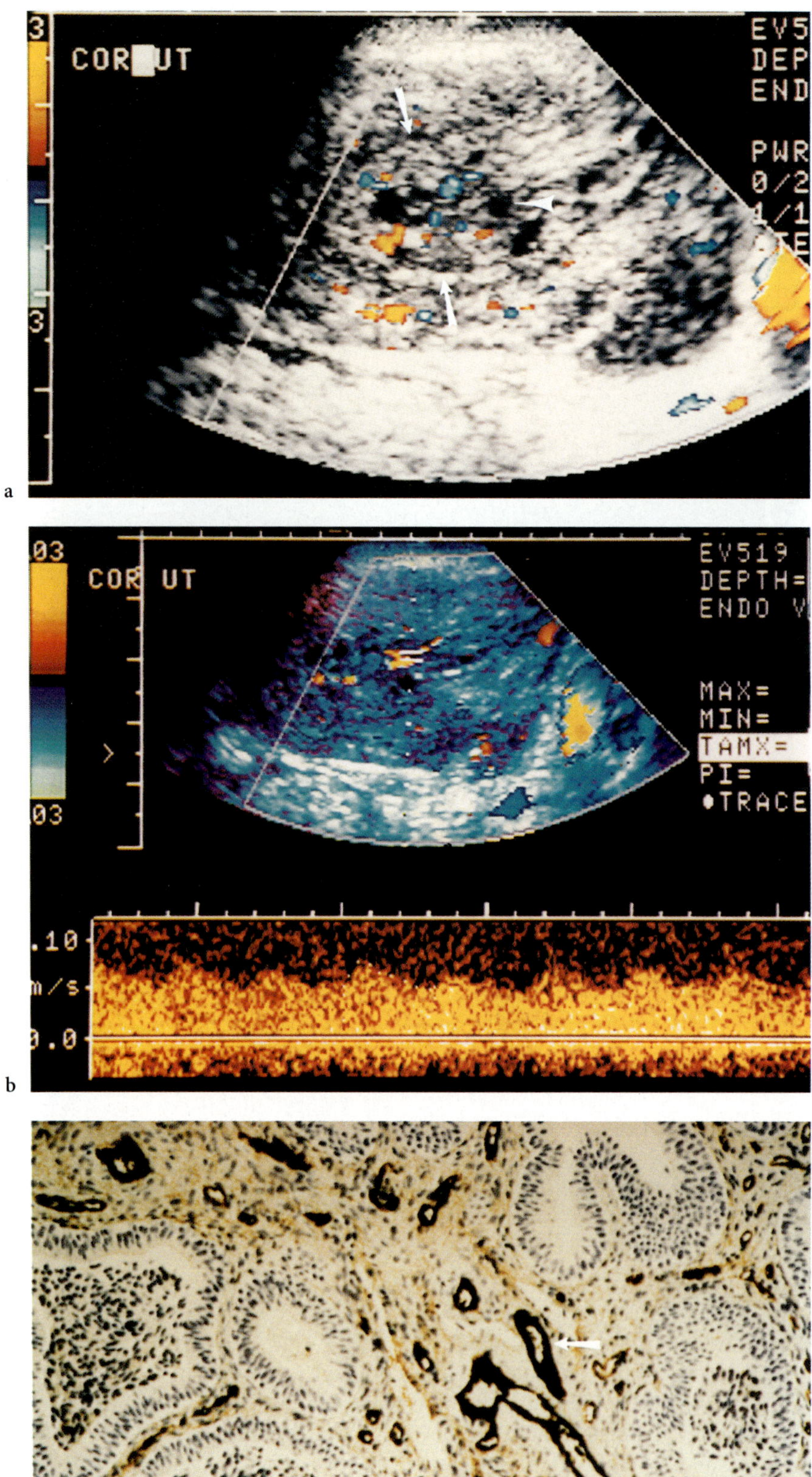
a
COR UT
b
COR UT
EV519
DEPTH=
MAX=
MIN=
TAMX=
PI=
TRACE
.10
m/s
c

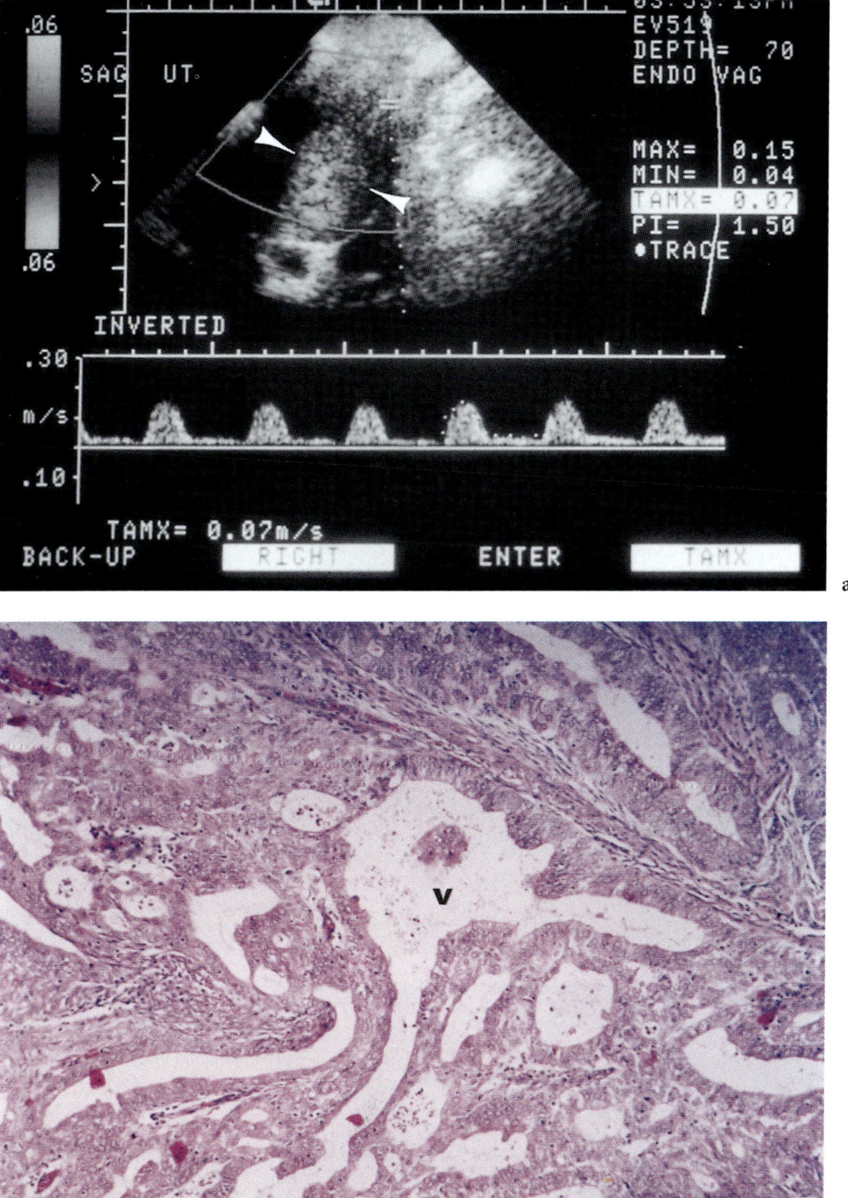


**Fig. 4.6.** **a** Sagittal CDEVS of the uterus from a 65-year-old woman with vaginal bleeding shows a thick echogenic endometrium (*arrowheads*). No vascularity is seen within the lesion. Doppler spectrum from the right uterine artery shows little diastolic flow. Endometrial carcinoma was found at histology. **b** Photomicrograph shows many thin-walled vessels within the tumor (*v*). Several vessels contain tumor thrombus. H&E; original magnification ×40. (From Sheth et al. 1995a)

**Fig. 4.5.** **a** Coronal CDEVS of the uterus from a 83-year-old woman with vaginal spotting shows a thickened endometrium (*arrows*) with several small cystic areas within it (*arrowhead*). Several vessels are seen within the lesion. Endometrial curettage revealed a benign endometrial polyp. **b** The Doppler spectrum shows low resistance, high diastolic flow with a PI of 0.44 and an RI of 0.38. **c** Photomicrograph of curettage specimens stained with factor VIII demonstrates the presence of numerous thin-walled vessels (*arrows*) interspersed with the dilated endometrial glands (*G*). Factor VIII stain; original magnification ×40. (From Sheth et al. 1995a).

flow in benign as well as malignant causes of endometrial thickening (SHETH et al. 1995a,b). There was an overlap in the PI and RI values of endometrial arteries across a spectrum of endometrial disease including endometrial cancer (Fig. 4.4), benign endometrial polyps (Fig. 4.5), hyperplasia, chronic endometritis, and submucous myoma. Assessment of lesion vascularity in histologic specimens correlated with color Doppler US results. All endometrial cancers with increase vascularity at CDEVS had characteristic thin-walled vessels in the center or periphery of the tumor (Fig. 4.4). However, thin-walled vessels were also found in several benign endometrial polyps, accounting for decreased impedance to flow in these lesions (Fig. 4.5). On the other hand, the lack of endometrial vascularity should not lead to a false sense of security. In our series, some endometrial cancers were avascular at CDEVS. At histology, this

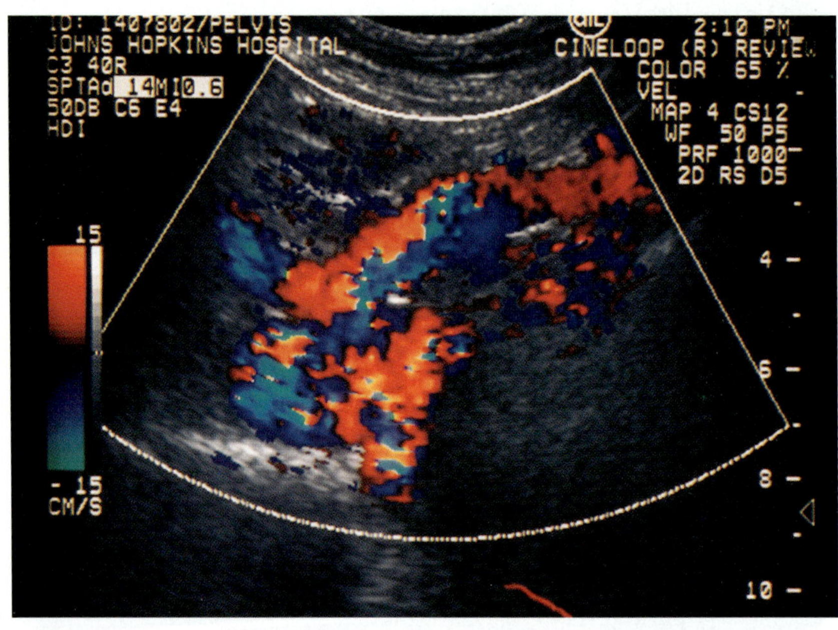

a

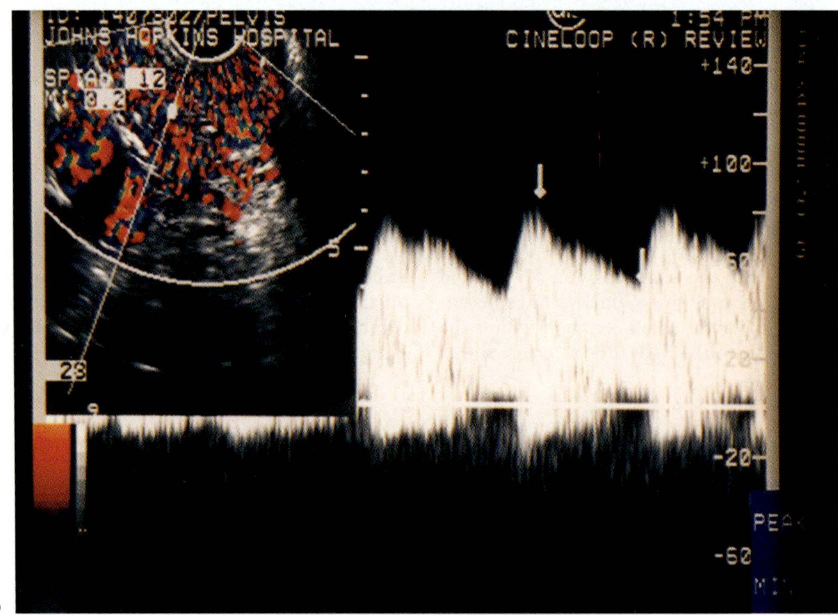

b

**Fig. 4.7.** **a** Transabdominal color Doppler image of the pelvis demonstrates a large vascular structure near the iliac vessels. **b** Endovaginal image shows a complex cystic mass with a speckled color display of a "bruit" with a low-impedance arterial waveform characteristic of arteriovenous shunting

lack of vascularity correlated with the presence of tumor thrombi and lymphovascular invasion (Fig. 4.6). Similar observations were noted by CARTER and colleagues (1993).

Postmenopausal women with a history of breast cancer on long-term tamoxifen adjuvant therapy are considered at risk for endometrial cancer. Although it was initially reported that CDEVS might be helpful in this group of patients (KEDAR et al. 1994), it appears that this technique is not effective in the assessment of endometrial pathology related to tamoxifen. TEPPER and colleagues (1994) were unable to demonstrate uterine artery PI changes associated with tamoxifen intake. ACHIRON and his group (1995) found that tamoxifen produces alteration of endometrial blood flow and appearance that can mimic endometrial cancer in patients with a histologically benign endometrium.

In summary, EVS is quite sensitive in depicting endometrial abnormalities, but lacks specificity as there is an overlap in the sonographic appearance of benign and malignant lesions of the endometrium. Initial results using CDEVS in the evaluation of postmenopausal endometrium have also been disappointing (SHETH et al. 1995a,b) and we would agree with BOURNE's comment that at this point there are not enough data to recommend evaluation or screening for endometrial cancer with CDEVS (BOURNE 1995). Perhaps an area worthwhile investigating is whether CDEVS might be of value in assessing the depth of myometrial invasion by demonstrating increased vascularity in the myometrium in patients with known endometrial cancer.

## 4.4 Miscellaneous Applications

Color Doppler US plays a significant role in confirming or suggesting the benign nature of an adnexal or uterine mass. Hemorrhagic cysts, abnormal fallopian tubes, ovarian torsion, vascular malformations, and pedunculated masses are benign processes which can be diagnosed with Doppler US. It can also be helpful in the diagnosis of recurrent trophoblastic disease.

Hemorrhagic corpus luteum cyst is a common complication of ovulation. In the appropriate clinical setting, the diagnosis is easily made. However, the echoes within a hemorrhagic cyst may be nearly isoechoic with the adjacent ovarian tissue such that it can simulate a solid mass. Color Doppler US can help confirm the diagnosis by demonstrating the absence of flow in the center of these lesions (GRANT 1992; REYNOLDS et al. 1986; BALTAROWICH et al. 1987).

Fallopian tube abnormalities should be considered in the differential diagnosis of a complex cystic adnexal mass. Pyosalpinx can present as a complex

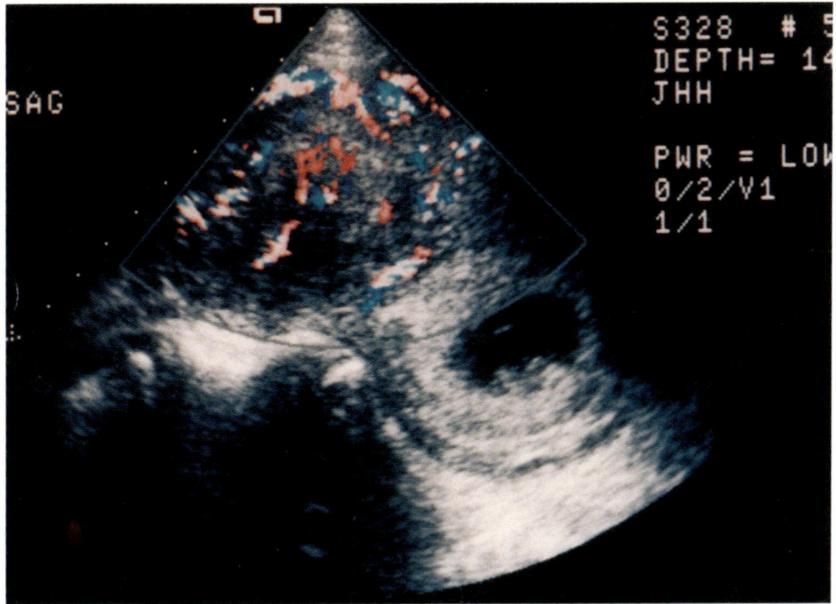


**Fig. 4.8.** A fundal uterine leiomyoma in a patient with an early uterine pregnancy is demonstrated to be highly vascular with color flow imaging

cystic mass with septations and/or debris. The diagnosis is usually aided by the clinical history of pain, fever, and vaginal discharge. Low-impedance flow patterns have been described in pyosalpinges and tubo-ovarian abscesses, reflecting their inflammatory nature (Tinkaneu and Kujansuu 1993).

Ovarian torsion can simulate a solid adnexal mass. In addition, ovarian torsion can be precipitated by a mass such as an ovarian dermoid (Warner et al. 1985). Although the absence of color or pulsed Doppler flow is useful in detecting this abnormality, the presence of arterial flow has been reported in surgically proven ovarian torsion (Rosado et al. 1992).

Pelvic varicosities are a common entity which may be a cause of chronic pelvic pain. Easily identified by their serpentine appearance, pelvic varices are rarely mistaken for a neoplasm. However, in the problematic case, the use of color Doppler US can be useful in confirming their venous origins.

Arteriovenous malformations of the uterine and pelvic vessels are uncommon lesions (Eberhardt et al. 1988; Abu Musa et al. 1989; Jain et al. 1991). Pelvic arteriovenous malformations can present as a complex predominately cystic adnexal mass on endovaginal imaging. Color and pulsed Doppler US can demonstrate the vascular origin of these lesions with color flow evidence of increased vascularity, a

a 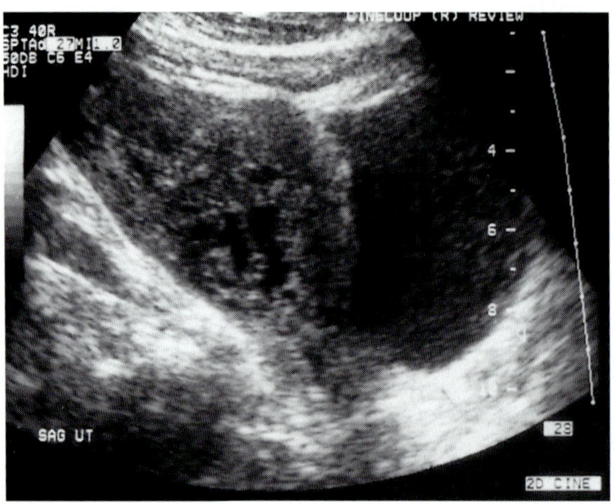


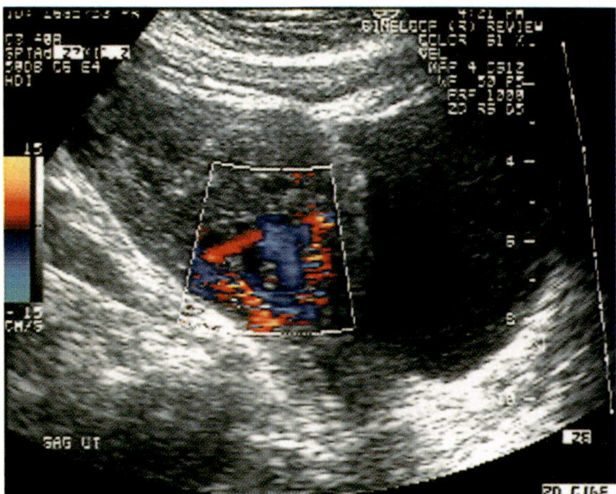 b


**Fig. 4.9.** **a** Gray-scale and **b** color Doppler images of a recurrent mole with myometrial invasion

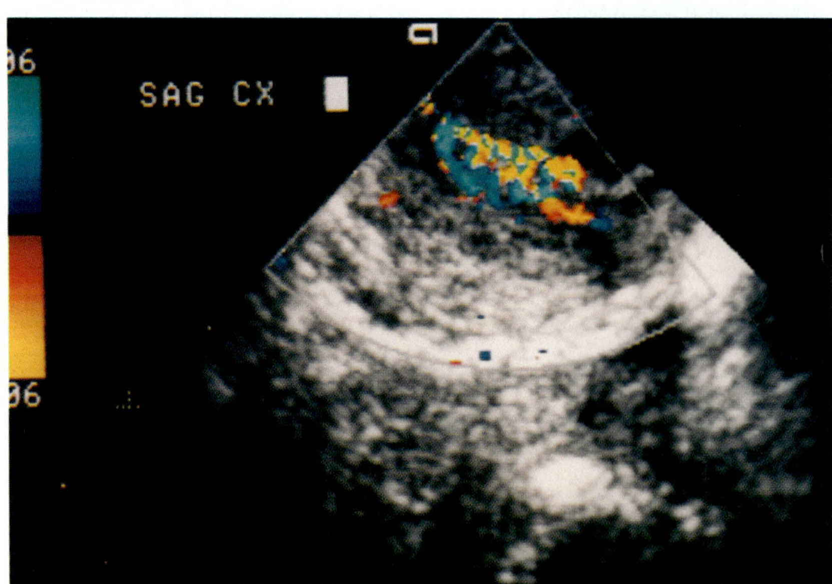


**Fig. 4.10.** Pedunculated polyp prolapsing in the cervix demonstrating increased flow with color Doppler imaging

speckled color pattern of turbulence, and a low-impedance waveform of arteriovenous shunting (Fig. 4.7).

Pedunculated uterine leiomyomas can also simulate an adnexal mass (FLEISCHER et al. 1992). Uterine leiomyomas are common benign neoplasms which can present as a cystic, solid, or complex uterine or adnexal mass. Color Doppler US can be useful in demonstrating the origin of these masses by demonstrating the vascular stalk of subserosal lesions. A low-impedance flow pattern has been demonstrated in very vascular uterine fibroids (Fig. 4.8).

Color and pulsed Doppler US may be useful in the evaluation of recurrent gestational trophoblastic disease and choriocarcinoma. Markedly increased flow in the intramyometrial vessels has been described (Fig. 4.9).

Pedunculated uterine polyps or submucosal fibroids may protrude to the cervix to simulate a mass. Transvaginal color flow imaging can be useful in demonstrating the increased vascularity of these lesions as well as the associated vascular pedicle (Fig. 4.10).

## References

Abu Musa A, Hata T, Hata K, Kitao M (1989) Pelvic arteriovenous malformation diagnosed by color flow Doppler imaging. AJR 152:1311–1312

Achiron R, Lipitz S, Sivan E, Goldenberg M, Horovitz A, Frenkel Y, Mashiach S (1995) Changes mimicking endometrial neoplasia in postmenopausal, tamoxifen-treated women with breast cancer: a transvaginal Doppler study. Ultrasound Obstet Gynecol 6:116–120

Aleem F, Predanic M, Calame R, Moukhtar M, Pennisi J (1995) Transvaginal color and pulsed Doppler sonography of the endometrium: a possible role in reducing the number of dilatation and curettage procedures. J Ultrasound Med 14:139–145

Andolf E, Svalenius E, Astedt B (1986) Ultrasonography for early detection of ovarian carcinoma. Br J Obstet Gynaecol 93:1286–1289

Andolf E, Jorgensen C, Svalenius E, Sunden B (1987) Ultrasound measurement of the ovarian volume. Acta Obstet Gynecol Scand 66:387–389

Averette HE, Donato DM (1990) Ovarian carcinoma. Advances in diagnosis, staging, and treatment. Cancer 65:703–708

Baltarowich OH, Kurtz AB, Pasto ME, Rifkin MD, Needleman L, Goldberg BB (1987) The spectrum of sonographic findings in hemorrhagic ovarian cysts. AJR 148:901–905

Bourne TH (1995) Evaluating the endometrium of postmenopausal women with transvaginal ultrasonography. Ultrasound Obstet Gynecol 6:75–80

Bourne T, Campbell S, Steer C, Whitehead MI, Collins WP (1989) Transvaginal color flow imaging: A possible new screening technique for ovarian cancer. BMJ 299:1367–1370

Bourne TH, Campbell S, Whitehead MI, Royston P, Steer CV, Collins WP (1990) Detection of endometrial cancer in postmenopausal women by transvaginal ultrasonography and colour flow imaging. BMJ 301:369

Bourne TH, Jurkovic D, Waterstone J, Campbell S, Collins WP (1991a) Intrafollicular blood flow during human ovulation. Ultrasound Obstet Gynecol 1:53–59

Bourne TH, Campbell S, Steer CV, Royston P, Whitehead MI, Collins WP (1991b) Detection of endometrial cancer by transvaginal ultrasonography with color flow imaging and blood flow analysis: a preliminary report. Gynecol Oncol 40:253–259

Bourne TH, Reynolds K, Campbell S (1991c) Ovarian cancer screening. Eur J Cancer 27:655–659

Brown DL, Frates MC, Laing FC, et al. (1994) Ovarian masses: can benign and malignant lesions be differentiated with color and pulsed Doppler US? Radiology 190:333–336

Campbell S, Goessens L, Goswamy R, Whitehead M (1982) Real-time ultrasonography for determination of ovarian morphology and volume. A possible early screening test for ovarian cancer? Lancet I:425–426

Campbell S, Bhan V, Royston P, Whitehead MI, Collins WP (1989) Transabdominal ultrasound screening for early ovarian cancer. Br Med J 299:1363–1389

Cancer facts and figures (1998) American Cancer Society, pp 11–13

Carter JR, Fowler JM, Carlson JW, Carson LF, Adcock LL, Twiggs LB (1993) Prediction of malignancy using transvaginal color flow Doppler in patients with gynecologic tumors. Int J Gynecol Cancer 3:279–284

Coleman BG, Arger PH, Langer JE, et al. (1994) Power color Doppler US versus conventional color Doppler US of the ovary. Radiology 193(P):145

De Ziegler D, Bessis R, Frydman R (1991) Vascular resistance of uterine arteries: physiological effects of estradiol and progesterone. Fertil Steril 55:775–779

Eberhardt H, Cyr DR, Easterling TR, Nyberg DA, Mack LA (1988) Diagnosis of a uterine arteriovenous malformation by duplex sonography. J Diagn Med Sonogr 4:130–132

Einhorn N, Sjovall K, Knapp RC, Hall P, Scully RE, Bast RC Jr, Zurawski VR Jr (1992) Prospective evaluation of serum CA 125 levels for early detection of ovarian cancer. Obstet Gynecol 80:14–18

Flam F, Almstrom H, Hellstrom AC, Moberger B (1995) Value of uterine artery Doppler in endometrial cancer. Acta Oncol 34:779–782

Fleischer AC, Kepple DM (1992) Benign conditions of the uterus, cervix, and endometrium. In: Nyberg DA, Hill LM, Bohm-Velez, Mendelson EB (eds) Transvaginal ultrasound. Mosby-Year Book, St. Louis, pp 21–41

Fleischer AC, Rodgers WH, Rao BK, Kepple DM, Worrell JA, Williams L, Jones HW 3d (1991a) Assessment of ovarian tumor vascularity with transvaginal color Doppler sonography. J Ultrasound Med 10:563–568

Fleischer AC, Rogers WH, Rao BK, Kepple DM, Jones HW (1991b) Transvaginal color Doppler sonography of ovarian masses with pathological correlation. Ultrasound Obstet Gynecol 1:279–283

Fleischer AC, Rodgers WH, Kepple DM, Williams LL, Jones HW 3d, Gross PR (1992) Color Doppler sonography of benign and malignant ovarian masses. Radiographics 12:879–885

Fleischer AC, Rodgers WH, Kepple DM, Williams LL, Jones HW 3d (1993) Color Doppler sonography of ovarian masses: a multiparameter analysis. J Ultrasound Med 12:41–48

Folkman J, Watson, K, Ingber D, Hanahan D (1989) Induction of angiogenesis during the transition from hyperplasia to neoplasia. Nature 339:58–61

Goldstein SR, Nachtigall M, Snyder JR, Nachtigall L (1990) Endometrial assessment by vaginal ultrasonography before endometrial sampling in patients with postmenopausal bleeding. Am J Obstet Gynecol 163:119–123

Goswamy RK, Campbell S, Royston JP, et al. (1988) Ovarian size in postmenopausal women. Brit J Obstet Gynaecol 95:795–801

Grant EG (1992) Benign conditions of the ovaries. In: Nyberg DA, Hill LM, Bohm-Velez M, Mendelson EB (eds) Transvaginal ultrasound. Mosby-Year Book, St. Louis, pp 187–208

Hamper UM, Sheth S, Abbas FM, Rosenshein NB, Aronson D, Kurman RJ (1993) Transvaginal color Doppler sonography of adnexal masses: differences in blood flow impedance in benign and malignant lesions. AJR 160:1225–1228

Hata K, Hata T, Manabe A, Sugimura K, Kitao M (1992a) A critical evaluation of transvaginal Doppler studies, transvaginal sonography, magnetic resonance imaging, and CA 125 in detecting ovarian cancer. Obstet Gynecol 80:922–926

Hata K, Hata T, Manabe A, Makihara K, Kitao M (1992b) New pelvic sonoangiography for detection of endometrial carcinoma: a preliminary report. Gynecol Oncol 45:179–184

Hata T, Hata K, Senoh D, Makihara K, Aoki S, Takamiya O, Kitao M (1989) Doppler ultrasound assessment of tumor vascularity in gynecologic disorders. J Ultrasound Med 8:309–314

Hulka CA, Hall DA, McCarthy K, Simeone JF (1994) Endometrial polyps, hyperplasia, and carcinoma in postmenopausal women: differentiation with endovaginal sonography. Radiology 191:755–758

Jain KA (1994) Prospective evaluation of adnexal masses with endovaginal gray-scale and duplex and color Doppler US: correlation with pathologic findings Radiology 191:63–67

Jain KA, Jeffrey RB Jr (1994) Evaluation of pelvic masses with magnetic resonance imaging and ultrasonography. J Ultrasound Med 13:845–853

Jain KA, Jeffrey RB Jr, Sommer FG (1991) Gynecologic vascular abnormalities: diagnosis with Doppler US. Radiology 178:549–551

Kawai M, Kano T, Kikkawa F, Maeda O, Oguchi H, Tomoda Y (1992) Transvaginal Doppler ultrasound with color flow imaging in the diagnosis of ovarian cancer. Obstet Gynecol 79:163–167

Kedar RP, Bourne TH, Powles TJ, Collins WP, Ashley SE, Cosgrove DO, Campbell S (1994) Effects of tamoxifen on uterus and ovaries of postmenopausal women in a randomised breast cancer prevention trial. Lancet 343:1318–1321

Kurjak A, Zalud I (1991) The characterization of uterine tumors by transvaginal color Doppler. Ultrasound Obstet Gynecol 1:50–52

Kurjak A, Zalud I (1992) Doppler and color flow imaging. In: Nyberg DA, Hill LM, Bohm-Velez M, Mendelson EB (eds) Transvaginal ultrasound. Mosby-Year Book, St. Louis, pp 28–38

Kurjak A, Zalud I, Alfirevic Z (1991) Evaluation of adnexal masses with transvaginal color Doppler ultrasound. J Ultrasound Med 10:295–297

Kurjak A, Predanic M, Kupesic-Urek S, Jukic S (1993a) Transvaginal color and pulsed Doppler assessment of adnexal tumor vascularity. Gynecol Oncol 50:3–9

Kurjak A, Shalan H, Sosic A, Benic S, Zudenigo D, Kupesic S, Predanic M (1993b) Endometrial carcinoma in postmenopausal women: evaluation by transvaginal color Doppler ultrasonography. Am J Obstet Gynecol 169:1597–1603

Kurjak A, Shalan H, Kupesic S, et al. (1994) An attempt to screen asymptomatic women for ovarian and endometrial cancer with transvaginal color and pulsed Doppler sonography. J Ultrasound Med 13:295–301

Levine D, Gosink BB (1992) The postmenopausal pelvis. In: Nyberg DA, Hill LM, Bohm-Velez M, Mendelson EB (eds) Transvaginal ultrasound. Mosby-Year Book, St. Louis, pp 223–231

Mann WJ, Patsner B, Cohen H, Loesch M (1988) Preoperative serum CA-125 levels in patients with surgical stage I invasive ovarian adenocarcinoma. J Natl Cancer Inst 80:208–209

Mendelson EB, Bohm-Velez M, Joseph N, Neiman HL (1988) Endometrial abnormalities: evaluation with transvaginal sonography. AJR 150:139–142

Mogavero G, Sheth S, Hamper UM (1993) Endovaginal sonography of the nongravid uterus. RadioGraphics 13:969–981

Nasri MN, Coast GJ (1989) Correlation of ultrasound findings and endometrial histopathology in postmenopausal women. Br J Obstet Gynaecol 96:1333–1338

Nasri MN, Shepherd JH, Setchell ME, Lowe DG, Chard T (1991) Sonographic depiction of postmenopausal endometrium with transabdominal and transvaginal scanning. Ultrasound Obstet Gynecol 1:279–283

Patsner B (1991) How serum Ca-125 serves as tumor marker? Cont Ob/Gyn, pp 37–52

Reynolds T, Hill MC, Glassman LM (1986) Sonography of hemorrhagic ovarian cysts. J Clin Ultrasound 14:449–453

Rosado WM Jr, Trambert MA, Gosink BB, Pretorius DH (1992) Adnexal torsion: diagnosis by using Doppler sonography. AJR 159:1251–1253

Ross LD (1988) Pelvic ultrasound – should it be used routinely in the diagnosis and screening of postmenopausal bleeding? Discussion paper. J R Soc Med 81:723–724

Sassone AM, Timor-Tritsch IE, Artner A, Westhoff C, Warren WB (1991) Transvaginal sonographic characterization of ovarian disease: evaluation of a new scoring system to predict ovarian malignancy. Obstet Gynecol 78:70–76

Sheth S, Hamper UM, Kurman RJ (1993) Thickened endometrium in the postmenopausal woman: sonographic-pathologic correlation. Radiology 187:135–139

Sheth S, Hamper UM, McCollum ME, Caskey CI, Rosenshein NB, Kurman RJ (1995a) Endometrial blood flow analysis in postmenopausal women. Can it differentiate benign versus malignant causes of endometrial thickening? Radiology 195:661–665

Sheth S, Hamper UM, Caskey CI, Rosenshein NB (1995b) Sonographic appearance of the endometrium in women on tamoxifen therapy. Radiology 197(P):229

Sparks JM, Varner RE (1991) Ovarian cancer screening. Obstet Gynecol 77:787–792

Steer CV, Campbell S, Pampiglione JS, Kingsland CR, Mason BA, Collins WP (1990) Transvaginal colour flow imaging of the uterine arteries during the ovarian and menstrual cycles. Hum Reprod 5:391–395

Stein SM, Laifer-Narin S, Johnson MB, Roman LD, Muderspach LI, Tyszka JM, Ralls PW (1995) Differentiation of benign and malignant masses: relative value of gray scale color Doppler, and spectral Doppler sonography. AJR 164:381–386

Taylor KJ, Burns PN, Wells PN, Conway DI, Hull MG (1985) Ultrasound Doppler flow studies of the ovarian and uterine arteries. Br J Obstet Gynaecol 92:240–246

Taylor KJ, Ramos I, Carter D, Morse SS, Snower D, Fortune K (1988) Correlation of Doppler US tumor signals with neovascular morphologic features. Radiology 166(1 Pt 1):57–62

Tepper R, Cohen I, Altaras M, Shapira J, Cordoba M, Dror Y, Beyth Y (1994) Doppler flow evaluation of pathologic endometrial conditions in postmenopausal breast cancer patients treated with tamoxifen. J Ultrasound Med 13:635–640

Timor-Tritsch LE, Lerner JP, Monteagudo A, Santos R (1993) Transvaginal ultrasonographic characterization of ovarian masses by means of color flow-directed Doppler measurements and a morphologic scoring system. Am J Obstet Gynecol 168:909–913

Tinkanen H, Kujansuu E (1993) Doppler ultrasound findings in tubo-ovarian infectious complex. J Clin Ultrasound 21:175–179

Warner MA, Fleischer AC, Edell SL, Thieme GA, Bundy AL, Kurtz AB, James AE Jr (1985) Uterine adnexal torsion; sonographic findings. Radiology 154:773–775

Weiner Z, Thaler I, Beck D, Rottem S, Deutsch M, Brandes JM (1992) Differentiating malignant from benign ovarian tumors with transvaginal color flow imaging. Obstet Gynecol 79:159–162

Wolf SI, Gosink BB, Feldesman MR, Lin MC, Stuenkel CA, Braly PS, Pretorius DH (1991) Prevalence of simple adnexal cysts in postmenopausal women. Radiology 180:65–71

Zalud I, Conway C, Schulman H, Trinca D (1993) Endometrial and myometrial thickness and uterine blood flow in postmenopausal women: the influence of hormonal replacement therapy and age. J Ultrasound Med 12:737–741

# 5 Magnetic Resonance Imaging of Cervical Cancer

Y. YAMASHITA and M. TAKAHASHI

CONTENTS



## 5.1 Introduction

Accurate staging of cervical carcinoma is essential to the selection of the best form of treatment. In fact, a high percentage of patients with advanced local carcinoma (FIGO stage Ib through IVa) may be cured by optimal surgery or radiation therapy. An accuracy of 50%–75% has been reported with regard to the correlation of clinical FIGO stage with histopathologic results (NAGELL et al. 1971). Although the diagnosis of cervical carcinoma needs to be established histologically, magnetic resonance (MR) imaging has an important role in the preoperative staging of disease, as shown by a number of studies. High-field MR imaging has been shown to be particularly useful in its evaluation (TOGASHI et al. 1986, 1989; RUBENS et al. 1988; HRICAK et al. 1988) because it has an inherently higher signal-to-noise ratio and can have higher resolution, especially when the phased array coil is used. However, it has not been demonstrated that high-resolution imaging with a high-field MR unit has significant advantages in tumor detection and staging. A number of studies have demonstrated MR imaging to be an excellent means of depicting either stromal and parametrial or vaginal invasion (TOGASHI et al. 1986, 1989; HRICAK et al. 1988; SIRONI et al. 1992; KIM et al. 1990).


Y. YAMASHITA, MD, Associate Professor, Department of Radiology, Kumamoto University School of Medicine, 1-1-1 Honjo, Kumamoto, 860, Japan
M. TAKAHASHI, MD, Professor and Chairman Department of Radiology, Kumamoto University School of Medicine, 1-1-1 Honjo, Kumamoto, 860, Japan


## 5.2 Anatomic Considerations

To understand the extension of cervical carcinoma, knowledge of the anatomy of the uterine cervix is of the utmost importance. The cervix is the lowest portion of the uterus, and protrudes into the vagina surrounded by the vaginal fornices (Fig. 5.1). The internal os is the beginning of the cervix; this is demarcated by a histologic change from glandular to columnar epithelium. Cervical carcinoma develops almost exclusively within the transition zone between the internal os and the squamocolumnar junction (FERENCZY and WINKLER 1987).

The vaginal fornices divide the cervix into the supravaginal cervix and the vaginal portion. The vaginal portion is also called the cervical lips and protrudes into the vagina, being separated from the parametrium by the vaginal fornix. The supravaginal cervix above the vaginal fornix is directly adjacent to the parametrium, contiguous with the cardinal ligament. Supravaginal lesions, which are commonly involved by cancer in older women, tend to be located directly adjacent to the parametrium (Fig. 5.2). On the other hand, lesions developing on the cervical lips (usually in young women) tend to be separated from the parametrium by the vaginal fornix.

## 5.3 Imaging Techniques

Magnetic resonance imaging is used to visualize cervical masses as well as associated myometrial or vaginal abnormalities, enlarged lymph nodes, or

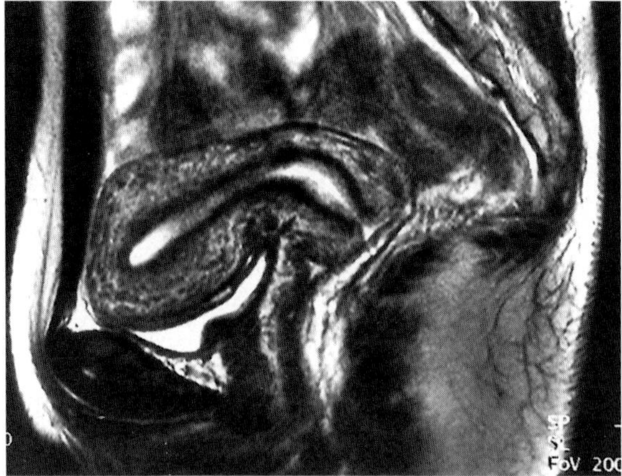

Fig. 5.1. Sagittal T2-weighted image showing the normal cervix at the inferior aspect of the uterus. The high-signal endocervical canal, which is thickest at its center, is demonstrated between the internal os and the external os. The anterior and posterior vaginal fornices can also be seen

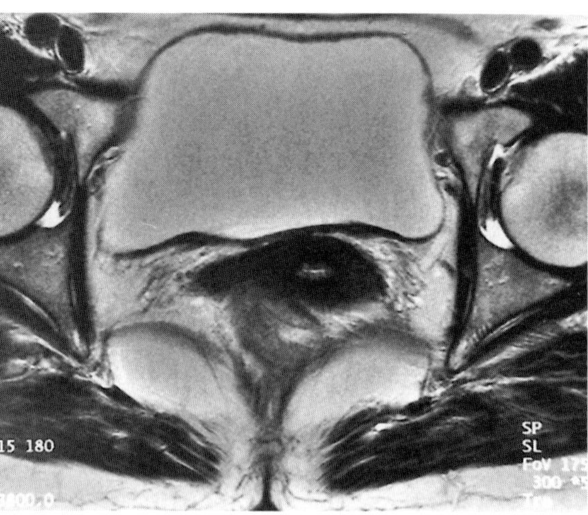

Fig. 5.2. Axial T2-weighted image at the level of the supravaginal cervix, demonstrates the low-signal cervical stroma and the high-signal endocervical canal

direct invasion of other organs. T2-weighted imaging has been reported to be the optimal pulse sequence for the visualization of cervical carcinomas (Togashi et al. 1986; 1989; Rubens et al. 1988; Hricak et al. 1988). Because cervical cancers have long T2 values in comparison with the cervical stroma, the tumor generates a higher signal intensity than normal cervix on this pulse sequence. Sagittal images are considered essential for the depiction of intrauterine abnormalities because they most clearly display the uterine and vaginal anatomy, whereas transverse images are helpful in defining stromal invasion and parametrial or intrapelvic spread of cervical lesions. On T1-weighted images, the lesion will appear as a nodular mass enlarging the normal cervical contour. The signal intensity of the tumor is usually isointense to the cervical stroma. Transverse T1-weighted images may be adequate for the evaluation of lymphadenopathy.

Using a 1.5-T MR unit, a long repetition time (TR) will allow for clear visualization of the normal zonal anatomy of the cervix. The spin-echo (SE) sequence has been used for T2-weighted imaging with a long TR (2500 ms) and long echo time (TE; 80 ms). Fast spin echo (FSE) is an alternative to the SE sequence. The FSE sequence use multiple 180° pulses during T2 decay, to acquire multiple echoes. If there are 15 180° pulses, the scan acquisition can be reduced by a factor of 15. This allows for the matrix and number of signal averages to be increased, thus improving the signal-to-noise ratio and resolution. On FSE images, the contrast between the cervical stroma and tumor is somewhat less than on SE images. Application of the FSE sequence and a phased array coil may produce excellent image quality of the female pelvis (Figs. 5.1, 5.2) (Smith et al. 1992). An extremely high resolution image can be obtained by using an endorectal surface coil; however, staging of disease is sometimes difficult due to the small field of view.

Intravenous contrast medium, most commonly gadopentetate dimeglumine (Gd-DTPA), is often useful in demonstrating endometrial adnormalities (Hricak et al. 1991; Yamashita et al. 1993a). However, the role of contrast-enhanced images in the cervical cancer has not been established. Superficial lesions may be underestimated because of (a) poor contrast between the high signal intensity of the tumor and the cervical epithelium and (b) the presence of surface blood clot. The early phase of dynamic imaging demonstrates significantly better contrast than T2-weighted images (Fig. 5.3) (Yamashita et al. 1992).

The enhancement of normal fibrocervical stroma is gradual and less intense in comparison with myometrium or cervical epithelium (Figs. 5.3, 5.4) (Hricak et al. 1991; Yamashita et al. 1992). On delayed images of patients with cervical cancer, considerable enhancement of the cervical stoma is seen. Cervical congestion, increased vascularity, and edema associated with tumor may be responsible for such enhancement. In contrast to the normal fibrocervical stroma, most cervical carcinomas show prominent enhancement in the early phase of a dy-

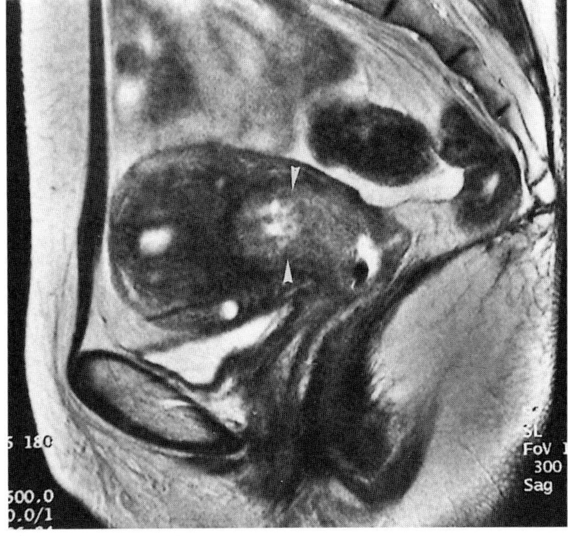


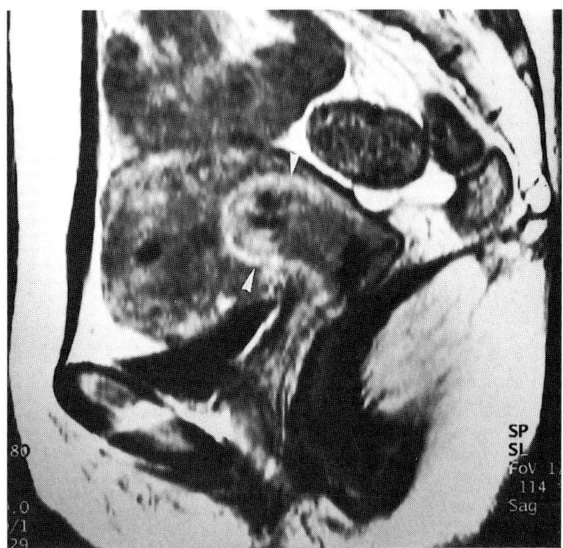


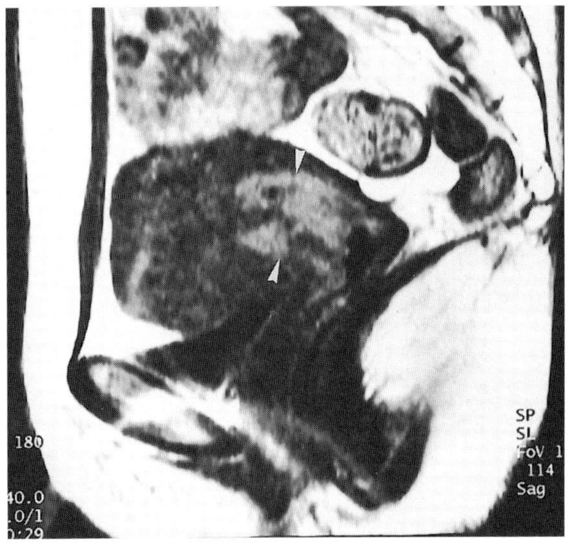


**Fig. 5.3.** **a** A high signal intensity mass (*arrowheads*) located in the uterine cervix is seen on this T2-weighted image. **b** Early stage of the sagittal Gd-DTPA dynamic study shows selective enhancement of the mass. The early phase of dynamic imaging demonstrated significantly better contrast than did T2-weighted images. **c** At the delayed phase, there is inhomogeneous enhancement of the uterine corpus as well as the tumor. The central area of mass is poorly enhanced due to necrosis

namic study (Figs. 5.3, 5.4). In the delayed phase, the contrast between the cervical stroma and the tumor diminishes (Fig. 5.4) (YAMASHITA et al. 1992).

Our current imaging protocol is as follows: Before administration of Gd-DTPA, T1-weighted SE images are obtained with a TR of 580 ms, TE of 14 ms, a 256 × 512 matrix, and one averaging without use of the fat saturation technique. T2-weighted fast SE images are obtained with a TR of 4000–5000 ms, a TE of 120 ms, a 210 × 512 matrix, echo train length of 15, (high resolution, rectangular field of view technique), and two averagings. Images are obtained in the sagittal and axial planes with a section thickness of 5 mm and 0.3% interslice spacing, typically with 21 × 28 cm fields of view.

Gd-DTPA is usually given as a bolus, most commonly in a does of 0.1 mmol/kg. Images are obtained dynamically, using a T1-weighted FSE sequence (TR of 330 ms, TE of 12 ms and echo train length of 3). Greater contrast between the abnormal tissue and normal cervix is obtained in the dynamic study, while greater resolution is obtained in the post-contrast fat-saturated T1-weighted SE images (YAMASHITA et al. 1993b).

## 5.4 Normal MR Appearance of the Cervix

Axial and sagittal images, which take advantage of the usual anatomic relationship of the cervix to surrounding structures, are important for the visualization and staging of cervical carcinomas. On sagittal T2-weighted images, the characteristic zonal

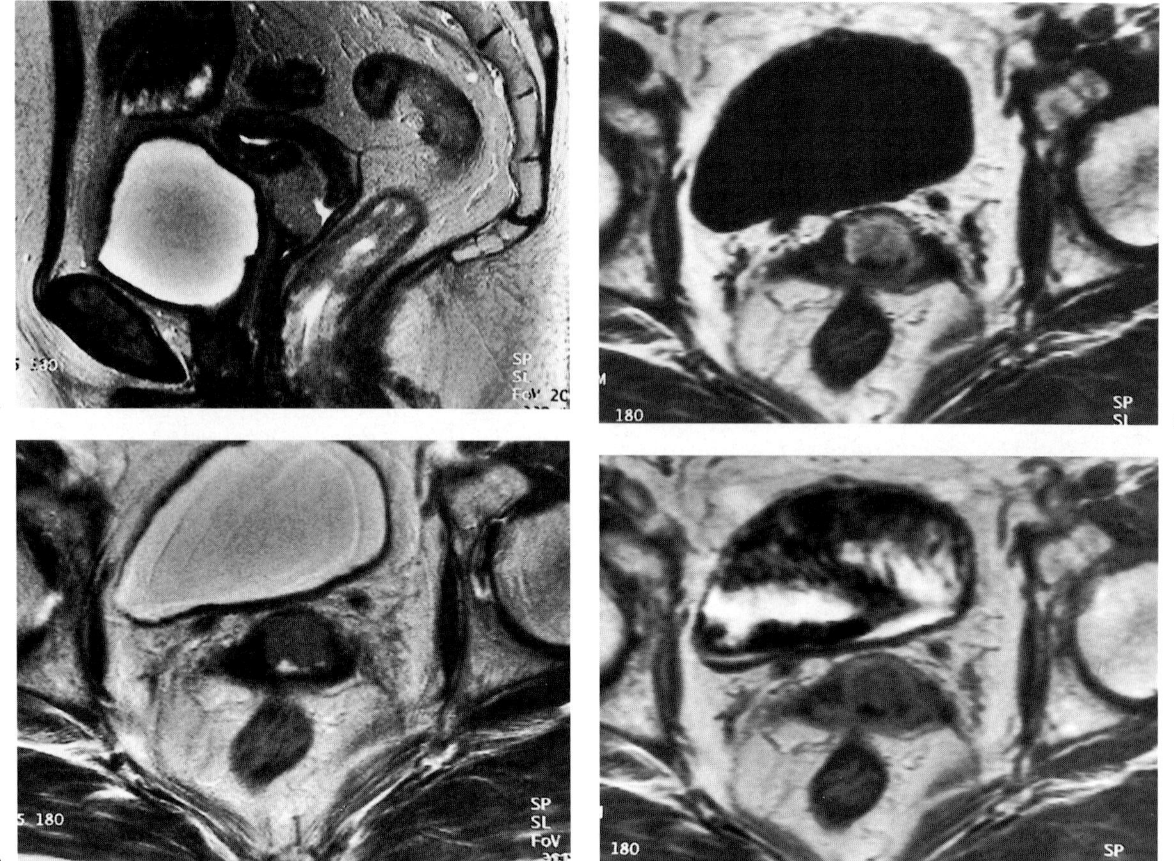

**Fig. 5.4.** **a** Sagittal T2-weighted FSE image demonstrating a moderately high signal intensity mass on the anterior cervical lip which protudes slightly into the vagina and invades the cervical stroma. Note the excellent demonstration of the anterior and posterior vaginal fornices. **b** Axial T2-weighted image at the vaginal cervix level shows the same mass within the anterior aspect of the cervical stroma ring. The intact cervical stroma between the mass and the parametrium indicates an absence of parametrium invasion. **c** Early phase Gd-DTPA dynamic study provides good contrast between the mass and the cervical stroma because of the moderately enhanced mass and the unenhanced normal stroma, further proving the absence of parametrial invasion. **d** Decreased contrast is observed at the delayed phase because of the washout of the contrast medium from the mass and gradual enhancement of the cervical stroma

architecture of the cervix is well defined (Fig. 5.1). The high signal intensity central stripe corresponds to the endocervical gland (mucus and epithelium), and the surrounding low signal intensity stripe contiguous to the junctional zone represents the fibrous stroma (Scoutt et al. 1993). Using recent MR units with the phased array coil system, the fibrous stroma appears to have two layers, an inner one that is of very low signal intensity and an outer intermediate layer (Smith et al. 1992; Hricak et al. 1983; Heiken and Lee 1988). The exact histologic counterparts of these layers are not known. On axial images, the fibrous stroma appears as very low signal intensity ring, surrounded by an outer layer of intermediate signal intensity (Fig. 5.2).

## 5.5 Pathology

Histologically, most cervical carcinomas are squamous cell carcinomas (SCCs). Various factors have been shown to be related to prognosis, and some are important in planning therapy (Ferenczy and Winkler 1987). These factors are as follows: tumor volume, gross tumor configuration, vaginal and endometrial cavity extension, histologic grade of tumor, depth of myometrial invasion, vascular invasion, regional and distant lymph node metastases, and distant metastases. In the diagnosis of cervical cancer with MR imaging, all of these factors should be taken into account; the following are of particular importance:

1. *Tumor volume and gross tumor configuration.* In all stages of cervical carcinoma, tumor volume is an important factor in predicting the spread of disease and in determining the best method of therapy. There are two types of gross tumor configuration: exophytic and endophytic. Bulky exophytic and endophytic lesions, especially those that are barrel shaped, have a poor prognosis.

2. *Depth of tumor invasion.* It has been shown that the depth of stromal invasion is correlated with the involvement of pelvic lymph nodes and pelvic recurrence (THOMPSON 1992). Although the depth of stromal invasion is not analyzed for FIGO staging, correct preoperative evaluation of invasion may be of the utmost importance in optimizing treatment planning. It should be noted that cases with full-thickness stromal invasion have shown a relatively high incidence of microscopic parametrial invasion (TOGASHI et al. 1986).

3. *Vaginal extension.* When vaginal extension of cervical carcinoma occurs, even with no parametrial involvement, the incidence of pelvic lymph node metastases will be higher. In stage IIa lesions, the incidence of lymph node metastases is 42% (THOMPSON 1992).

4. *Uterine corpus and endometrial cavity extension.* Previously, uterine corpus and endometrial cavity extension were considered to have significance as a poor prognostic factor: stage Ib or IIb cervical cancers with uterine corpus and endometrial cavity extension were believed to have a worse prognosis (PEREZ et al. 1981). In recent years, the significance of such extension has gradually been discounted.

5. *Lymph node metastases.* Cervical carcinoma spreads along the lymph node chain, first to the paracervical lymphatic chain, then to the obturator, hypogastric, and external iliac lymph nodes; subsequently para-aortic lymph node metastase occur. Pelvic or para-aortic lymph node metastases have proved to be one of the most reliable prognostic factors for patients with cervical cancer. The frequency of metastases to pelvic lymph nodes is less than 2% for stage Ia, 10%—15% for stage Ib, 20%–25% for stage IIb, greater than 35% for stage III, and greater than 50% for stage IV. Metastatic disease to para-aortic lymph nodes occurs in less than 5% of patients with stage I disease, in 10%–15% with stage II, in 25%–30% with stage III, and in more than 40% with stage IVa (THOMPSON 1992).

## 5.6 MR Appearances of Cervical Carcinoma

Detection and staging of cervical carcinomas by MR imaging requires: (a) delineation of the tumor in relation to the cervical stroma, (b) clear demonstration of the boundaries between the cervix and the parametrium, pelvic wall, bladder, rectum, and vagina, and (c) assessment of pelvic lymph nodes.

### 5.6.1 Tumor Volume and Stromal Invasion

Although tumor volume and stromal invasion are not included in the FIGO staging system, MR imaging can directly visualize these important prognostic factors. On T2-weighted images, cervical carcinoma with stromal invasion is demonstrated as a mass of high or heterogeneous signal intensity that invades the hypointense cervical stroma. Unenhanced T1-weighted images usually offer little additional information for the evaluation of cervical cancer.

Measurements of tumor size by MR imaging correlate well with measurements determined by histopathology (TOGASHI et al. 1989; HRICAK et al. 1988). Linear measurements of greatest tumor diameter have an error margin within 5 mm. Factors that limit the accuracy of tumor measurement include edema surrounding the tumor, cervicitis, postbiopsy changes, and nabothian cysts. Other pathologic conditions such as endometrial polyps and submucosal leiomyomas need to be differentiated. Some metastatic tumors may mimic the MR appearance of cervical carcinoma; we have experienced this with metastatic tumors from melanoma and ovarian cancer (Fig. 5.5).

The distinction between viable tumor and uterine secretion or necrotic tissue is often difficult on T2-weighted images. Contrast-enhanced MR, preferably a dynamic enhanced study, may be able to show tumor margins more accurately because of the higher contrast between tumor and cervical stoma or between tumor and parametrium (YAMASHITA et al. 1992). Dynamic enhanced MR imaging provides better enhancement of the myometrium than do postcontrast T1-weighted images (Figs. 5.3, 5.4).

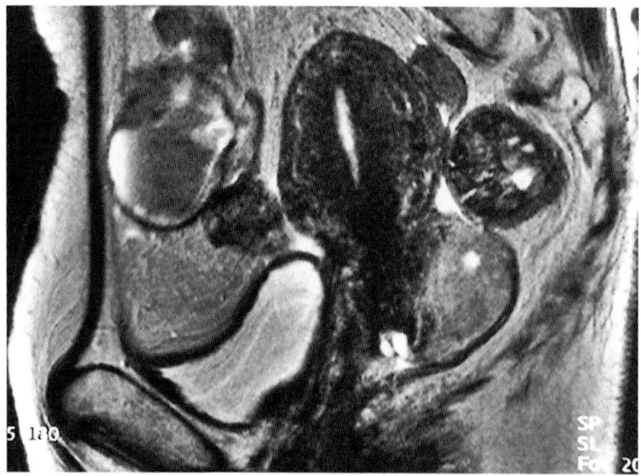

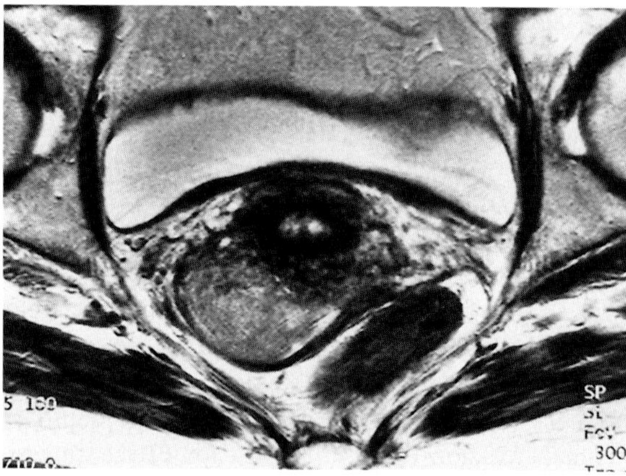

**Fig. 5.5.** **a** Sagittal T2-weighted image displaying a hyperintense metastatic lesion located at the posterior vaginal cuff, causing it to be widened. The superoanterior border between the mass and the posterior cervical lip is ambiguous whereas the posterior border is clear, being limited within the posterior vaginal wall. **b** Axial T2-weighted images shows the same mass located at the left posterior portion of the vaginal cuff. Part of the posterior vaginal wall is blurred, indicating the possibility of vaginal invasion, but there is no sign of parametrial invasion

## 5.6.2 Staging

### *5.6.2.1 Stage I*

In patients with stage Ia cervical cancer or carcinoma in situ, the cervix may appear entirely normal on MR examination, or the endocervical stripe may be widened but have a normal, homogeneous high signal intensity on T2-weighted images (Togashi et al. 1989). Occasionally a mass distends the endocervical cavity without disrupting the cervical stroma. In these cases, differentiation from cervical polyps may be impossible.

In the presence of superficial invasion in stage Ib, tumors may or may not detected. The deep stromal invasion in stage Ib is consistently identified on T2-weighted imaging because the hypointense cervical stroma provides excellent contrast in relation to the hyperintense tumor (Fig. 5.4). The percentage of the myometrial wall invasion correlates with findings on MR imaging (Togashi et al. 1989; Hricak et al. 1988). Cervical stromal invasion can be accurately evaluated on axial images. Lesions may be well marginated, remaining within the configuration of the ring and presenting with well-preserved signal intensity of the hypointense rim, or may be demonstrated as a fully expanded mass but without extension to the parametrium. Both forms can be stage Ib. On fast SE images, because signal contrast between tumor and residual myometrium is sometimes poor, assessment of the depth of invasion is often difficult. Contrast-enhanced MR imaging may be useful because it displays more marked contrast between tumor and residual cervical stroma (Fig. 5.4). An accuracy of 83%–93% has been reported for the evaluation of stromal invasion by means of T2-weighted MR images (Togashi et al. 1989; Hricak et al. 1988). Acquisition of high-resolution images may improve the accuracy.

Although it is difficult to establish a diagnosis of uterine corpus and endometrial cavity extension by clinical examination, and this factor is not included in the FIGO staging system. Sagittal MR imaging clearly shows such extension.

### *5.6.2.2 Stage II*

Stage IIa carcinoma (invasion of the upper two-thirds of the vagina) may be suspected on T2-weighted images when a high signal intensity mass replaces or invades the upper two thirds of the vaginal wall (see Fig. 5.15) (Worthington et al. 1986). False-positive diagnoses may result from large exophytic tumors distending the vaginal fornix. Stage IIb (deep cervical spread to the fibrous cervical stroma) is diagnosed on T2-weighted images when a mass invades and disrupts the low signal intensity of the fibrous cervical stroma (Figs. 5.6, 5.7). The accuracy of stage II detection by MR imaging is reported to be 88%–93% (Togashi et al. 1986, 1989; Hricak et al. 1988; Sironi et al. 1992; Kim et al. 1990).

Lesions with full-thickness stromal invasion have shown a relatively high incidence of microscopic

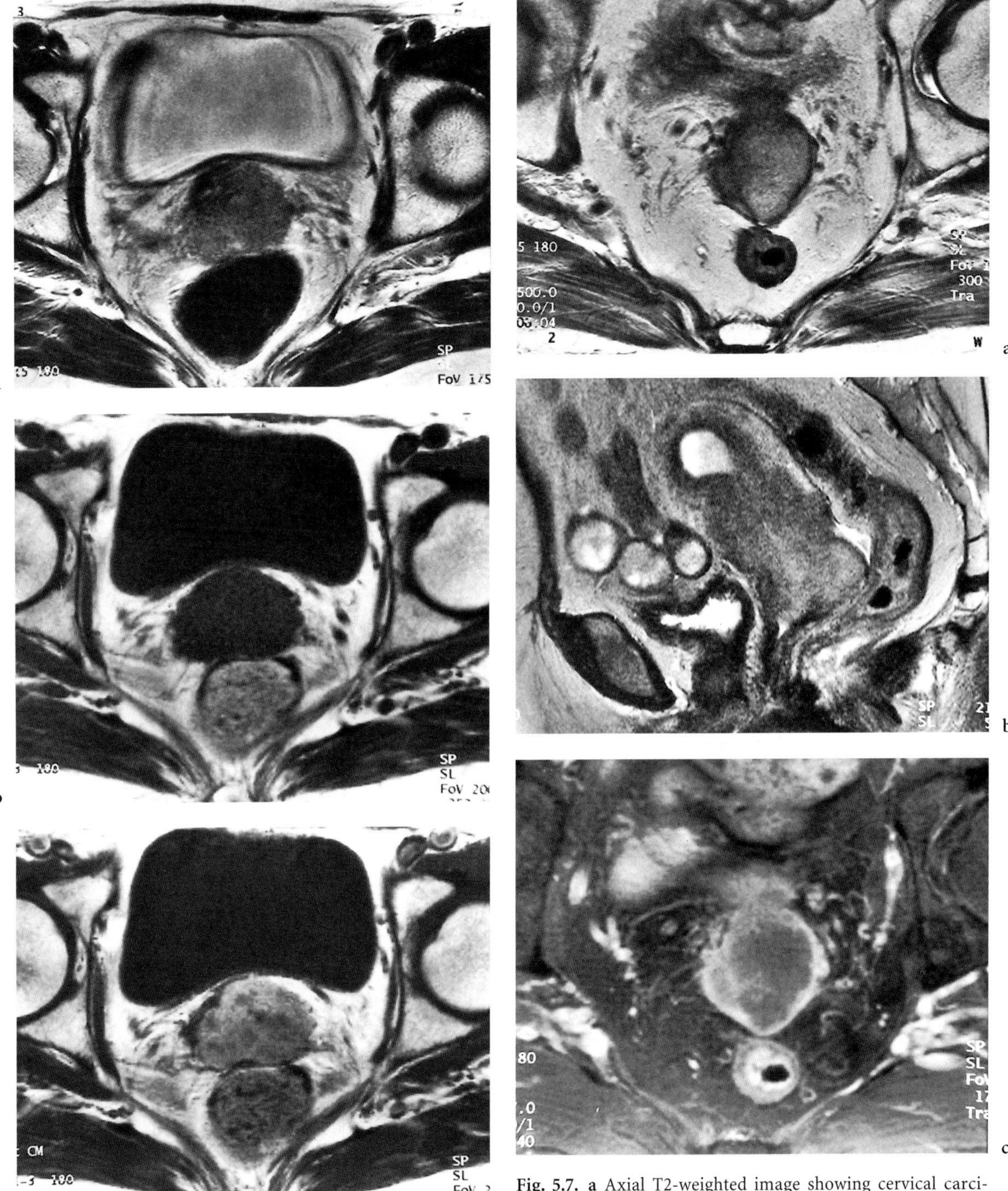

**Fig. 5.6.** **a** Cervical cancer with invasion through the entire cervical stromal ring in the supravaginal cervix, indicating parametrial invasion. **b** Isointense cervical cancer cannot be identified on the axial T1-weighted image. **c** Early phase dynamic study shows that the cervical mass is invading and disrupting the low signal intensity fibrous cervical stroma, producing the same finding as in **a**; however, there is no sign of invasion of adjacent organs

**Fig. 5.7.** **a** Axial T2-weighted image showing cervical carcinoma with invasion through the anterior aspect of the cervical stroma ring into the parametrium. **b** A supravaginal endocervical mass enlarges the cervical contour and extends to the upper portion of the vagina and the lower half of the uterine corpus, causing mucous accumulation in the endometrial cavity. The mass shows slightly higher intensity on T2-weighted image. **c** Contrast-enhanced axial image with fat saturation demonstrates enhancement of the mass, which protrudes anteriorly into the parametrium tissue

parametrial invasion, although KIM et al. (1990) showed that disruption of the low signal intensity stripe of cervical stroma alone, without an abnormal signal intensity lesion in the parametrium, does not convincingly indicate parametrial involvement. Relatively large tumors confined to the cervix often stretch and thin the remaining cervical stroma. On MR imaging, visualization of this thin stroma is often difficult.

### 5.6.2.3
### Stage III

Stage IIIa entails involvement of the lower third of the vagina, and stage IIb indicates extension to the pelvic side wall or hydronephrosis. Stage IIIa tumors are recognized on T2-weighted images as a high signal intensity mass replacing or invading the lower third of the hypointense vaginal wall (Fig. 5.8). However, direct clinical inspection is straightforward and MR diagnosis may not be critical (KIM et al. 1990). Stage IIIb tumors are recognized on T2-weighted images as a high signal intensity mass attaching to, replacing, or invading the pelvic side wall vessels and musculature (Fig. 5.9). Patients with dilated, obstructed ureters are also classified as having stage IIIb disease or higher. The sensitivity of MR imaging in respect of stage IIIb is reported to be 86% (HRICAK et al. 1988).

### 5.6.2.4
### Stage IV

Stage IV tumors extend outside the reproductive system and are subdivided into those that involve the mucosa of the bladder or rectum (stage IVa) and those with distant metastases or extension out of the true pelvis (stage IVb). T2-weighted sagittal and axial images show replacement of the usually hypointense bladder wall or rectal wall with high signal intensity tumor (Fig. 5.10). However, the MR criteria for stage IVa tumors and the accuracy of MR imaging are less clear because the number of patients reported is small. Inflammatory changes and edema are common causes of false-positive diagnosis.

Ovarian metastases most commonly appear as lobulated, triangular masses of intermediate signal intensity replacing the normal signal intensity of the ovarian stroma, and occasionally forming a large mass (Fig. 5.11) (JAVITT et al. 1987; HRICAK et al.

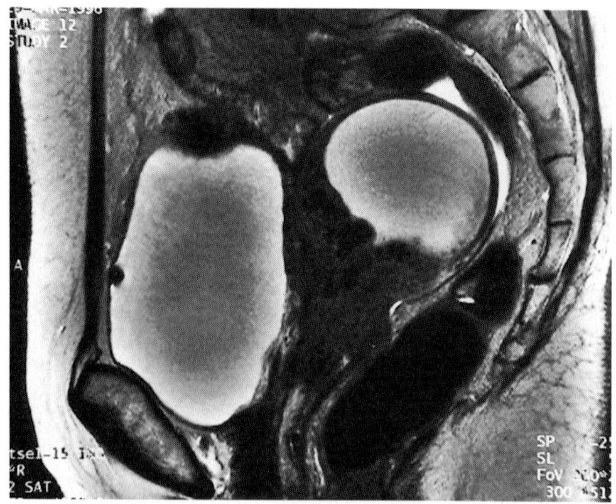


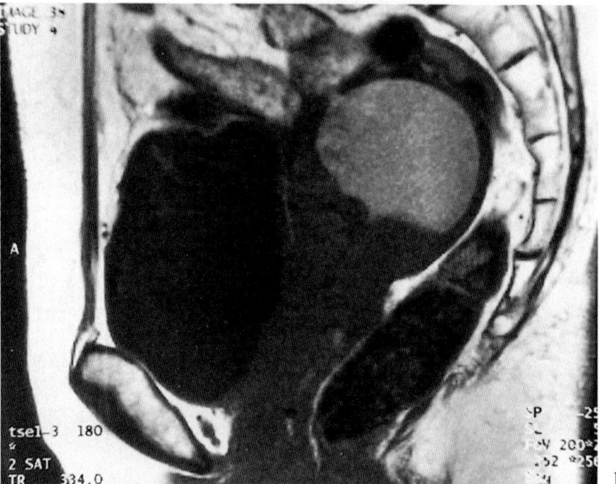


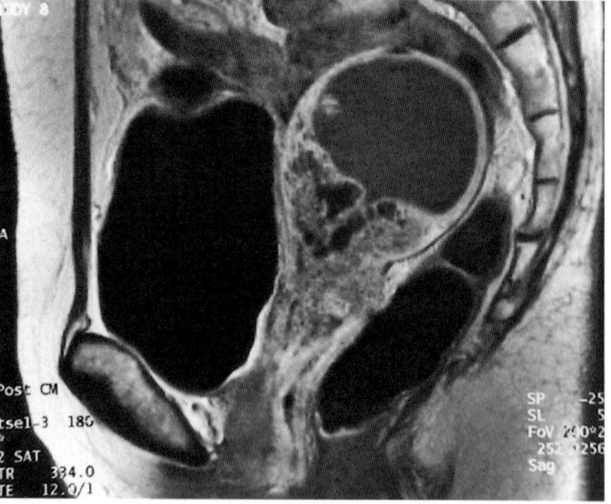


**Fig. 5.8.** **a** T2-weighted sagittal image demonstrating a large isointense cancer which was later proved by histology to extend inferiorly to the lower third of the vaginal wall and superiorly to the corpus, accompanied by obstructive mucous accumulation. **b** T1-weighted sagittal scan reveals the enlargement of the cervical contour but no difference in intensity between the mass and the surrounding tissue. The high signal intensity of obstructive mucus is caused by its viscosity. **c** After intravenous injection of Gd-DTPA, a reticular-appearing mass lesion is seen

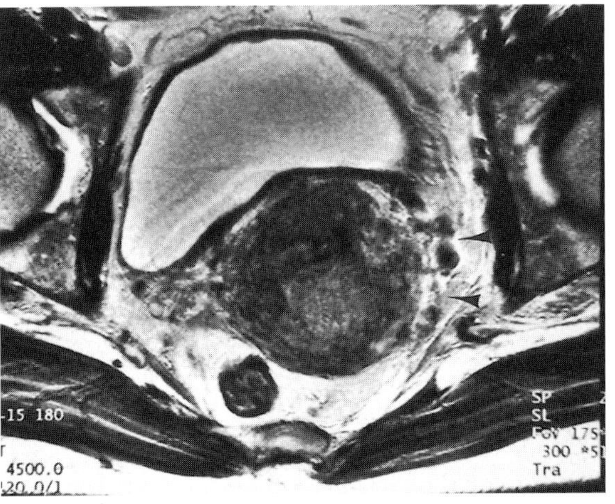
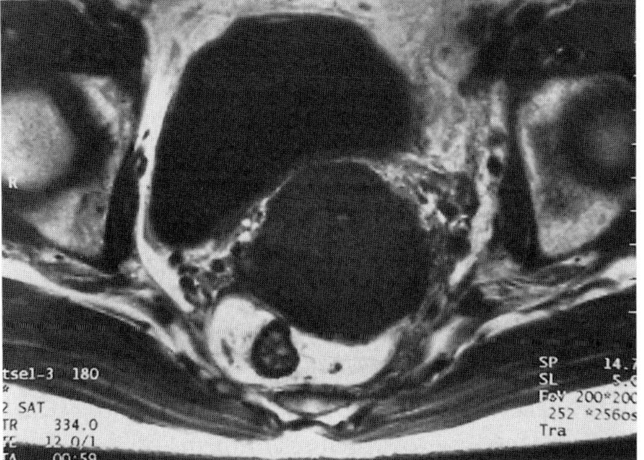
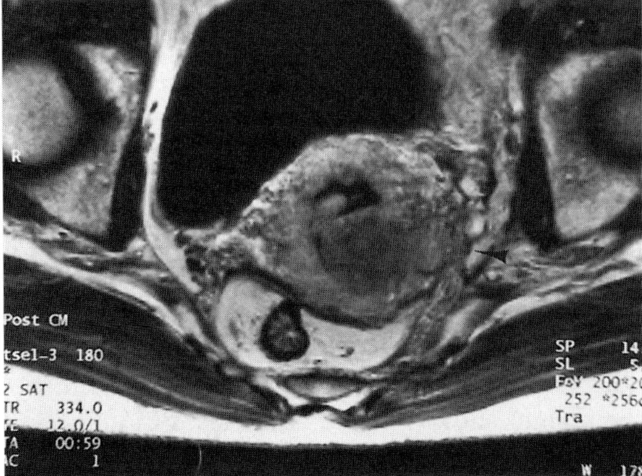

**Fig. 5.9. a** T2-weighted axial scan showing a large, heterogeneous mass of slightly increased intensity that is located at the cervix and attached to the pelvic wall on the left side (*arrowheads*). **b** On the axial T1-weighted image at the same level, the fat plane between the lesion and the pelvic wall disappears, and the left margin of the lesion is attached to the left-sided pelvic wall, suggesting pelvic side wall invasion. Note the bilateral multiple nodular lesions, which may be lymph nodes or vascular structures. **c** Postcontrast T1-weighted axial image reveals a heterogeneously enhanced mass with comparatively low-intensity nodules in its center, while along its left aspect there is invasion of the left-sided pelvic wall (*arrowhead*)

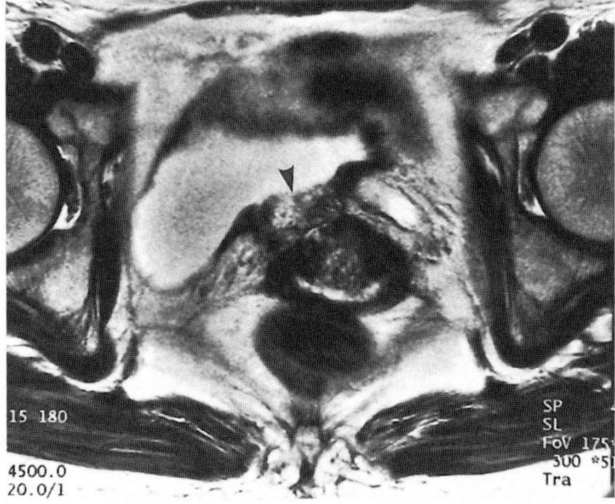
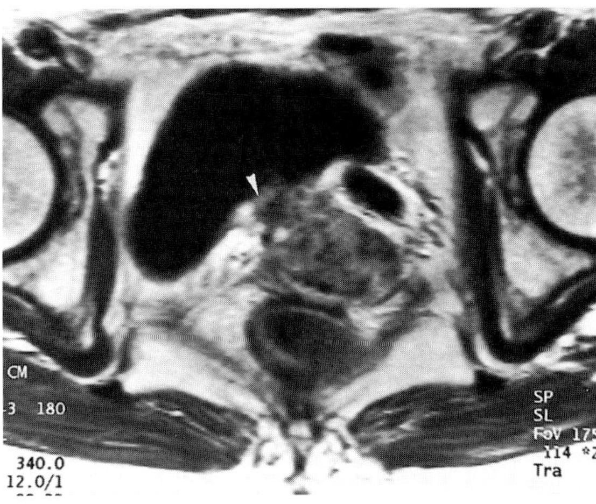

**Fig. 5.10. a** On this T2-weighted axial image, a large cervical mass of slightly high intensity protrudes anteriorly and invades the posterior bladder wall, causing interruption of the low-intensity bladder wall (*arrowhead*). **b** Postcontrast T1-weighted axial image shows the tumor to enhance heterogeneously and to infiltrate the posterior bladder wall (*arrowhead*)

1987; Posniak et al. 1990). Peritoneal or omental tumor implants usually have an intermediate signal intensity on T1-weighted images and higher signal intensity on T2-weighted images. The presence of normal pelvic fat planes does not exclude extrauterine spread of microscopic foci of tumor. The criterion for diagnosis of lymph node metastases by tumor is enlargement of lymph nodes to more than 1.5 cm in the pelvic or periaortic region. The determination of lymphadenopathy is by size and number, with criteria similar to those used with computed tomography (CT) – and with a similar lack of accuracy.

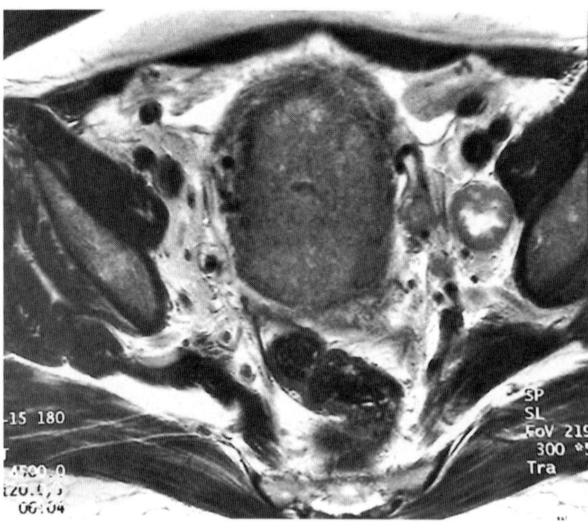


**Fig. 5.11.** Axial T2-weighted image showing a round metastatic lesion of moderate intensity that involves the left ovary. The border is sharply delineated. Multiple necrotic components are present within the tumor

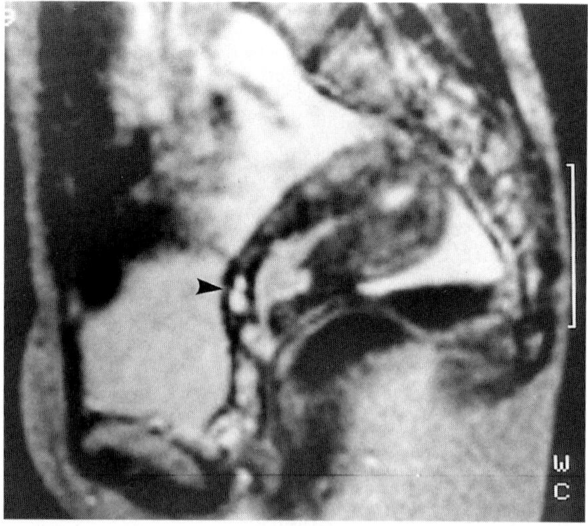


**Fig. 5.12.** Sagittal T2-weighted image. Adenoma malignum appears as multiple irregular, very high signal intensity lesions in the cervix (*arrowhead*), suggesting mucin-rich components. The tumor shows an endophytic growth pattern and widening of the internal os could be observed (Permission of Yamashita et al., AJR 162:649–650)

## 5.7 Adenocarcinoma

Adenocarcinoma of the cervix is becoming more common, especially in young women. This increase in frequency has occurred worldwide (Thompson 1992). Adenocarcinoma of the cervix accounts for 5%–15% of all carcinomas of the cervix (Rosai 1989). It usually arises from the columnar epithelium of the endocervical canal and may grow within the cervix and not be obvious on external inspection (Ferenczy and Winkler 1987). The primary endocervical location of this tumor may lead to later detection and poorer prognosis. Therefore, accurate preoperative diagnosis and accurate staging are very important.

The pathologic and clinical features of adenocarcinoma of the cervix are well documented (Ferenczy and Winkler 1987; Thompson 1992; Rosai 1989; Kurman et al. 1992; Saigo et al. 1986; Eifel et al. 1990; Berek et al. 1981). Adenocarcinomas tend to show an endophytic growth pattern on gross examination. Nearly 15% of patients have no gross lesion, because the carcinoma is located within the canal or deep within the endocervical clefts. Histologically, mucinous adenocarcinomas are the most common type of adenocarcinoma of the cervix (Fu et al. 1982). An uncommon variant of endocervical mucinous adenocarcinoma is adenoma malignum or minimal deviation adenocarcinoma (Kaku and Enjoji 1983; Kaminski and Norris 1983; Anderson 1987). Microscopically, these lesions are mainly composed of well-differentiated endocervical glands with mucin-rich cystic spaces, which extend from the surface to the deeper portion of the cervical wall (Figs. 5.12, 5.13). The MR appearance is usually indistinguishable from that of deep nabothian cysts (Fig. 5.14). Such lesions show early dissemination, a poor response to therapy, and an unfavorable prognosis (Fu et al. 1982; Kaku and Enjoji 1983).

The prognosis in adenocarcinoma of the cervix is generally less favorable than that of the SCC counterpart. Adenocarcinomas are usually resistant to chemotherapy or radiation. The incidence of residual tumor in hysterectomy specimens after intracavitary treatment is much higher than with SCC (Kjorstad and Bond 1984). The pattern of metastatic spread of adenocarcinomas differs from that of SCCs in that the former show a higher incidence of ascites and para-aortic spread (Eifel et al. 1990).

Although there is considerable overlap in MR the appearances of SCCs and adenocarcinomas, invasive adenocarcinoma of the cervix has some characteristic MR features due to the submucosal location and the relatively poor tumor vascularity (Torashima et al. 1997). Adenocarcinomas are typically seen as a mass with preservation of endocervical epithelium and a lower degree of contrast enhancement (Fig. 5.15). The preservation of endocervical epithelium in adenocarcinoma is well-appreciated on contrast-enhanced MR images. Most mucinous adeno-

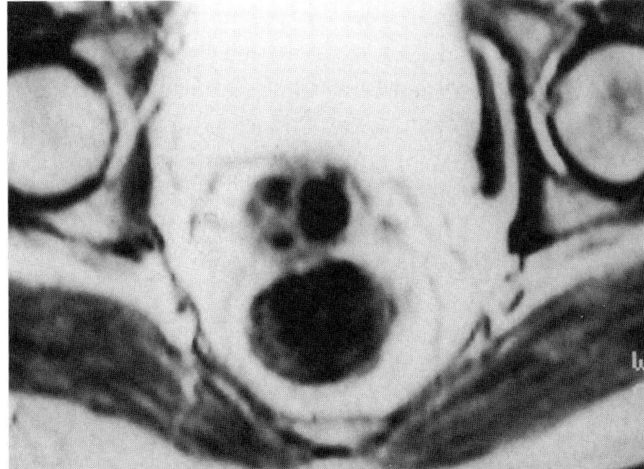
a

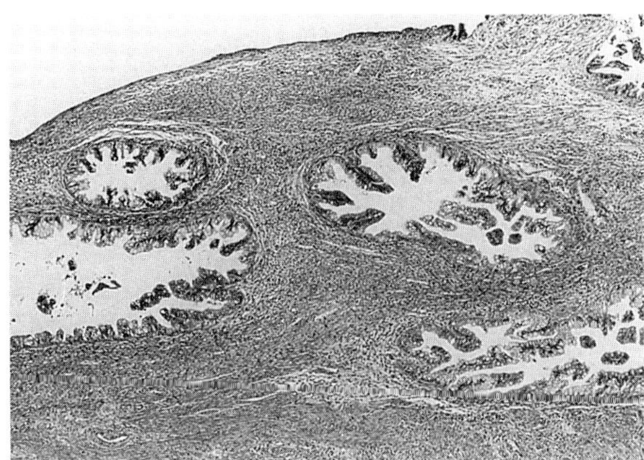
b

**Fig. 5.13.** **a** Axial post Gd-DTPA T1-weighted image showing multiple cystic lesions in the cervix. **b** Histologically, mucinous adenocarcinoma is composed of well-differentiated endocervical glands with mucin-rich cystic spaces and some connecting tissue (Permission of YAMASHITA et al., AJR 162: 649–650)

carcinomas are visualized as a hyperintense mass on T2-weighted MR imaging. Abundant mucin results in T2 elongation, but some tumors are not visualized because of their endophytic growth pattern. The endocervical canal tends to be preserved even in larger tumors involving the entire cervix.

When tumors involve predominantly the submucosal layer, histologic specimens need to be obtained from the deep cervical tissue. For evaluation of the degree of stromal invasion and parametrial invasion, radiologic assessment often has an important role.

The staging accuracy of MR imaging in respect of adenocarcinomas appears to be somewhat inferior to that for SCCs. Adenocarcinomas that have infiltrated the parametrial tissue may not be appreciated on MR imaging. The majority of tumors of stage Ib or less cannot be visualized, probably due to their infiltrative nature or the poor contrast between the tumor and the cervical stroma.

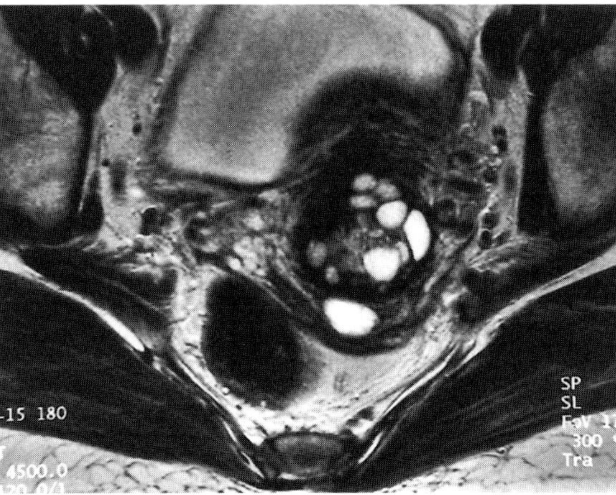


**Fig. 5.14.** Axial T2-weighted image demonstrating multiple high signal intensity nabothian cysts with a sharp border within the cervix, caused by the obstruction of the gland tubes

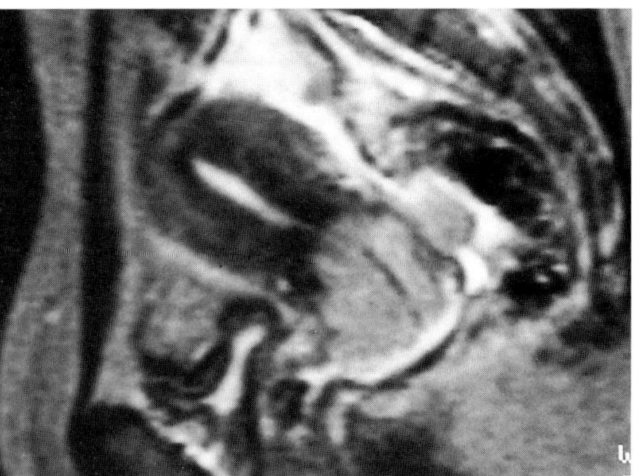
a

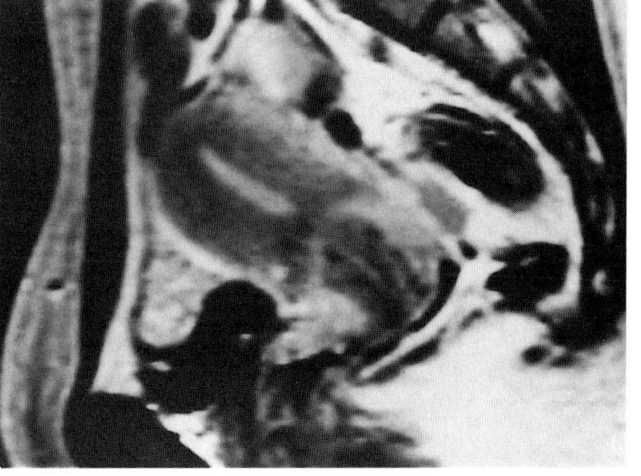
b

**Fig. 5.15.** **a** Sagittal T2-weighted image. Adenocarcinoma shows diffuse high signal intensity in the cervix with preservation of the endocervical epithelium. The anterior fornix and upper two-thirds of the vaginal wall are involved by tumor. **b** Gd-DTPA enhanced T1-weighted image. The adenocarcinoma shows little enhancement while the endometrium and cervical epithelium are enhanced; the endocervical canal is seen to be well preserved (Permission of TORASHIMA et al., Comp Med Imag Graphics 21:253–260)

## 5.8 Recurrent Cervical Carcinoma

Recurrent endometrial carcinomas are most frequently seen in the vagina, uterus, pelvic lymph nodes, para-aortic lymph nodes and lung. Recurrent lesions develop outside the pelvis in 75% of cases (CURRIE 1992); if they are confined to the pelvis, they produce symptoms of low back pain or sciatic pain, leg edema, or obstructing uropathy. CT has been the imaging modality of choice for the detection of persistent and recurrent carcinomas (WALSH et al.

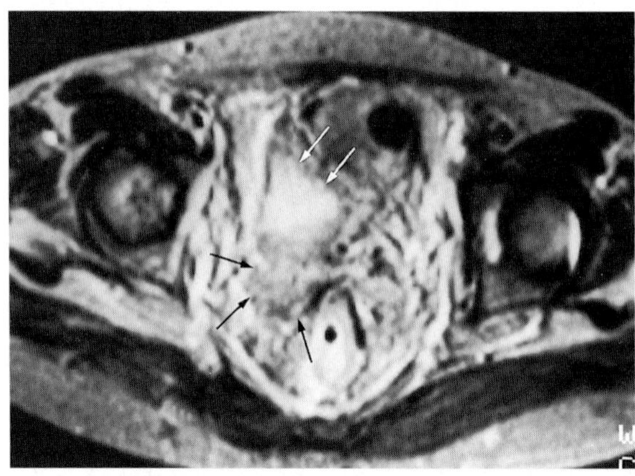

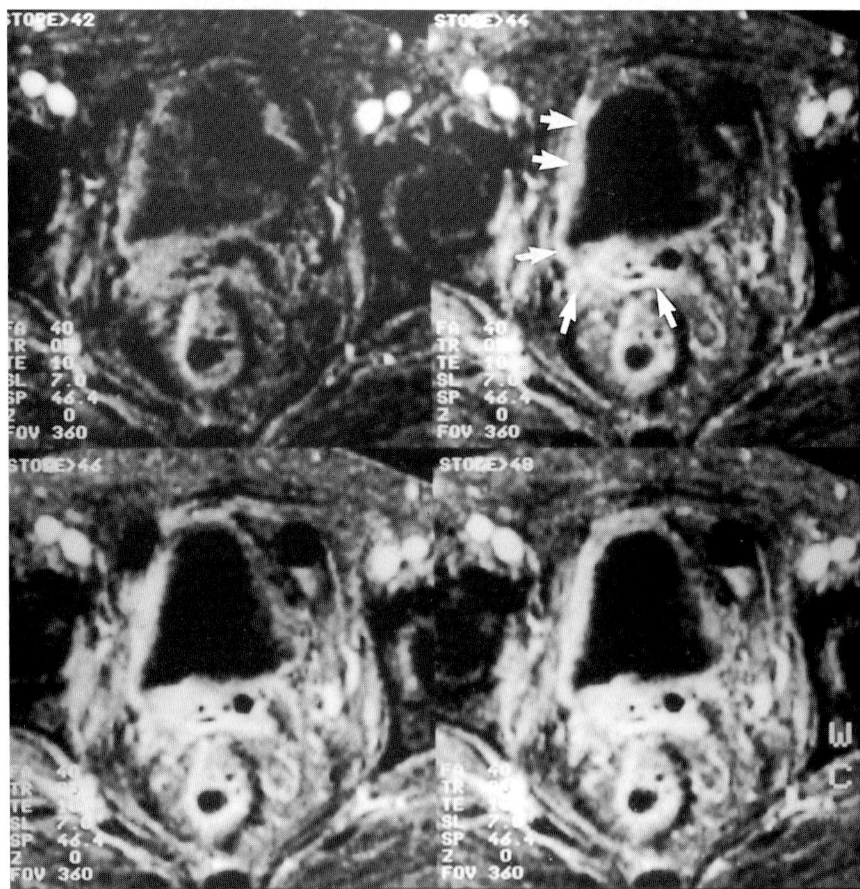


**Fig. 5.16.** **a** Axial T2-weighted image showing the appearance in a patient who had been operated on for cervical carcinoma. There is diffuse high signal intensity of the cervix and disappearance of the tissue plane between the bladder (*white arrows*) and cervix (*black arrows*). **b** Dynamic Gd-DTPA study reveals diffuse and intense enhancement of the cervix and bladder wall, indicating recurrence of cervical carcinoma and contiguous metastasis in the bladder (Permission from YAMASHITA et al., J Magn Reson Imaging 6:167–171)

1981). CT and MR imaging features include a central pelvic mass with or without an intact uterus, pelvic and para-aortic lymph node metastases, and mesenteric, peritoneal, omental, and liver metastases (YAMASHITA et al. 1996). MR imaging may be useful in distinguishing recurrent tumor from post-treatment fibrosis. Recurrent tumors may be seen as a mass of higher signal intensity than pelvic side wall or fat (EBNER et al. 1988). Recent radiation-induced change produces high signal intensity on T2-weighted images. With time, late fibrosis is expected to show lower signal intensity (EBNER et al. 1988). These findings are essential for choice of additional surgery, radiation therapy, or chemotherapy. Most false-positive results are related to post-radiation changes that simulate recurrent tumor. On T1-weighted and T2-weighted imaging, the signal intensity of radiation changes occasionally cannot be differentiated from that of recurrent tumor. Dynamic MR imaging may be useful for this purpose (Fig. 5.16) (YAMASHITA et al. 1996); however, further studies will be requried to establish its accuracy.

## 5.9 Summary

High-resolution MR imaging with the use of a phased array coil clearly visualizes cervical carcinomas and has a significant role in the accurate staging of disease. In general, dynamic contrast-enhanced studies have higher contrast than FSE images. However, it has not been clarified whether this increase in contrast resolution results in an increase in staging accuracy. Diagnosis of adenocarcinomas and recurrent disease is still difficult even with these new imaging techniques.

## References


Aderson MC (1987) Premalignant and malignant disease of the cervix. In: Fox H (ed) Haines and Taylor, obstetrical and gynecological pathology, 3rd edn, vol 1. Churchill Livingstone, Edinburgh, pp 255–301

Berek JS, Castaldo TW, Hacker NF, Petrilli ES, Lagasse LD (1981) Adenocarcinoma of the uterine cervix. Cancer 48:2734–2741

Currie JL (1992) Malignant tumors of the uterine corpus. In: Thompson JD, Rock JA (eds) Te Linde's operative gynecology. Lippincott, Philadelphia, pp 1253–1302

Ebner F, Kressel HY, Mintz MC, et al. (1988) Tumor recurrence versus fibrosis in the female pelvis: differentiation with MRI at 1.5T. Radiology 166:333–340

Eifel PJ, Morris M, Oswald MJ, Wharton JT, Delcos L (1990) Adenocarcinoma of the uterine cervix. Cancer 65:2507–2514

Ferenczy A, Winkler B (1987) Carcinoma and metastatic tumors of the cervix. In: Kurman RJ (ed) Blaustein's pathology of the female genital tract, 3rd edn. Springer, Berlin Heidelberg New York, pp 218–256

Fu YS, Reagan JW, Hsiu JG, Storaalsi JP, Wentz WB (1982) Adenocarcinoma and mixed carcinoma of the uterine cervix. Cancer 49:2560–2570

Heiken JP, Lee JKT (1988) MR imaging of the pelvis. Radiology 166:11–16

Hricak H, Crooks JE, Sheldon PE (1983) Magnetic resonance imaging of the female pelvis: initial experience. AJR 141:1119–1128

Hricak H, Stern JL, Fisher MR, Shapeero LG, Winkler MI, Lancey CG (1987) Endometrial carcinoma staging by MR imaging. Radiology 162:297–305

Hricak H, Lacey CG, Sandles LG, Chang YCF (1988) Invasive cervical carcinoma: comparison of MR imaging and surgical findings. Radiology 166:623–631

Hricak H, Hamm B, Semelka RC, et al. (1991) Carcinoma of the uterus: use of gadopentetate dimeglumine in MR imaging. Radiology 181:95–106

Javitt MC, Stein HL, Lovecchio L (1987) MRI in staging of endometrial and cervical carcinoma. Magn Reson Imaging 5:83–92

Kaku T, Enjoji M (1983) Extremely well-differentiated adenocarcinoma ("adenoma malignum") of the cervix. Int J Gynecol Pathol 2:28–41

Kaminski PF, Norris HJ (1983) Minimal deviation carcinoma (adenoma malignum) of the cervix. Int J Gynecol Pathol 2:141–152

Kim SH, Shoi BI, Lee HP, et al. (1990) Uterine cervical carcinoma: comparison CT and MR findings. Radiology 175:45–51

Kjorstad KE, Bond B (1984) Metastatic potential and patterns of dissemination. Am J Obstet Gynecol 64:553–556

Kurman RJ, Norris HJ, Wilkinson EJ (eds) (1992) Tumors of the cervix, vagina and vulva. Armed Forces Institute of Pathology, Washington, pp 37–139

Nagell JR, Roddick JW, Lowin DM (1971) The staging of cervical cancer: inevitable discrepancies between clinical staging and pathologic findings. Am J Obstet Gynecol 110:973–978

Perez CA, Camel HM, Askin F, et al. (1981) Endometrial carcinoma of the uterine cervix: prognostic factors that may modify staging. Cancer 48:170–180

Posniak HV, Olson MC, Dudiak CM, et al. (1990) MR imaging of uterine carcinoma: correlation with clinical and pathologic findings. Radiographics 10:15–27

Rosai J (1989) Female reproductive system/uterus-cervix. In: Rosai J (ed) Ackerman's surgical pathology, vol 2. Mosby, St. Louis, pp 1022–1049

Rubens D, Thornbury JR, Angel C, et al. (1988) Stage IB cervical carcinoma: comparison of clinical, MR and pathological staging. AJR 150:135–138

Saigo PE, Cain JM, Kim WS, Gaynor JJ, Johnson K, Lewis JL (1986) Prognostic factors in adenocarcinoma of the uterine cervix. Cancer 57:1548–1593

Scoutt LM, McCauley TR, Flynn SD, et al. (1993) Zonal anatomy of the cervix: correlation of MR imaging and histological examination of hysterectomy specimens. Radiology 186:159–162

Sironi S, Belloni C, Taccagni G, et al. (1992) Carcinoma of the cervix: value of MR imaging in detecting parametrial involvement. AJR 156:753–756

Smith RC, Reinhold C, McCauley TR, et al. (1992) Multicoil high-resolution fast spin-echo MR imaging of the female pelvis. Radiology 184:671–675

Thompson JD (1992) Cancer of the cervix. In: Thompson JD, Rock JA (ed) Te Linde's operative gynecology, 7th edn. Lippincott, Philadelphia, pp 1161–1252

Togashi K, Nishimura K, Itoh K, et al. (1986) Uterine cervical cancer: assessment with high-field MR imaging. Radiology 160:431–435

Togashi K, Nishimura K, Sagoh T, et al. (1989) Carcinoma of the cervix: staging with MR imaging. Radiology 171:245–251

Torashima M, Yamashita Y, Hatanaka Y, Takahashi M, Miyazaki K, Okamura H (1997) Invasive adenocarcinoma of the uterine cervic: MR imaging. Comp Med Imag & Graphics 21:253–260

Walsh JW, Amendola MA, Hall JT, Tisnado J, Goplerud DR (1981) Recurrent carcinoma of the cervix: CT diagnosis. AJR 136:117–122

Weber TM, Sostman DH, Spritzer CE, et al. (1995) Cervical carcinoma: determination of recurrent tumor extent versus radiation changes with MR imaging. Radiology 194:135–139

Worthington JL, Balfe DM, Lee JKT, et al. (1986) Uterine neoplasm: MR imaging. Radiology 159:725–730

Yamashita Y, Takahashi M, Sawada T, Miyazaki K, Okamura H (1992) Carcinoma of the cervix: dynamic MR imaging. Radiology 182:643–648

Yamashita Y, Mizutani H, Torashima M, et al. (1993a) Assessment of myometrial invasion by endometrial carcinoma: transvaginal sonography vs contrast-enhanced MR imaging. AJR 161:595–599

Yamashita Y, Harada M, Sawada T, Takahashi M, Miyazaki K, Okamura H (1993b) Normal uterus and FIGO stage I endometrial carcinoma: dynamic gadolinium-enhanced MR imaging. Radiology 186:495–501

Yamashita Y, Takahashi M, Katabuchi H, Fukumatsu Y, Miyazaki K, Okamura H (1994) Adenoma malignum: MR appearances mimicking nabothian cysts: AJR 162:649–650

Yamashita Y, Harada M, Torashima M, et al. (1996) Contrast-enhanced dynamic MR imaging of recurrent postoperative cervical cnacer. J Magn Reson Imaging 6:167–171

# 6 Assessment of Endometrial Carcinoma by Magnetic Resonance Imaging and Ultrasound

A. Del Maschio, A. Vanzulli, S. Sironi, F. De Cobelli, and D. Spagnolo

CONTENTS



## 6.1 Introduction

Endometrial carcinoma is the most common malignant neoplasm of the female genital tract (Berman et al. 1980; Boronow et al. 1984). The prognosis and treatment of the disease are mainly based on three factors: histologic grading of the neoplasm, the extent of myometrial invasion, and the presence of nodal metastases (Berman et al. 1980; Boronow et al. 1984).

The depth of myometrial involvement is one of the most important aspects, because the prevalence of pelvic and lomboaortic nodal metastases is directly related to this parameter (Berman et al. 1980; Boronow et al. 1984). The revised staging classification of the International Federation of Gynecology and Obstetrics (FIGO) for endometrial carcinoma considers three degrees of myometrial invasion: stage la = no invasion, stage Ib = endometrial carcinoma involving the inner half of the myometrium, and stage Ic = carcinoma reaching the outer half of the myometrium. If the myometrium is not invaded, nodal metastases are present in about 3% of patients. If the invasion is deep (stage Ic), nodal metastases are present in about 40% of cases (Boronow et al. 1984; Hricak et al. 1987).

Transabdominal sonography is not considered adequate in the assessment of patients with endometrial carcinoma owing to the poor resolution of the low-frequency transducers used. On the other hand, the liver and retroperitoneal nodal status can be evaluated with transabdominal sonography, though computed tomography is regarded as superior.

Many authors (Cruickshank et al. 1989; Mendelson et al. 1988) advocate the use of transvaginal high-frequency transducers for sonographic evaluation of gynecologic neoplasms. The reported accuracy of transvaginal sonography for determining the depth of myometrial involvement by endometrial carcinoma is 80%–84% (Gordon et al. 1990; Cacciatore et al. 1989).

Magnetic resonance (MR) imaging is also a reliable technique in the local staging of endometrial carcinoma. The reported MR accuracy in distinguishing superficial from deep myometrial invasion is about 78%–82% (Hricak et al. 1987; Belloni et al. 1990; Sironi et al. 1989; Yazigi et al. 1989).

## 6.2 Sonography

### 6.2.1 Technical Considerations

Transabdominal sonography has to be performed with the patient having fasted for 4 or 5 h before the examination, and the patients should also have a full bladder. The bladder must be moderately distended in order to displace the bowel loops and create an appropriate acoustic window. An overdistended bladder has to be avoided because it does not allow the application of appropriate pressure of the transducer on the abdominal wall and displaces the uterus away from the transducer itself. The uterus can be visualized in longitudinal, axial, and oblique planes by simply aligning the orientation of the transducer

A. Del Maschio, MD, Director; A. Vanzulli, MD; S. Sironi; F. De Cobelli, MD; D. Spagnolo, MD, Department of Radiology, Scientific Institute S. Raffaele, University Hospital, Olgettina 60, I-20132 Milan, Italy

on the abdomen of the patient. The transducer frequency has to be optimized to the habitus of the patient: for obese women a transducer operating at 2.5–3.5 MHz is the best option; for thin women the transducer frequency can be raised to 4–6 MHz.

Modern equipment offers a variety of transducer frequencies owing to the capability of using broad-band piezoelectric crystals. Furthermore, the capability of electronic focusing of the ultrasonographic beam has to be adapted to the patient's habitus in order to achieve the best spatial resolution in the region of interest.

In the evaluation of patients with a suspected endometrial carcinoma the transabdominal approach is indicated for the study of the para-aortic nodal status and for the examination of the liver. Local staging of the endometrial neoplasm is best accomplished with a transvaginal probe.

In our opinion the transvaginal examination (transvaginal sonography, TVS) should be performed only after a transabdominal exploration in order to complement the overview of the pelvic anatomy and to detect any pathologic condition that may be outside the field of view of the intracavitary transducer. It is also to be borne in mind that the maneuverability of the probe within the vagina is limited.

Every manufacturer of ultrasound equipment currently offers intravaginal probes. These transducers are almost always electronically focused sector probes which consist of either an array of crystals sequentially triggered to produce the sector image or, more commonly, a set of crystals shaped to produce the image (microconvex probes). Transducer frequencies vary from 5 to 7.5 MHz; most transducers are fixed at a single frequency, but dual or broad-band probes are offered by some manufacturers. As for transabdominal scanning, the highest frequency that allows adequate penetration should be chosen. For imaging of the endometrium, the best results are obtained with 7.5 MHz transducers.

Before the examination a brief description of transvaginal scanning and of the reasons for performing it should be given to the patients. For the examination the patient must have an empty bladder and lie in the supine position, with the thighs abducted and the knees flexed. The buttocks must be elevated to permit anterior angulation of the probe, when necessary. The probe should be covered by a condom containing a small amount of gel. It is of some help to introduce into the vagina a gloved finger with some jelly on the glove in order to facilitate probe insertion. When the transducer is inserted the cervix and the lower uterine segment are visualized initially. The probe is advanced and angulated anteriorly until the uterine fundus comes into view. The transducer is then oriented to obtain a longitudinal and a transverse view of the uterus and of the endometrium (Bohm-Velez and Mendelson 1992).

### 6.2.2 Normal Anatomy

The endometrium is depicted by TVS with great detail and appears as an echogenic structure in the center of the uterus (Fig. 6.1). Sonographic measurements of normal endometrial thickness vary with the phase of the menstrual cycle. In the proliferative phase the endometrial thickness varies from 4 to 8 mm, while in the secretory phase it can reach 14 mm (Fleischer et al. 1986). In postmenopausal women who are not on hormone replacement therapy (HRT), an endometrial thickness above 8 mm is considered pathologic, while in women on HRT a thickness of less than 10 mm is considered normal (Deicher et al. 1986). Sonographic measurements should include both layers of the endometrium, but should not include the hypoechoic halo that usually surrounds the endometrium itself, which probably is cast by the inner layer of the myometrium (Fig. 6.2) (Welker et al. 1989).

During menses the endometrium appears as a thin echogenic interface; in the proliferative phase it thickens and becomes isoechoic. As ovulation ap-

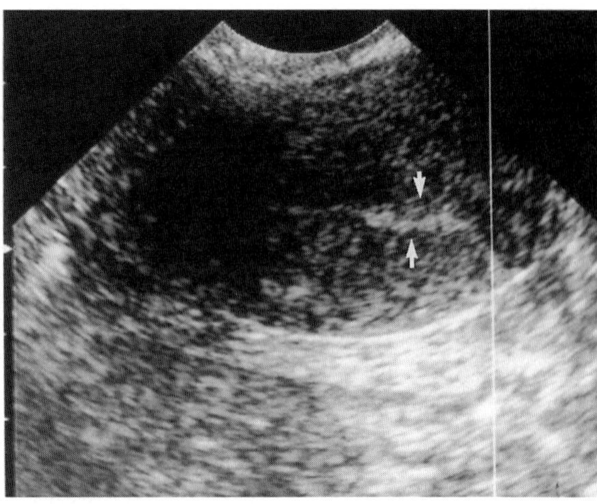

**Fig. 6.1.** Sagittal transvaginal sonogram of the uterus. The endometrium is identified as a central echogenic structure (*arrows*)

proaches the endometrium becomes more echogenic and a hypoechoic band develops within the inner endometrium. During the secretory phase the endometrium achieves its greatest thickness and echogenicity (WELKER et al. 1989; FLEISCHER et al. 1991).

Endometrial thickness, echotexture, and the margins between the endometrium and the myometrium have to be carefully evaluated.

### 6.2.3 Endometrial Carcinoma

An abnormally thickened endometrium may result from a variety of conditions such as early pregnancy and pregnancy-related complications, endometrial hyperplasia (Fig. 6.3), polyps, and endometrial carcinoma. In a series of 18 patients with endometrial carcinoma evaluated by sonography, the average endometrial thickness was 17.7 mm (GRANBERG et al. 1991; GOLDSTEIN et al. 1990). A similar degree of endometrial thickening has also been observed in patients with endometrial hyperplasia (MALPANI et al. 1990). Other sonographic aspects such as the presence of endometrial fluid or a lobular appearance of the endometrium may arouse suspicion of an endometrial carcinoma (Fig. 6.4). Color flow Doppler and duplex Doppler examinations may help in diagnosing this condition by demonstrating a low resistive index (BOURNE et al. 1990, 1991) but uterine curettage is recommended for diagnosing endometrial cancer in any patient with abnormal endometrial thickening, and particularly in those who are symptomatic.

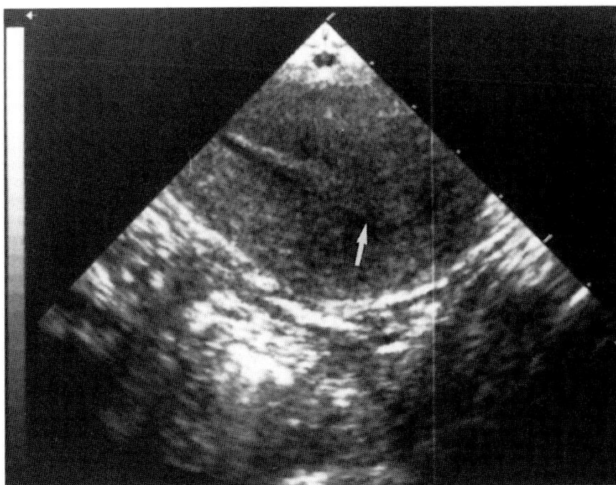

**Fig. 6.2.** Sagittal transvaginal sonogram: the hyperechoic endometrium is surrounded by a hypoechoic halo (*arrow*)

Transvaginal sonography is useful in the preoperative evaluation of patients with endometrial carcinoma since it permits the depth of myometrial invasion to be determined (GORDON et al. 1989, 1990; CACCIATORE et al. 1989; FLEISCHER et al. 1987). On the basis of accurate measurement of uterine wall thickness and of tumor invasion relative to myometrial thickness, the extent of invasion can be classified into superficial, intermediate, or deep. Preservation of the hypoechoic halo generally indicates no or only superficial invasion (Fig. 6.4); by contrast absence of the halo is associated with deep invasion (Fig. 6.5). The degree of invasion can be determined by measuring the myometrium thickness in an uninvolved region and the minimum myometrium thickness at the point of apparently deeper tumor invasion. By dividing the two measurements the precise percentage of tumor invasion can be obtained (FLEISCHER et al. 1987). In a study by GORDON et al. (1990), 25 patients with endometrial carcinoma underwent TVS 1 week before hysterectomy. In 21 cases (84%) the depth of invasion of the myometrium was predicted correctly on the basis of the sonographic findings. Using the same technique, CACCIATORE et al. (1989) correctly detected myometrial invasion in 80% of cases.

The margins of endometrial carcinoma may be difficult to distinguish from the adjacent myometrium when the echogenicity of each is similar (TEEFEY et al. 1996). Sometimes large endocavitary tumors that produce myometrial thinning can be confused for invasive tumors (Fig. 6.6) (GORDON et al. 1989). Preexisting conditions such as leiomyoma and adenomyosis also contribute to difficulties in delineating the precise extent of myometrial invasion. Moreover bulky tumors can be examined only partially and sometimes it may be difficult to appreciate the extrauterine component of the tumor itself, with consequent understaging of the neoplasm (GORDON et al. 1989).

## 6.3 MR Imaging

### 6.3.1 Technical Considerations

Patients are usually supine and breathing quietly during the examination. Partial distention of the bladder is preferred, as this displaces small bowel loops from the pelvis.

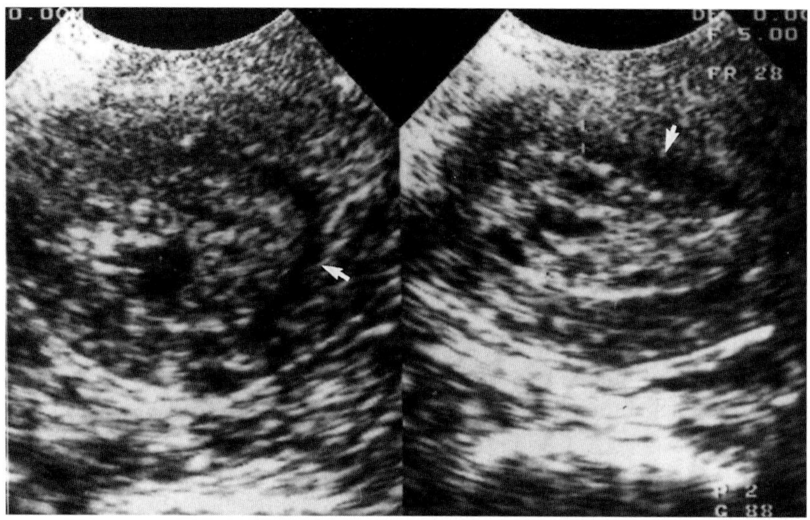

**Fig. 6.3.** Longitudinal (*left*) and transverse (*right*) transvaginal sonograms of a patient with endometrial hyperplasia secondary to tamoxifen treatment. Note the regular hypoechoic halo (*arrows*) which surrounds the endometrium

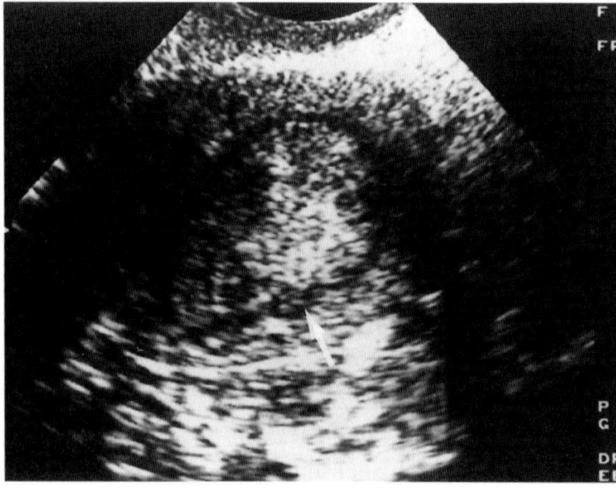

**Fig. 6.4.** Transverse transvaginal sonogram of a patient with endometrial carcinoma: the endometrium is abnormally thickened and the margins of the endometrial cavity are lobulated (*arrow*)

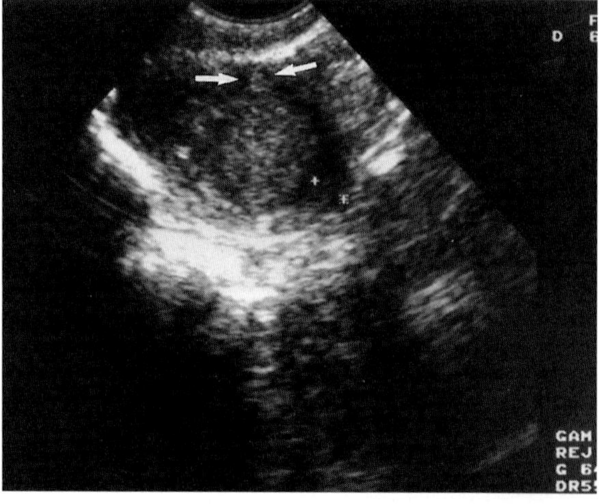

**Fig. 6.5.** Transverse transvaginal sonogram of a patient with endometrial carcinoma. The hyperechoic cancer is infiltrating the myometrium in the anterior portion, where the hypoechoic halo is disrupted (*arrows*)

Glucagon (1 mg intramuscularly or intravenously) may be administered to reduce motion artifacts produced by bowel peristalsis. Routine use of a vaginal tampon is not necessary and may obscure details of the vaginal anatomy. Occasionally additional information may be obtained by imaging the patient prone with rectal air insufflation.

A complete examination requires both T1- (short repetition and echo times) and T2-weighted (long repetition and echo times) pulse sequences. T2-weighted MR images delineate the internal anatomy of the uterus, cervix, and vagina. T1-weighted images are useful in detecting tumor extension into adjacent fat and lymph node enlargement. Evaluation of the signal intensity of pelvic masses on these two pulse sequences aids in tissue characterization. The use of fat suppression pulse sequences may be helpful in some patients to differentiate subacute hemorrhage from fat (Hricak et al. 1987, 1991a,b; Chen et al. 1990; Brown et al. 1990).

Imaging is performed in more than one plane. We generally obtain axial T1-weighted MR images and

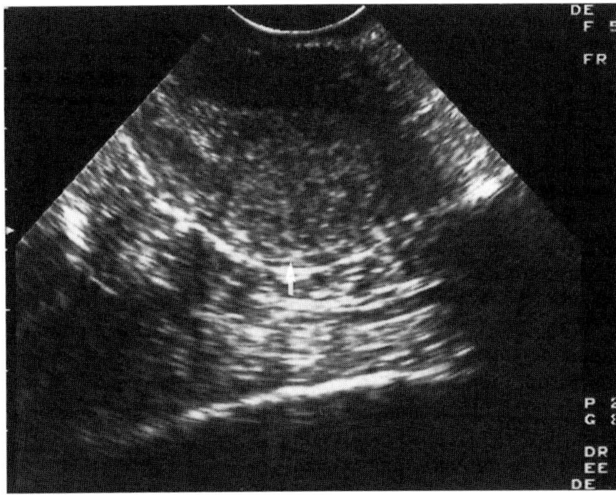

**Fig. 6.6.** Longitudinal transvaginal sonogram of a patient with endometrial carcinoma. The lesion expands the endometrial cavity and causes thinning of the myometrium posteriorly (*arrow*). At histologic evaluation of the hysterectomy specimen the myometrium was found not to be involved

sagittal T2-weighted images in all patients. Additional T2-weighted images in the axial, coronal, or oblique plane are obtained depending on the purpose of the examination. The uterus, cervix, vagina, cul-de-sac, and tumor extension into the bladder or rectum are best evaluated sagittally. Coronal or axial images are best for evaluating the ovaries, parametria, and adnexae. Axial images are most useful for evaluating the lymph nodes and developmental anomalies of the vagina. Oblique images that are parallel or perpendicular to the axis of the uterus may be useful in some cases.

Recently, it has been demonstrated that the use of a paramagnetic contrast agent (Gd-DTPA) may be useful in the evaluation of normal or pathologic uterine structures. The contrast medium is injected with the bolus technique (0.1 mmol/kg over 10–15 s) and then (SE/GRE) T1-weighted sequences are performed (Hricak et al. 1992; Hirano et al. 1992; Hricak 1991; Sironi et al. 1989; Lien et al. 1991; Yazigi et al. 1989; Javitt et al. 1987; Belloni et al. 1990).

## 6.3.2 Normal Anatomy

On T1-weighted MR images, the normal uterus has homogeneous low to medium signal intensity. Uterine zonal anatomy is appreciated on T2-weighted images with three discernible signal intensities. The endometrium has a high signal intensity similar to or greater than that of fat. The myometrium has medium signal intensity. Between them lies the thin, low signal intensity junctional zone that is thought to correspond to the innermost portion of the myometrium. The junctional zone may not be visible as a distinct structure in premenarchal and postmenopausal patients.

The MR appearance of the normal uterus is variable and is influenced by the hormonal status of the patient. During the reproductive years, there is a distinct temporal variation in uterine appearance in different phases of the menstrual cycle. During the follicular phase, endometrial width is typically 1–3 mm. The endometrial zone is widest during the middle of the secretory phase, when it usually measures 5–7 mm but may increase to 10 mm. Myometrial signal intensity varies during the menstrual cycle and is maximal during the secretory phase. In patients taking oral contraceptives, uterine zonal anatomy is less distinct and the endometrial width is usually 4 mm or less. This appearance is similar to that seen in premenarchal and postmenopausal patients. Postmenopausal women taking exogenous estrogen may have an endometrial width greater than 4 mm.

After injection of Gd-DTPA, the zonal anatomy of the corpus uterus is almost always demonstrated. The enhancement of the myometrium and normal endometrium is similar in both pre- and postmenopausal women.

## 6.3.3 Endomentrial Carinoma

Carcinoma of the endometrium is the fourth most common female cancer. Because the stage of the disease, the depth of myometrial invasion, and the lymph node status are crucial prognostic factors, surgical staging of this neoplasm has been recommended. While surgical staging offers a gold standard of diagnosis, it may not be suitable for every patient, and furthermore may make radiation therapy more difficult.

With present MR techniques, endometrial carcinoma cannot be consistently visualized or differentiated from blood clot, benign tumor (submucosal leiomyoma or endometrial polyp), or adenomatous hyperplasia. On nonenhanced T2-weighted images, endometrial carcinoma and normal endometrium are usually of similarly high signal intensity; therefore, small lesions confined to the endometrium can be detected only by demonstration of an increased thickness or lobulation of the uterine cavity (Figs. 6.7, 6.8). In some cases, however, tumors are of a lower signal intensity than the remaining normal endometrium, facilitating their detection. This limitation of unenhanced T1- or T2-weighted spin-echo MR imaging can in part be overcome by the use of Gd-DTPA. Following injection of Gd-DTPA, the endometrial carcinoma demonstrates an enhancement similar to or lower than that of the myometrium and less than that of the endometrium (Figs. 6.9, 6.10). The contrast between tumor and endometrium is therefore improved. Furthermore, while a nonenhanced scan often cannot differentiate between retained debris (e.g., hematometra, pyometra) and tumor as the cause for an enlarged uterus, this distinction is possible after Gd-DTPA administration, leading to an overall improvement in tumor evaluation, including tumor depiction and assessment of tumor growth pattern and location.

The MR staging classification for endometrial carcinoma can follow the guidelines in respect of surgical staging. Imaging is not applicable to stage 0 (Tis) cancer. In stage I endometrial carcinoma, the tumor is confined to the uterine corpus. Stage I tumors are further divided into stage Ia (tumor confined to the endometrium), stage Ib (tumor invasion to the inner half of the myometrium), and stage Ic (tumor invasion extending into the outer half of the myometrium). Tumors are considered to be confined to the endometrium when the junctional zone is preserved or there is a sharp tumor–myometrium interface. Stage Ib disease is indicated by disruption of the junctional zone with an irregular myometrial–endometrial interface and/or by increased tumor signal intensity in the inner half of the myometrium.

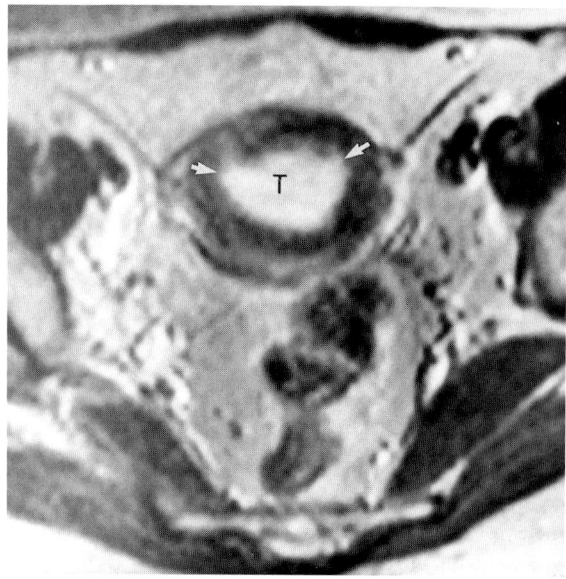


**Fig. 6.8.** Axial SE T2-weighted MR image shows a central area of high signal intensity corresponding to neoplastic tissue which infiltrates the inner layer of myometrium (*arrows*)

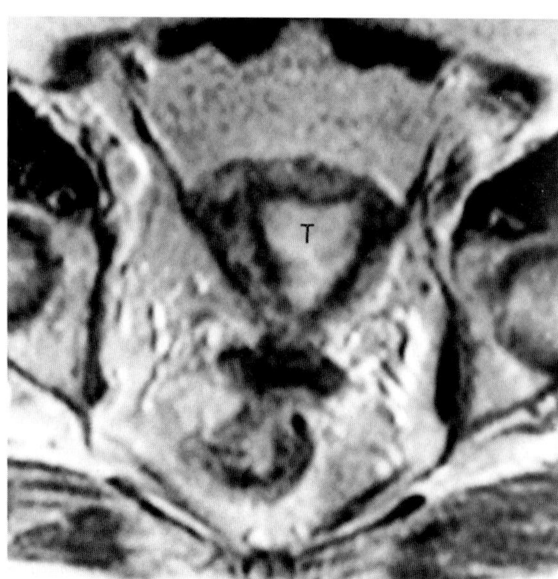


**Fig. 6.7.** Axial SE T2-weighted MR image shows a large endometrial tumor (*T*) limited to the endometrium. The junctional zone of low signal intensity appears to be intact, and no myometrial invasion is present

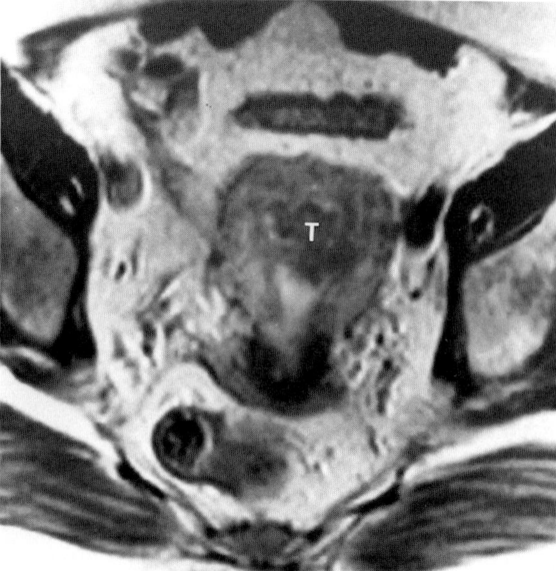


**Fig. 6.9.** Axial SE T1-weighted gadolinium-enhanced MR image shows an endometrial tumor (*T*) and infiltration of the inner myometrum on the left side

Deep myometrial invasion is suggested by high signal intensity tumor extending in the outer half of the myometrium. An accuracy rate of 82% has been reported by an NCI multicenter study in the differentiation between superficial and deep myometrial invasion (Hricak et al. 1991b).

Stage II endometrial cancer is diagnosed when the tumor extends into the cervix. The differentiation between stage IIa disease (cervical stroma not invaded) and stage IIb disease (cervical stroma invaded) is possible by MR imaging. The uninvolved cervical stroma in stage IIa disease remains of low signal intensity on T2-weighted images.

Magnetic resonance imaging can also be used in the evaluation of stage III and stage IV disease. The bladder and rectum are considered to be invaded when their wall demonstrates focal or diffuse loss of normal low signal intensity on T2-weighted images. The accuracy of MR imaging in the detection of lymph nodes relies on assessment of nodal size; MR imaging cannot distinguish between malignant and hyperplastic nodes, nor can it diagnose malignant disease within nodes of normal size.

The reported overall staging accuracy for MR imaging is between 83% and 92%. The usefulness of MR imaging in staging endometrial cancer, including direct tumor visualization, assessment of the depth of myometrial invasion, and detection of extrauterine tumor spread, has been established. Indications for the use of MR imaging include patients in whom physical examination is limited by obesity, patients who are unsuitable for surgical FIGO staging, and patients in whom the extend of tumor may alter the surgical approach. MR imaging is also useful in monitoring patients before and after radiotherapy.

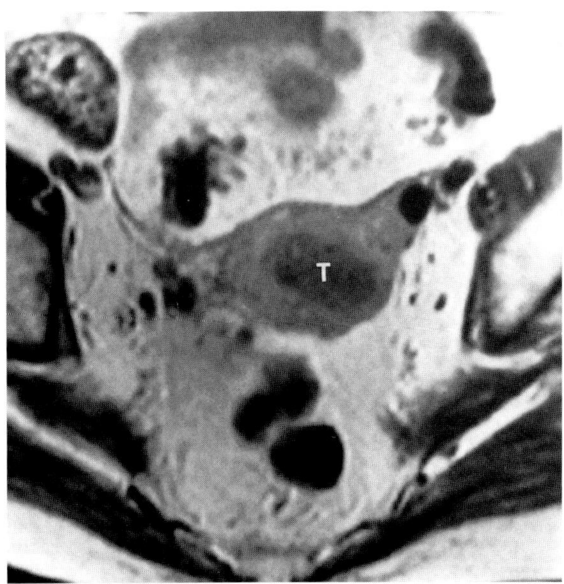


**Fig. 6.10.** Axial SE T1-weighted gadolinium-enhanced MR image shows a large endometrial tumor (*T*) limited to the endometrium

## 6.4 Conclusions

Cure of endometrial carcinoma is based on early identification of the tumor and on correct staging of the disease. When the tumor is infiltrating the myometrium only superficially or when there is no myometrial involvement, surgery can be limited to hysterectomy because the likelihood of lymph node invasion is very low. Conversely, when myometrial involvement is deep, a lymph node dissection is usually performed.

The diagnosis of myometrial carcinoma is usually not initially made by sonography or MR imaging. A cytologic evaluation of endometrial lavage or a uterine curettage is recommended for the diagnosis of endometrial cancer in any women with abnormal uterine bleeding, particularly after the menopause (Berman et al. 1980). However, identification of a thickened endometrium on TVS calls for further evaluation and may lead to the detection of endometrial carcinoma (Granberg et al. 1991; Goldstein et al. 1990).

The main purpose of abdominal sonography is the detection of distant metastases (liver, lymph nodes) and of bulky pelvic disease outside the uterus.

Transvaginal sonographic examination and MR imaging are accurate in the evaluation of the depth of myometrial involvement particularly in young patients, in whom the myometrium is relatively thick and the hypoechoic halo or the junctional zone is easily detected. In older patients and in patients with other pathologic conditions such as myomas or endometrial polyps, imaging evaluation is less accurate.

In a previous study (Del Maschio et al. 1993) we compared the accuracy of staging patients with endometrial carcinoma with TVS and with MR imaging, according to the staging classification of the International Federation of Gynecology and Obstetrics: stage la-tumor limited to endometrium; stage Ib-invasion of less than half of the myometrium; stage Ic-invasion of more than half of the myometrium. The results were analyzed using the

McNemar test, the chi-square test, and 95% confidence intervals. Histologic examination showed that four of the 34 patients had tumors confined to the endometrium (stage la), 12 had involvement of the inner half of the myometrium (stage Ib), and 18 had involvement of the outer half of the myometrium (stage Ic). Overall staging based on sonography was correct in 22 cases (sensitivity for staging, 65%). Four tumors (12%) were understaged and eight (24%) were overstaged. Staging based on MR findings was correct in 24 cases (sensitivity for staging, 71%). Four tumors (12%) were understaged and six (18%) were overstaged. Statistical analysis with the McNemar test revealed that the overall staging sensitivity of TVS and MR imaging were not significantly different.

In our opinion TVS and MR imaging are quite accurate in detecting patients with no myometrial involvement who can be cured with simple hysterectomy, but are less accurate in the precise determination of the depth of myometrial invasion. On the other hand, MR imaging is particularly useful when higher stages of disease are examined, particularly during follow-up after chemo- or radiotherapy.

Regarding the evaluation of pelvic and para-aortic lymph nodes, MR imaging is superior to transabdominal sonography, especially in obese patients. However, MR imaging can detect only enlarged lymph nodes, i.e., it is unable to detect pathologic changes in normal-sized lymph nodes.

In conclusion, even though the diagnosis of endometrial carcinoma must be confirmed on cytologic or histologic specimens, TVS may indicate that this diagnosis is likely on the basis of a thickened endometrium in the appropriate clinical setting. The staging of a young patient can be done with transabdominal and transvaginal sonography. After these examinations, the patient can undergo surgery for diagnostic and therapeutic purposes. In the case of obese elderly women, staging is better done using contrast-enhanced MR imaging, which permits more accurate local and nodal evaluation and thus may avoid unnecessary surgery.

## References


Belloni C, Vigano R, Del Maschio A, Sironi S, Taccagni GL, Vignali M (1990) Magnetic resonance imaging in endometrial carcinoma staging. Gynecol Oncol 37:172–177

Berman ML, Ballan SC, La Gasse LK, Watring WG (1980) Prognosis and treatment of endometrial cancer. Am J Obstet Gynecol 136:679–688

Bohm-Velez M, Mendelson EB (1992) Transvaginal sonography: applications, equipment, and technique. In: Nyberg DA, Hill LM, Bohm-Velez M, Mendelson EB (eds) Transvaginal Ultrasound. Mosby Year Book, St. Louis, pp 1–20

Boronow RC, Morrow CP, Creasman WT, et al. (1984) Surgical staging in endometrial cancer: clinical-pathological findings of a prospective study. Obstet Gynecol 63:825–832

Bourne TH, Campbell S, Whitehead MI, et al. (1990) Detection of endometrial cancer in postmenopausal women by transvaginal ultrasonography and colour flow imaging. BMJ 30:369

Bourne TH, Campbell S, Steer CV, et al. (1991) Detection of endometrial cancer by transvaginal ultrasonography with color flow imaging and blood flow analysis: a preliminary report. Gynecol Oncol 40:253–259

Brown JJ, Thurnher S, Hricak H (1990) MR imaging of the uterus: low signal intensity abnormalities of the endometrium and endometrial cavity. Magn Reson Imaging 8:309–313

Cacciatore B, Lehtovirta P, Wahlstrom T, Ylostalo P (1989) Preoperative sonographic evaluation of endometrial cancer. Am J Obstet Gynecol 60:133–137

Chen SS, Rumancik WM, Spiegel G (1990) Magnetic resonance imaging in stage I endometrial carcinoma. Obstet Gynecol 75:274–277

Cruickshank DJ, Randall JM, Miller ID (1989) Vaginal endosonography in endometrial cancer. Lancet 1:445–446

Deicher U, Hackeloer BJ, Daume E (1986) The sonographic and endocrinologic evaluation of the endometrium in the luteal phase. Hum Reprod 1:219–222

Del Maschio A, Vanzulli A, Sironi S, Spagnolo D, Belloni C, Garancini P, Taccagni GL (1993) Estimating the depth of myometrial involvement by endometrial carcinoma: efficacy of transvaginal sonography vs MR imaging. AJR 160:533–538

Fleischer AC, Kalemeris GC, Entman SS (1986) Sonographic depiction of the endometrium during normal cycles. Ultrasound Med Biol 12:271–277

Fleischer AC, Dudley BS, Entman SS, et al. (1987) Myometrial invasion by endometrial carcinoma: sonographic assessment. Radiology 162:307–310

Fleischer AC, Herebert CM, Hill GA, Kepple DM, Worrel JA (1991) Transvaginal sonography of the endometrium during induced cycles. J Ultrasound Med 10:93–95

Goldstein SR, Nachtigall M, Snyder JR, Nachtigall L (1990) Endometrial assessment by vaginal ultrasonography before endometrial sampling in patients with postmenopausal bleeding. Am J Obstet Gynecol 163:119–123

Gordon AN, Fleischer AC, Dudley BS, et al. (1989) Preoperative assessment of myometrial invasion of endometrial adenocarcinoma by sonography (US) and magnetic resonance imaging (MR). Gynecol Oncol 34:174–179

Gordon AN, Fleischer AC, Reed GW (1990) Depth of myometrial invasion in endometrial cancer: preoperative assessment by transvaginal ultrasonography. Gynecol Oncol 39:321–327

Granberg S, Wikland M, Karlsson B, et al. (1991) Endometrial thickness as measured by endovaginal ultrasonography for identifying endometrial abnormality. Am J Obstet Gynecol 164:47–52

Hirano Y, Kubo K, Hirai Y, et al. (1992) Preliminary experience with gadolinium-enhanced dynamic MR imaging for uterine neoplasms. Radiographics 12:243–256

Hricak H (1991) Carcinoma of the female reproductive organs. Value of cross-sectional imaging. Cancer 67(Suppl 4):1209–1218

Hricak H, Stern JL, Fisher MR, et al. (1987) Endometrial carcinoma staging by MR imaging. Radiology 162:297–305

Hricak H, Hamm B, Semelka RC, et al. (1991a) Carcinoma of the uterus: use of gadopentetate dimeglumine in MR imaging. Radiology 181:95–106

Hricak H, Rubinstein L, Gherman GM, Karstaedt N (1991b) MR imaging evaluation of endometrial carcinoma: results of an NCI cooperative study. Radiology 179:829–832

Hricak H, Finck S, Honda G, Goranson H (1992) MR imaging in the evaluation of benign uterine masses: value of gadopentetate dimeglumine-enhanced T1 weighted images. AJR 158:1048–1050

Javitt MC, Stein HL, Lovecchio JL (1987) MRI in staging of endometrial and cervical carcinoma. Magn Reson Imaging 5:83–92

Lewit N, Thaler I, Rottem S (1990) The uterus: a new look with transvaginal sonography. JCU J Clin Ultrasound 18:331–336

Lien HH, Blomlie V, Tropé C, Kaern J, Abeler VM (1991) Cancer of the endometrium: value of MR imaging in determining depth of invasion into the myometrium. AJR 157:1221–1223

Malpani A, Singer J, Wolverson MK, Merenda G (1990) Endometrial hyperplasia: value of endometrial thickness in ultrasonographic diagnosis and clinical significance. J Clin Ultrasound 18:173–177

Mendelson EB, Bohm-Velez M, Joseph N, Neiman HL (1988) Endometrial abnormalities: evaluation with transvaginal sonography. AJR 150:139–142

Sironi S, Mellone R, Vanzulli A, et al. (1989) Myometrial infiltration in stage I–II (FIGO) endometrial carcinoma. MR (1.5 T) accuracy. Radiol Med (Torino) 77:386–390

Teefey SA, Stahl JA, Middleton WD, et al. (1996) Local staging of endometrial carcinoma: comparison of transvaginal and intraoperative sonography and gross visual inspection. AJR 166:547–552

Welker BG, Gembruch U, Diedrick K, al-Hasani S, Krebs D (1989) Transvaginal sonography of the endometrium during ovum pickup in stimulated cycles for vitro fertilization. J Ultrasound Med 8:549–553

Yazigi R, Cohen J, Munoz AK, Sandstad J (1989) Magnetic resonance imaging determination of myometrial invasin in endometrial carcinoma. Gynecol Oncol 34:94–97

# 7 Assessment of Therapeutic Response and Recurrence of Malignancies of the Female Pelvis

K.H. KIM

CONTENTS



## 7.1 Introduction

The monitoring of the response of malignancies of the female pelvis to treatment is a central issue in oncology. Assessment of tumor size and extent of invasion is crucial in planning the further treatment of recurrent pelvic malignancies.

To evaluate tumor response and to detect recurrence, most previous studies have relied on the results of gynecologic examination. However, the estimation of disease extent by pelvic examination may be limited and difficult due to induration of the pelvic floor in patients who have undergone radical hysterectomy or radiation therapy. Conventional radiographic evaluation including excretory urography and barium enema examination does not aid in post-treatment assessment due to the inaccuracy of these techniques in detecting early pelvic recurrence.

## 7.2 Imaging Modalities

Over the past decade, evaluation of the female pelvis has greatly improved with the advances in ultrasonography (US), computed tomography (CT), and magnetic resonance imaging (MRI). The choice of imaging modality depends on the information required, the equipment available, local expertise, and patient and physician preference.

### 7.2.1 Ultrasonography

Although pelvic US remains a standard diagnostic procedure for the examination of patients with pelvic masses, the diagnostic value is limited in patients with previous radical hysterectomy (SQUILLACI et al. 1988). An accurate study is not possible in the postoperative patient due to inadequate bladder filling, which precludes proper through-transmission, descending bowel loops, which impede ultrasonic transmission (Fig. 7.1), and scar tissue, which decreases the quality of the image (HEIKEN and LEE 1985). In recurrent ovarian cancer, abdominal US has not been shown to be superior to rectal or vaginal examination in the detection of metastases (BUIST et al. 1994). Furthermore, the detection of peritoneal metastases with US is often very difficult.

Endovaginal sonography is gaining acceptance as a reliable technique for evaluating postmenopausal bleeding and screening for pelvic malignancy. It has not, however, proved useful in determining the

K.H. KIM, MD, Director, Department of Diagnostic Radiology, Korea Cancer Center Hospital, 215-4 Gongneung-dong, Nowon-gu, Seoul, 139-706, Korea

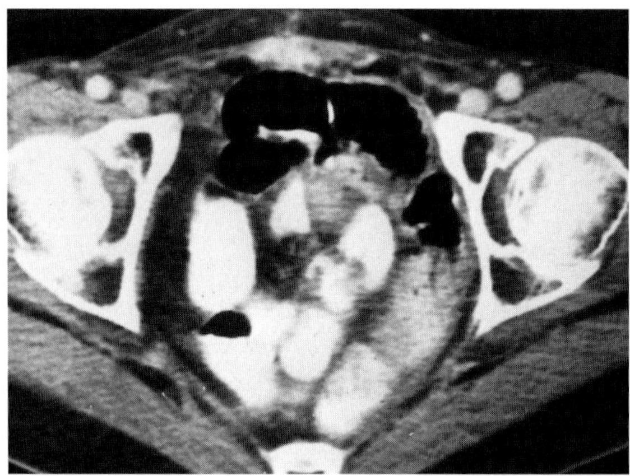

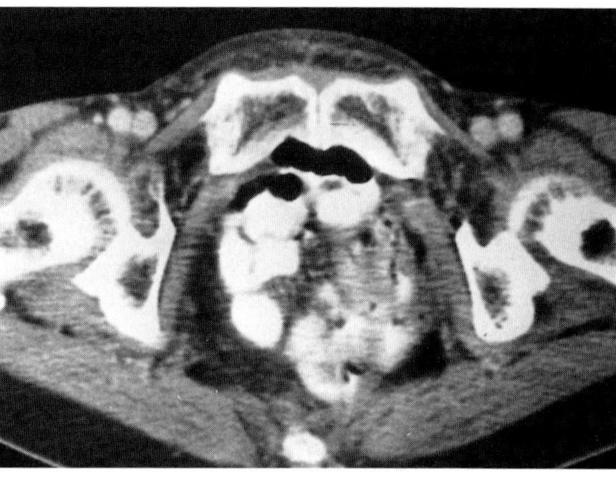

**Fig. 7.1 a,b.** A 52-year-old woman who underwent total exenteration for recurrent cervical carcinoma. **a** Axial contrast-enhanced CT demonstrates small bowel loops in the pelvic cavity filled with oral contrast medium. The lateral margin of the pelvic side wall is smooth, without any tumor mass. **b** CT at a lower level shows no pelvic organs such as the bladder or rectum. The small bowel abuts the posterior margin of the symphysis pubis

presence of recurrent disease after total hysterectomy or in evaluating lymph node metastases.

Nevertheless, US is relatively easy to perform and can be useful in confirming the findings of physical examination. US is an alternative imaging technique in the thin patient to detect a central pelvic or side wall mass, pelvic adenopathy, and hydronephrosis. Transrectal US has been reported to be useful in the evaluation of patients for recurrent pelvic neoplasms (SQUILLACI et al. 1988).

### 7.2.2 Computed Tomography

Computed tomography is the imaging method of choice for the detection of recurrent pelvic malignancies. The roles of CT in evaluating pelvic malignancies after treatment are to monitor tumor response, to detect metastases in unsuspected and clinically inaccessible areas, to evaluate the extent of recurrence, and to assist in assessment of the resectability of recurrent tumor (WALSH et al. 1981; REUTER et al. 1989; JOHNSON 1993).

Abundant oral contrast medium must be given to the patient to adequately opacify the gastrointestinal tract so that unopacified bowel loops are not mistaken for recurrent tumor (Fig. 7.1). Intravenous contrast medium is helpful in differentiating vascular structures from lymphadenopathy and the advent of thin-section CT has increased the overall accuracy in the detection of recurrent disease (BUY et al. 1988; REUTER et al. 1989).

Computed tomography has limited ability to distinguish radiation fibrosis from recurrent tumor, such as when defining the underlying cause of ureteral obstruction (WALSH et al. 1981). In equivocal cases, CT-guided percutaneous biopsy should be performed to differentiate between these conditions.

In uterine cancer, tumor volume assessment by CT is hindered by the similarity of attenuation values for tumor and normal uterus. This is exacerbated by the problem of imaging an obliquely positioned organ in the axial plane. The latter makes it difficult to detect tumor invasion of the lower uterus or upper vagina (HAWNAUR et al. 1994). CT is inadequate for detecting bladder or rectal involvement of recurrent disease, so cystoscopy and sigmoidoscopy are necessary to establish tissue diagnosis (WALSH et al. 1981).

A baseline study after initial radiation therapy can be helpful for comparison to reduce the false-positive rate of CT when patients have symptoms suggesting recurrent disease.

The use of cross-sectional images in the preoperative evaluation of ovarian cancer is controversial and not universally accepted. However, in the postsurgical assessment of residual disease and in the evaluation of response to subsequent therapy, CT remains the primary imaging modality (REUTER et al. 1989; JOHNSON 1993).

### 7.2.3 Magnetic Resonance Imaging

Magnetic resonance imaging has the benefit of a large field of view, high contrast with T2-weighted images, lack of ionizing radiation, and direct multiplanar imaging capability. Hence it is able to demonstrate lesions in locations that are obscure even for CT (Kim et al. 1990; Sironi et al. 1991). MRI provides not only valuable information in the assessment of changes in signal intensity and extent of tumor but also an assessment of the adjacent soft tissue that is inaccessible to clinical examination (Ramsey and Zacharias 1985; Sugimura et al. 1990; Stevens et al. 1990). MRI can demonstrate pelvic recurrences, which may invade the pelvic floor and pelvic side walls, more effectively than can CT, and frequently it is capable of showing more extensive disease. This information may be helpful for determining the optimal approach to management (Williams et al. 1989).

Magnetic resonance imaging is limited by chemical shift artifacts, which may significantly impair the image quality, most prominently along the urinary bladder. It is possible, however, to avoid this artifact at the region of interest by changing the direction of the frequency-encoding gradient. Although sagittal images demonstrate well the relationship of the pelvic organs, it may be difficult to interpret the image when the uterus is tilted to one side. Axial images avoid this but they have the problem of partial volume averaging, which may be lessened by adequate distention of the urinary bladder, so that the axis of the uterus becomes perpendicular to the imaging plane (Kim et al. 1990).

## 7.3 Normal Post-treatment Changes

In evaluating the pelvic cavity in patients who have undergone hysterectomy or radiation therapy, it is essential to understand the surgical procedure, the postoperative anatomy, and radiation changes as reflected on imaging. Many changes in the postoperative and irradiated pelvis can be recognized with CT or MRI.

### 7.3.1 Postoperative Change

Simple hysterectomy results in a very high likelihood of cure in cervical carcinoma of stage Ib or less. More advanced lesions, when confined to the uterus, can usually be treated by radical hysterectomy. The operation involves removal of the uterus, the upper third of the vagina, the entire uterosacral and uterovesical ligaments, and the entire parametrium on each side. It also includes pelvic node dissection including the ureteral, obturator, hypogastric, and iliac chains (Mezrich 1994). The primary treatment of endometrial carcinoma is total abdominal hysterectomy and bilateral salpingo-oophorectomy with or without radiation therapy. In addition, extirpation of the involved nodes combined with postoperative irradiation can lead to good local control (Yamashita et al. 1993). A definitive staging procedure for ovarian carcinoma requires total abdominal hysterectomy with bilateral salpingo-oophorectomy and surgical cytoreduction (Wagner et al. 1994). Most patients with stage III or IV ovarian carcinomas undergo second-look laparotomy after chemotherapy to assess whether residual disease is present, although this procedure is controversial (Hoskins 1993). Pelvic exenteration, performed in patients with recurrent disease, consists in radical hysterectomy, lymph node dissection, removal of the bladder (anterior exenteration), removal of the rectosigmoid colon (posterior exenteration), or both (total exenteration).

After hysterectomy the vaginal cuff is located posterior to the bladder and anterior to the rectum at the level of the acetabula. It has a roughly rectangular or oblong shape and should be symmetric and sharply marginated from the surrounding fat. The upper limit of normal size of the vaginal cuff is 2.1 cm in the anteroposterior diameter (Squillaci et al. 1988). The bladder and small intestine occupy the space just superior to the vaginal cuff.

Postoperative hematomas, lymphoceles, abscesses, fistulas, and venous thromboses can be detected and characterized with CT or MRI (Fig. 7.2). Lymphoceles develop over months after lymphadenectomy and manifest as sharply marginated cystic masses along the lymphatic chains. Postoperative abscesses appear as irregularly enhancing masses with infiltrative borders; typical tubo-ovarian abscesses have a different multicystic appearance.

### 7.3.2 Postradiation Change

The development of high-energy megavoltage beams and intracavitary irradiation techniques has improved the effects of radiation therapy. The aim of radiation therapy is to precisely deliver a uniform dose to the tumor, but radiation is invariably associated with damage to normal tissue (Hricak et al. 1993).

Radiation changes are dependent on the radiation dose delivered and time elapsed since radiation

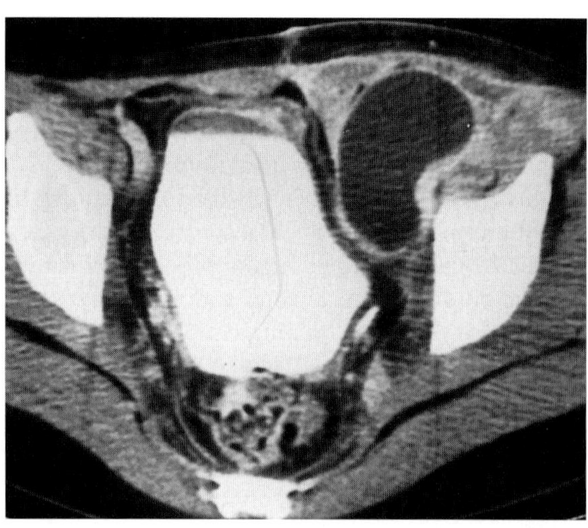

**Fig. 7.2.** A 28-year-old woman with a history of radical hysterectomy for cervical carcinoma. Contrast-enhanced axial CT shows a well-defined ovoid mass with fluid density just anterior to the left external iliac vein, representing a typical site and shape of lymphocele

therapy (SUGIMURA et al. 1990. STEVENS et al. 1990). The total incidence of radiation damage is about 2%–5% (TAYLOR et al. 1990), which increases as the dose surpasses 4500 cGy (HRICAK 1994). Large bowel damage is seen from 6 months to 20 years after treatment, while urinary tract injuries appear in 1–3 years (TAYLOR et al. 1990).

The dose received by each organ during intracavitary treatment is related to its proximity to the radiation source. The close relationship of the bladder, ureters, rectosigmoid, and pelvic small bowel to the uterus explains the high incidence of damage to these structures (TAYLOR et al. 1990).

Changes are typically seen in rapidly renewing tissue and are caused by a combination of the effects of radiation on the endothelium and on stromal cells (SUGIMURA et al. 1990). Individual variation exists in the development of tissue toxicity and symptoms vary from mild damage without symptoms to severe damage with life-threatening episodes (SUGIMURA et al. 1990). The severity of the radiation injury is not related to the interval from the start of therapy. Prior surgery or chemotherapy can increase the risk of radiation toxicity (HRICAK 1994).

Radiation changes can be divided into acute (up to several weeks after therapy) and chronic (more than 1 year after therapy) depending on the time elapsed since radiation therapy. An acute reaction results in symptoms similar to cystitis and enteritis and is self-limiting as the mucosal injuries heal in 4–6 weeks. Such a reaction is caused by endarteritis resulting in the formation of interstitial edema and congestion. Damage to the stroma of tissues results in weakening of tissue integrity that can cause acute necrosis with ulceration and perforation. A minority of patients develop bowel obstruction or perforation during this phase (TAYLOR et al. 1990). Chronic changes are caused by ischemia and subsequent fibrosis, resulting in fibrotic stricture (HRICAK 1994).

Conventional imaging modalities cannot detect acute radiation changes, whereas chronic fibrotic changes such as radiation-induced strictures of the gastrointestinal and urinary tracts are easily recognized (TAYLOR et al. 1990).

Radiation-induced changes affect many organs corresponding to the radiation port: the urinary bladder and rectum, uterosacral ligament, presacral space, adipose tissue, skeletal muscle, and bone marrow. The sensitivity of individual organs to radiation is variable. The small bowel is more radiosensitive than the rectosigmoid, and the ureter and bladder are relatively radioresistant (TAYLOR et al. 1990). These differences mean that the presence or absence of damage to one organ cannot serve as a basis on which to predict the state of other organs.

Magnetic resonance imaging is superior to other modalities in demonstrating radiation-induced changes in all pelvic tissues (ARRIVE et al. 1989; KRESTIN et al. 1988; HRICAK 1994). The radiological changes in individual organs and systems are described below.

#### *7.3.2.1* *Genital Organs*

The mechanism of uterine changes is a direct radiation effect on the uterus and ovarian hypofunction that causes reduced hormonal stimulation (SUGIMURA et al. 1990; ARRIVE et al. 1989).

The radiation changes of the uterus are observed as early as 3 months after the treatment and are characterized by bilateral poorly defined irregular parametrial "whiskers" without pelvic side wall extension (WALSH 1992). The irradiated uterus may show a decrease in size and a loss of zonal anatomy of the corpus and cervix. Both myometrium and endometrium undergo atrophy and demonstrate a diffuse decrease in signal intensity on T2-weighted images (ARRIVE et al. 1989). The cervix shows a wide cervical canal and hyperintense stroma, correlating with radiation-induced inflammatory changes (HRICAK et al. 1993).

The wall of the vagina shows an increased signal intensity on T2-weighted images in the acute phase, probably as a result of edema and inflammation (Fig. 7.10b) (HRICAK 1994). In the chronic phase, however, the vagina is atrophic and its wall demonstrates homogeneous low signal intensity. Finally the development of fibrosis results in low signal intensity of the vagina on all image sequences (SUGIMURA et al. 1990). Constrast study shows enhancement of the vaginal tissue even 2 years after radiation, presumably due to increased capillary permeability and interstitial edema (HRICAK et al. 1993).

In women of reproductive age the radiation effects on the ovaries are as pronounced as those on the uterus. The ovaries become smaller and show a homogeneously decreased signal intensity on T2-weighted images and the follicular cysts become atrophic owing to increased fibrosis and vascular sclerosis (HRICAK 1994).

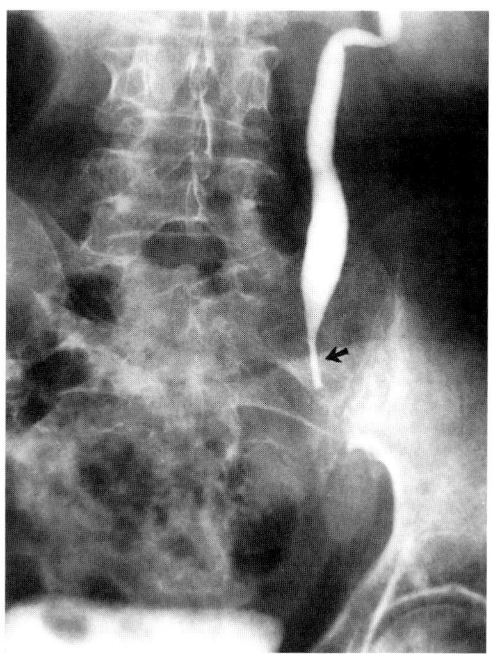

**Fig. 7.3.** An antegrade ureterogram demonstrating the typical concentric narrowing of the ureter (*arrow*) corresponding to the level of external ports. Avascular necrosis and secondary stricture resulted from excessive radiation dose

### *7.3.2.2*
### *Urinary System*

Ureteric strictures due to radiation fibrosis appear smooth and tapered (Fig. 7.3). Their appearance is, however, similar to that of strictures caused by recurrent tumor, and this poses a diagnostic problem. Strictures at the level of the pelvic brim are usually a result of metastases in the iliac lymph nodes (TAYLOR et al. 1990).

Various degrees of radiation change in the urinary bladder can be seen, in correlation with the severity of histologic features. MRI changes will always be detectable in the presence of moderate or severe clinical symptoms, but high signal intensity of the mucosa also can be detected in one-half of asymptomatic patients (SUGIMURA et al. 1990). With more severe radiation injury, the bladder wall increases in thickness when fully distended (Fig. 7.4). MRI demonstrates either uniformly high signal intensity or, characteristically, low signal intensity in its inner layer with high signal intensity at the periphery (SUGIMURA et al. 1990). Bladder wall thickening due to radiation may be difficult to differentiate from other causes such as tumor infiltration, cystitis, or outlet obstruction. The most extreme form of radiation change is the formation of a fistula.

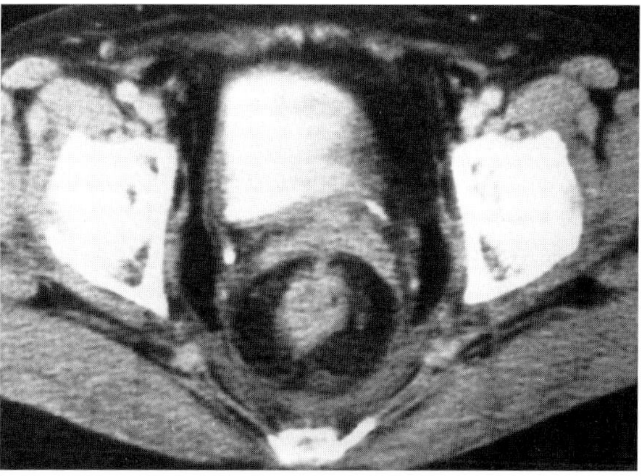

**Fig. 7.4.** A 52-year-old woman who had received radiation therapy for cervical carcinoma. Axial CT shows a diffusely thickened uterosacral ligament and a thickened bladder and rectal wall. The patient had urinary urgency

Contrast-enhanced studies show enhancement of the bladder wall regardless of the cystoscopic or clinical findings of bladder pathology. Such enhancement can be noted for as long as $2^1/_2$ years after irradiation (HRICAK 1994).

Patients treated with radiation are likely to have associated cystitis while those with recurrent tumor are likely to have pelvic pain, but the distinction between these two conditions is difficult (TAYLOR et al. 1990).

### 7.3.2.3
### Rectum and Sigmoid Colon

On barium enema X-ray examination, the presence of a smooth and tapered stricture is the most important finding in the diagnosis of radiation change (Taylor et al. 1990). A smooth muscle relaxant can be used to enhance subtle findings such as segments of minimally reduced caliber.

On MRI, there is initially an increase in the thickness of the rectal wall on T1-weighted images, predominantly involving the submucosal layer. The outer muscle layer retains its normal low signal intensity on T2-weighted images (Sugimura et al. 1990). The changes in the wide presacral space are dependent on the time since radiation. In the acute phase, the presacral space often demonstrates high signal intensity, probably due to edema. In the chronic phase, by contrast, a low signal intensity is predominant on T2-weighted images (Sugimura et al. 1990). As with bladder injury, minor rectal changes also may be seen in an asymptomatic patient. These early changes are more likely to cause rectal urgency and frequency, rather than bleeding, which is a major clinical criterion for the diagnosis of radiation-induced damage (Sugimura et al. 1990).

The effects of pelvic irradiation are most prominent in the perirectal area. There is thickening of the perirectal fascia over 3 mm at the level of the S4–5 vertebral bodies with an increase in the perirectal fat in the subacute and chronic phases (Doubleday and Bernadino 1980; Sugimura et al. 1990). These findings can produce a halo effect about the rectum (Fig. 7.4). A wide presacral space measuring greater than 1 cm consists of a large amount of fat and a lesser amount of fibrous tissue. The symmetrically thickened perirectal fibrous tissue represents postradiation change, while an asymmetric lesion is usually related to recurrent tumor (Fig. 7.13).

### 7.3.2.4
### Pelvic Side Wall

Recognition of the normal changes in the muscle is important when searching for recurrent tumor. The differentiation relies on morphologic changes as well as changes in signal intensity. The normal striated muscle is of medium signal intensity on T1-weighted images and decreases in signal intensity on T2-weighted images. Within 6 months after radiation there is a diffuse, usually bilateral, symmetric, high signal intensity of the muscles on T2-weighted images (Sugimura et al. 1990). In the late phase, the pelvic side wall muscles and other soft tissues of the pelvis show decreased signal intensity. After contrast administration, diffuse enhancement is seen in the muscle of the radiation field (Hricak et al. 1993).

### 7.3.2.5
### Bone and Bone Marrow

After the first year following radiation therapy, demineralization can be seen that often progresses with time (Libshitz 1994). Two to 3 years after therapy, multiple small foci of aseptic necrosis can be observed. With progression, small lytic areas are noted with thickening of the remaining trabecula. If the lytic areas grow larger, the appearance may resemble that of metastatic disease (Libshitz 1994). CT can demonstrate radiation changes, particularly in the pelvis, which are less obvious on conventional radiographs. Osteonecrosis is demonstrated with low signal intensity on T1-weighted images and with heterogeneous high signal intensity on T2-weighted images (Hricak 1994). The lesion is usually focal and can be distinguished from diffuse radiation changes.

The bone marrow demonstrates high signal intensity on T1-weighted images around the radiation port (Fig. 7.5). This alteration in signal intensity is secondary to the replacement of hematopoietic marrow by fatty marrow, which begins as early as 2 weeks after radiation at a dose of approximately 1600 cGy (Ramsey and Zacharias 1985). These changes are permanent in adults, but reversible in children (Stevens et al. 1990). After administration of contrast material, the irradiated bone marrow shows enhancement, especially in the acute phase (Hricak 1994). It is important to differentiate the changes of radiation therapy from other pathologic conditions. Metastatic disease in bones within the irradiated field is extremel unusualy (Libshitz 1994). Tumor replacement of the marrow results in a relatively low signal intensity on T1-weighted images.

### 7.3.2.6
### Fistula

Radiation therapy for cervical cancer is the most frequent factor predisposing to vaginal fistula in

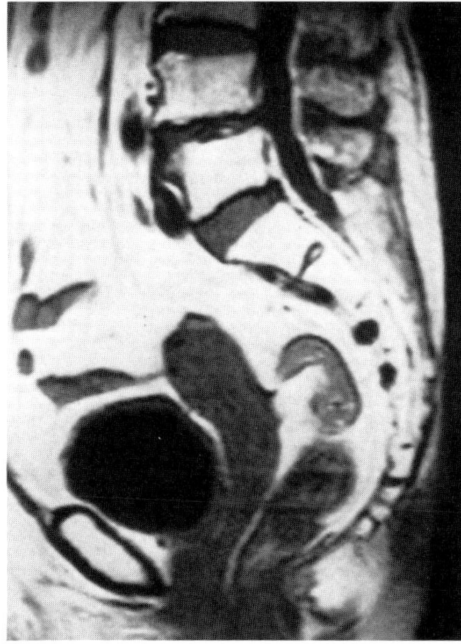

**Fig. 7.5.** A 63-year-old woman with a history of previous radiation therapy for cervical carcinoma. On the sagittal T1-weighted image, bone marrow of the lumbosacral and coccygeal region is replaced by diffuse homogeneous high signal intensity corresponding to the radiation port. The uterus appears small. Note the focal thickening of the posterior bladder wall

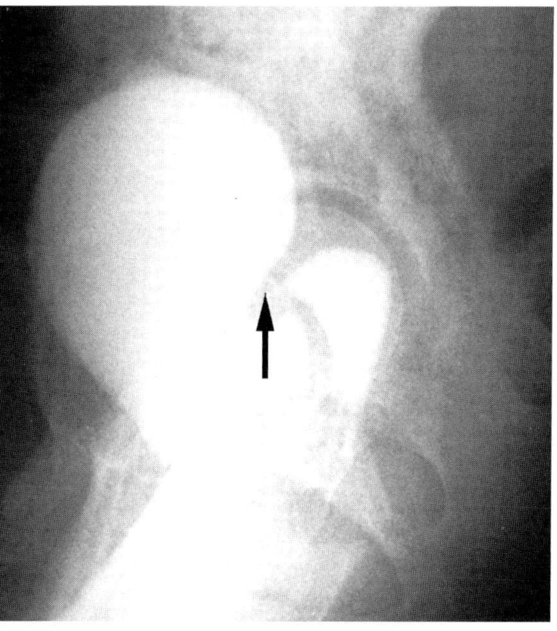

**Fig. 7.6.** A 43-year-old woman with a history of radiation therapy for cervical carcinoma. Lateral view of retrograde cystography shows leakage of contrast medium from the posterior wall of the urinary bladder to the vaginal canal through a narrow fistulous tract (*arrow*)

patients with gynecologic neoplasms: vaginal fistulas develop in 1%–10% of patients so treated (Kuhlman and Fishman 1990). Vesicovaginal and rectovaginal fistulas are the most common types due to the anatomic location of the vagina between the bladder and rectum.

A history of passage of urine, feces, or foul-smelling air through the vagina usually indicates the presence of a rectovaginal or vesicovaginal fistula. However, demonstration of the fistulous tract and its cause is often difficult by conventional radiography (Kuhlman and Fishman 1990). Intravenous urography, cystography, and barium enema X-ray examination may be undertaken to confirm the presence of a fistula, but these studies frequently fail to detect the fistulous tract, because many fistulas are small, tortuous, and obliquely oriented (Fig. 7.6). A further complication is the inability of the bladder to distend after an operation or radiation therapy and the difficulty of performing a barium enema in a painful narrowed rectum. Another limitation of conventional studies is their inability to determine the nature and extent of the extraluminal disease process causing the vaginal fistula, whether resulting from radiation therapy or from recurrent tumor.

Computed tomography is an effective imaging modality for detecting fistulas and their underlying causes. Evaluation of the disease extent on CT may determine not only what kind of surgical repair should be done but also whether surgical repair is possible (Thorvinger et al. 1990).

In suspected cases of enterovaginal fistula, administration of oral contrast medium to opacify distal bowel loops is essential. Intravenous contrast medium is avoided, so that if contrast medium is identified within the vagina, its origin from the bowel can be definitely established. If the rectosigmoid area is not yet opacified, rectal contrast medium can also be given. Delayed scanning is useful in detecting small communications and in demonstrating contrast medium within the vagina.

In a suspected case of vesicovaginal fistula, intravenous contrast medium but no oral contrast medium is administered. Again, delayed scanning has proved helpful in detecting such fistulas. Caution must be applied because contrast medium may spill into the vagina from the bladder in an incontinent patient (Kuhlman and Fishman 1990). Delayed enhanced MRI may help in the detection of fistula, although its efficacy is untested.

## 7.4 Assessment of Therapeutic Response

### 7.4.1 Radiation Therapy

The primary treatment of choice for many pelvic cancers is radiation therapy. MRI has been the most useful tool in assessing the effect of radiation therapy. The value of MRI depends on the time interval between the start of radiation therapy and imaging. The poorest correlation is seen in images obtained 3–6 months after radiation therapy. After radiation therapy, the signal intensity of the tumor decreases due to progressive replacement of the tumor by scar tissue, which is most precipitous during the first 3 months and is almost complete by 6 months (Fig. 7.7) (Flueckiger et al. 1992). Sometimes, the signal intensity still may be relatively high 3 months after radiation therapy due to the presence of residual but devitalized tumor tissue, surrounding tissue edema, bleeding, or prominent inflammation (Flueckiger et al. 1992).

An early decrease in the signal intensity and volume of the tumor indicates a good response to radiation therapy and a high probability of complete regression (Fig. 7.8). Large tumors show a delayed response to radiation therapy. The late response suggests that a decision regarding nonresponsiveness in patients with residual tumor cannot be made until 9 months (Flueckiger et al. 1992).

After tumor regression the newly formed cervix appears as a signal-poor area on T2-weighted images (Fig. 7.7b). Such areas correspond to fibrosis and chronic inflammatory reaction at pathologic examination (Flueckiger et al. 1992). This reconstitution of the thin stripe of cervical stroma is a reliable indicator that the cervix is free of cancer (Kim et al. 1994). In contrast, the presence of a measurable high signal intensity tumor on T2-weighted images indicates recurrence with a probability of 86% (Flueckiger et al. 1992). From a clinical point of view, a recurrent tumor after radiation therapy is defined as renewed tumor growth in a reformed, normally epithelialized ectocervix.

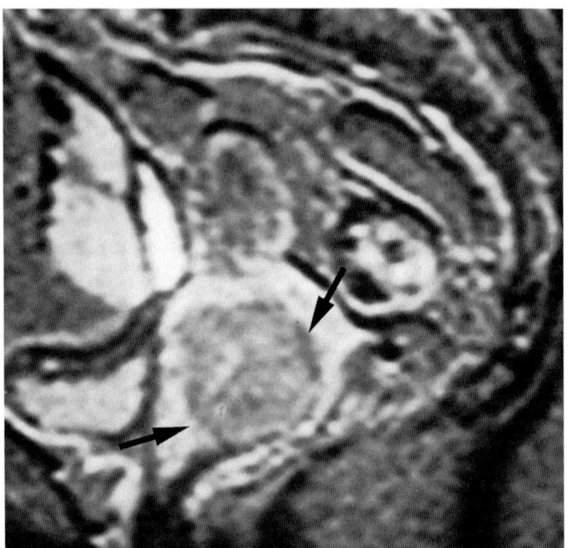
a

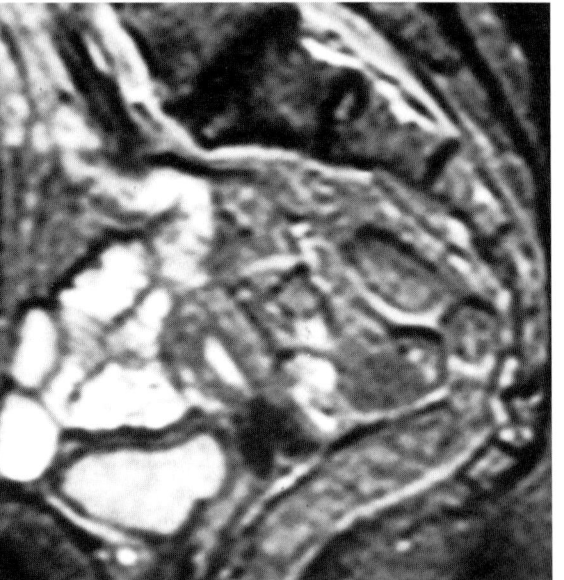
b

**Fig. 7.7 a,b.** A 67-year-old patient with squamous cell carcinoma of the cervix. **a** Sagittal T2-weighted image shows a large tumor (*arrows*) with surrounding high signal intensity presumed to be peritumoral inflammatory reaction. **b** About 4 months after radiation therapy, sagittal T2-weighted image shows almost complete disappearance of the tumor. Low signal intensity of cervical stromal tissue is restored.

### 7.4.2 Postradiation Fibrosis Versus Recurrence

The distinction between recurrent tumor and radiation-induced fibrosis is often difficult and may result in a delay in the diagnosis of recurrent disease.

Follow-up CT in cases of postoperative granuloma or fibrosis shows a progressive decrease in size (Fig. 7.9), while in recurrent tumor the lesion grows with time.

Magnetic resonance imaging is useful in distinguishing recurrent tumor from fibrosis. Fibrosis typically shows low signal intensity on both T1-weighted and T2-weighted images, while recurrent

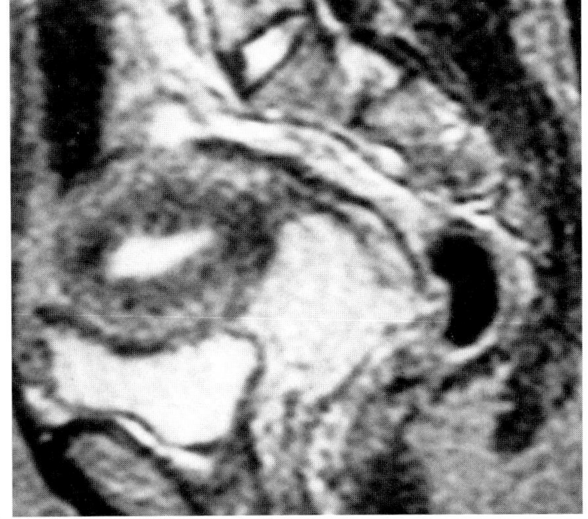

a

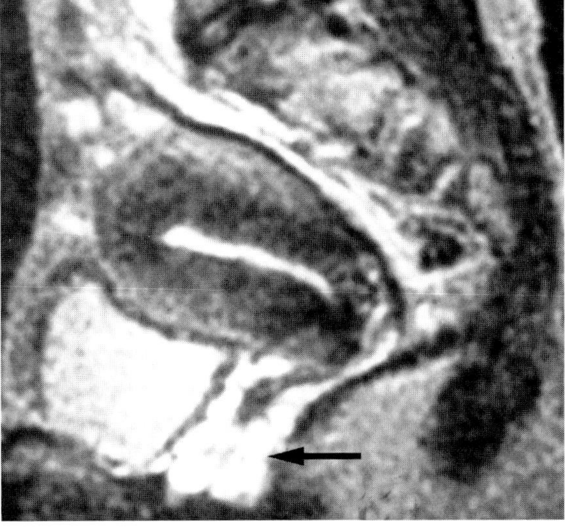

b

**Fig. 7.8 a,b.** A 55-year-old patient with stage IIb cervical carcinoma. **a** Sagittal T2-weighted image shows a homogeneous bulky tumor in the uterine cervix invading the upper vagina and lower uterine segment. **b** No residual tumor is seen on MRI 2 months after radiation therapy. The diffuse wide band of junctional zone in the uterine body represents adenomyosis. Note the very high signal intensity of vaginal tissue (*arrow*) in this early period following radiation therapy

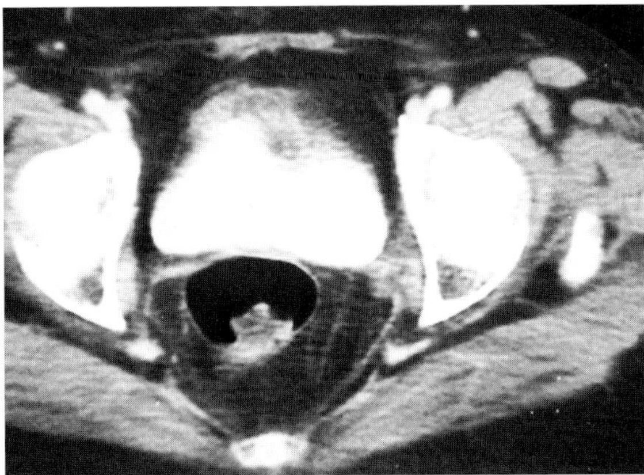

a

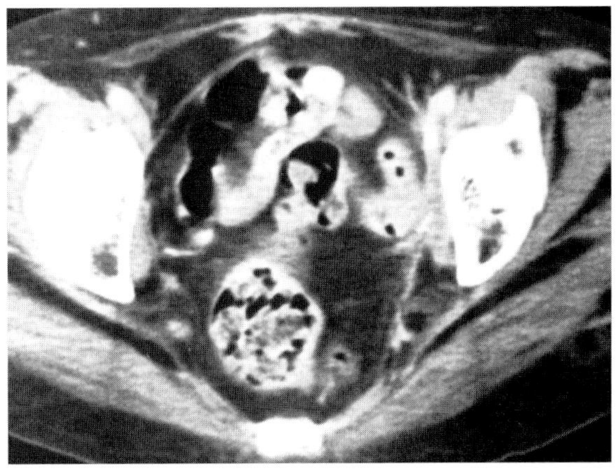

b

**Fig. 7.9 a,b.** A 57-year-old woman who underwent radical hysterectomy for cervical carcinoma. **a** Three months after surgery CT shows a slightly enhancing solid lesion along the left pelvic side wall. **b** Six months later, CT shows a decrease in the extent of the previously noted pelvic side wall lesion without any treatment during the course; this was a benign granulomatous lesion

tumor shows a higher signal intensity than that of the adjacent muscle and fat on T2-weighted images (Ebner et al. 1988). However, there are some difficulties in distinguishing recurrent tumor from radiation changes during the first 6 months after therapy, because early postradiation fibrosis produces high signal intensity on T2-weighted images (Ebner et al. 1988). The accuracy (69% vs 88%) and specificity (46% vs 81%) of MRI for the detection of recurrence are lower in the first 6 months after radiation therapy than more than 6 months thereafter (Hricak et al. 1993). Therefore it is important to know the history of the radiation therapy as well as the expected radiation changes at that point when evaluating for possible recurrent carcinoma.

Diagnosis based on signal intensity alone may be misleading. In some cases the tumor mass may be extremely subtle. If the pelvic fat as a contrasting background is replaced by fibrosis, a mass may not be clearly definable on the T1-weighted images. Similarly, if the fat is acutely radiated, a mass may not be evident on the T2-weighted images. In these cases, chemically fat-suppressed T2-weighted images may help to improve the detectability of the lesion.

Edema and inflammation in scar tissue also show high signal intensity on T2-weighted images and may persist for up to 18 months after surgery or irradiation (HAWIGHORST et al. 1995). Tumor producing a desmoplastic reaction, in contrast, will demonstrate low signal intensity on T2-weighted images.

When necrosis in the peripheral tumor is accompanied by a change in MR signal intensity the diagnosis of recurrent tumor is likely. However, the usefulness of MRI varies with the primary site of the tumor. In cases of infiltrative tumor growth in the rectum or bladder, differentiation may not be accurate (DELANGE et al. 1989; TAVARES et al. 1988). Findings attributed to radiation-induced changes are more frequently demonstrated on MRI rather than is residual tumor (SUGIMURA et al. 1990). There is also a problem in the differentiation between radiation necrosis and tumor recurrence. In patients in whom CT or MRI findings are equivocal, a CT-guided aspiration biopsy is an accurate way to differentiate recurrent tumor from fibrosis (Fig. 7.10).

The problem posed by the coexistence of tumor and fibrosis depends on the amount of interspersed tumor tissue (FLUECKIGER et al. 1992). Low signal intensity on T2-weighted images indicates prominent fibrosis and low cellularity, whereas high signal intensity indicates benign or malignant hypercellularity or edema (DELANGE et al. 1989). In these patients, nests of tumor cells surrounded by dense fibrous tissue cannot be aspirated successfully to confirm recurrence.

### 7.4.3 Systemic and Intra-arterial Chemotherapy

Recent trials of various regimens of neoadjuvant systemic chemotherapy before definitive irradiation for patients with stage IIb and III carcinoma of the cervix have been reported to be effective with high response rates (PARK et al. 1995). In evaluating tumor response following systemic chemotherapy, clinical examination or CT is used to evaluate tumor regression in most cases, but both are imprecise, particularly in the assessment of tumor volume. MRI provides a more valuable, precise estimate of volume than does clinical palpation or coposcopic examination. Tumor volume can be calculated by the product of the anteroposterior, transverse, and craniocaudal diameters of the tumor on T2-weighted images. The tumor response can be classified into four groups according to volume reduction: complete response is defined as total disappearance of tumor; partial response as a more than 50% reduction in tumor volume; minor response as a less than 50% reduction; and progressive disease as an increase in tumor volume (KIM et al. 1994). Correlation between the MRI and the pathologic measurement is good (KIM et al. 1994; HAWNAUR et al. 1994).

a

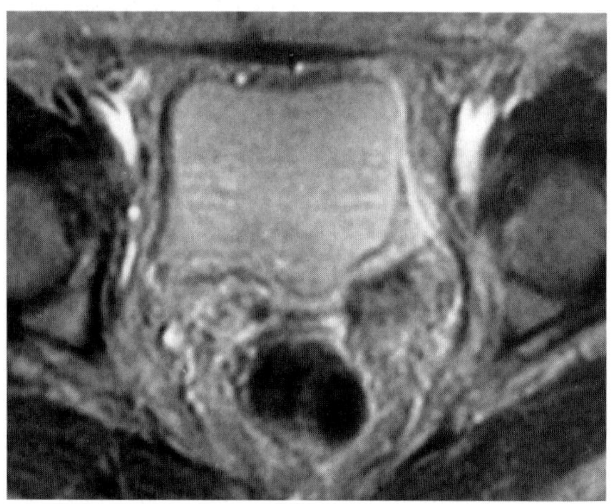

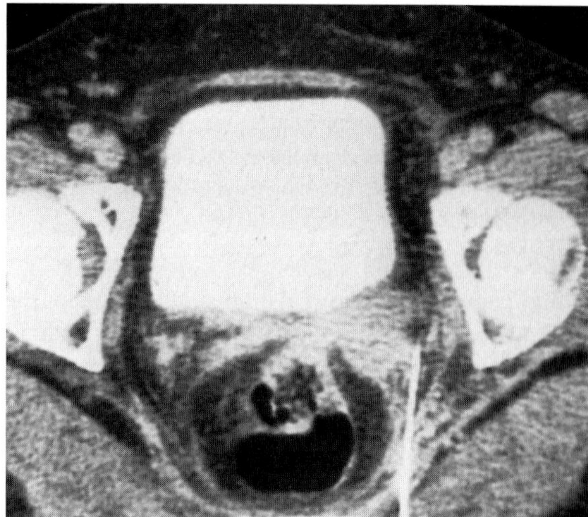

b

**Fig. 7.10 a,b.** A 55-year-old patient with stage Ib cervical carcinoma who had undergone radical hysterectomy. **a** Axial T2-weighted image shows an irregular mass of intermediate signal intensity in the left parametrial region with extension to the ipsilateral pelvic side wall; whether this represents recurrence or fibrosis is uncertain. **b** CT-guided biopsy of the mass was performed, and confirmed the lesion to be recurrent disease

Some discrepancies in absolute values may exist, these being attributable to various factors. MRI measurements may overestimate tumor volume due to the inclusion of inflammatory reaction and edema in addition to neoplastic tissue. Recent cone biopsy produces distortion of normal cervical anatomy on MRI with or without small high signal intensity areas which are difficult to differentiate from residual tumor. It is difficult to define the entire tumor margin in patients during pregnancy, in the postpartum period, or in patients taking the oral contraceptive pill.

Besides tumor volume, tumor volume reduction rate, change in tumor stage, and change in tumor signal intensity can be evaluated on MRI (Fig. 7.11) (Kim et al. 1994).

The tumor signal intensity decreases with tumor regression due to intratumoral necrosis and fibrosis. The necrotic areas show low signal intensity on T2-weighted images and are readily distinguished from high signal intensity of tumor (Sironi et al. 1991). Decreased signal intensity in the regions of necrosis may be related to hemosiderin deposits in necrotic tissue.

Microscopically, ablation or regression of tumor, disappearance of surface ulceration with healing of the epithelium and fibrosis, and areas of chronic inflammatory exudate localized around tumor islands have been noted. In patients with complete response, the areas of previous cancerous tissue show a low signal intensity corresponding to fibrosis and extensive foreign body reaction with an increased tendency for keratinization and foci of calcification (Kim et al. 1994).

Pelvic intra-arterial chemotherapy has been used by many investigators in patients with recurrent cervical carcinoma or inoperable stage IIb uterine cervical carcinoma (Fig. 7.12). This provides higher efficacy and fewer side-effects compared with systemic chemotherapy. Intra-arterial vincristine, mitomycin C, and cisplatin chemotherapy shows an excellent response rate (94.7%) and remarkable tumor volume reduction (88.5%) (Kim et al. 1994). MRI is useful in the assessment of tumor response to intra-arterial chemotherapy and provides criteria for decision-making with regard to further radiation or surgical therapy. On arteriography, vascular change after chemotherapy is not meaningful because most cervical carcinomas do not show hypervascularity. The uterine arteries gradually narrow and uterine vascularity decreases when intra-arterial chemotherapy is repeated. At surgery, most of the pelvic vessels are fragile and oozing is frequent. Pathologic examination reveals arteritis with perivascular

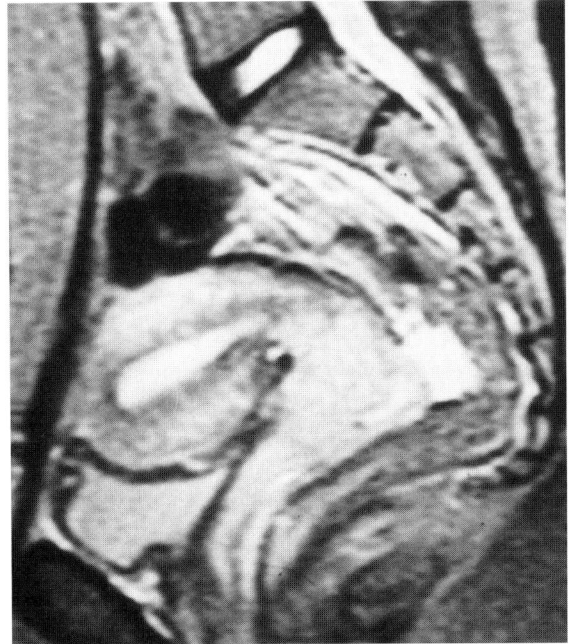

a

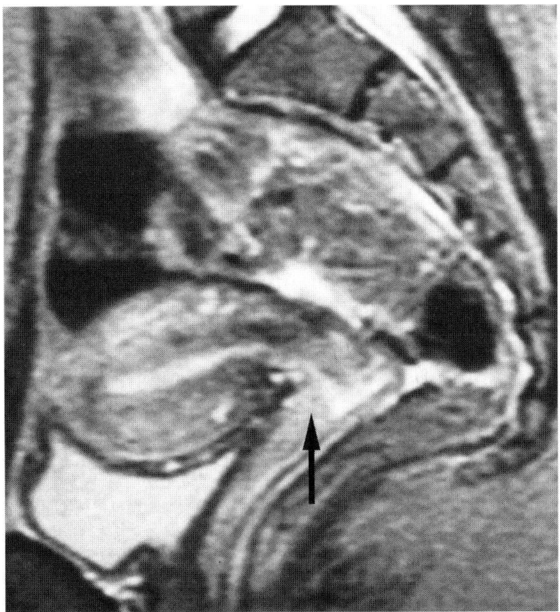

b

**Fig. 7.11 a,b.** A 26-year-old patient with stage IIb cervical carcinoma. **a** Sagittal T2-weighted image showing bulky uterine cervical tumor invading the upper vagina. **b** Two months after systemic chemotherapy including cisplatin, MRI shows a remarkably reduced tumor volume. However, a focal high signal intensity lesion is still noted in the cervical portion (*arrow*). The patient received additional radiation therapy

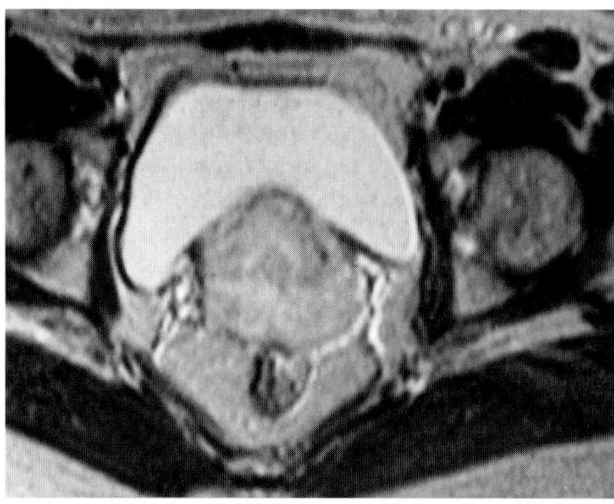

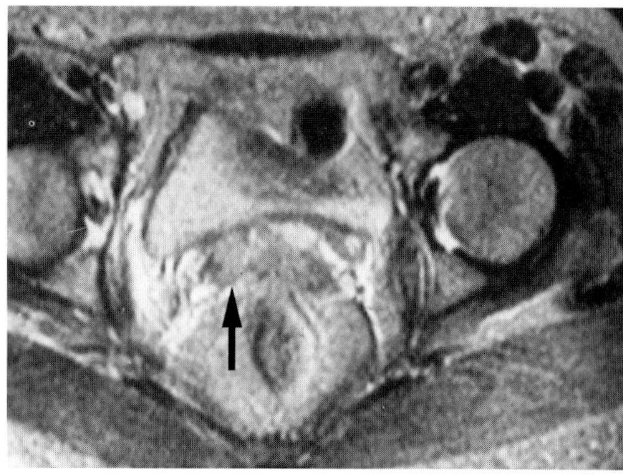

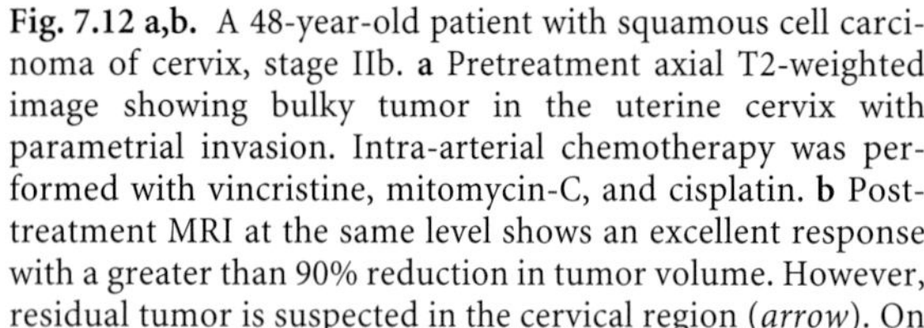

**Fig. 7.12 a,b.** A 48-year-old patient with squamous cell carcinoma of cervix, stage IIb. **a** Pretreatment axial T2-weighted image showing bulky tumor in the uterine cervix with parametrial invasion. Intra-arterial chemotherapy was performed with vincristine, mitomycin-C, and cisplatin. **b** Post-treatment MRI at the same level shows an excellent response with a greater than 90% reduction in tumor volume. However, residual tumor is suspected in the cervical region (*arrow*). On subsequent radical hysterectomy, many tumor emboli were noted within the vascular space in the ecto- and endocervix without any definable mass. The only noted morphologic changes were related to the chemotherapeutic effect, e.g., extensive fibrosis and foreign body reaction. The focal high signal intensity lesion on post-treatment MRI turned out to be inflammatory change

fibrotic change induced by the chemotherapeutic agent (Kim et al. 1994).

## 7.5 Evaluation of Recurrent Malignancies

The most important factors determining the incidence of recurrence in patients with pelvic malignancy are the stage and bulk of disease at presentation. The degree of differentation of the tumor also has an influence on survival. Patients with well-differentiated lesions have a better prognosis than do those with poorly differentiated ones.

Because additional operative or radiation therapy is feasible in patients with recurrent disease, early detection of recurrence is extremely important. Long-term cure can be expected in patients with isolated plevic or vaginal recurrences with appropriate management. It is, therefore, necessary to know the regional extent of tumor recurrence before the institution of therapy (Ng et al. 1992).

### 7.5.1 Recurrent Cervical Carcinoma

Treatment with radical surgery or radiation therapy usually carries a good cure rate. However, approximately 32–35% of patients treated for cervical carcinoma develop a recurrence and 80% of recurrences develop within the first 2 years after treatment (Perez et al. 1983; Flueckiger et al. 1992). This makes the first 2 years following treatment the most important period for the detection of a recurrence.

Most recurrences after radiation therapy occur in patients with large solid tumors, whose hypoxic central zones are relatively radioresistant, or patients with undetected spread to regional lymph nodes. The cardinal symptoms and signs of recurrent cervical carcinoma are low back and sciatic pain, leg edema, and hydronephrosis.

Sites of recurrence may be multiple or single; they are usually confined to the pelvis and are often centrally located. About 7% of patients treated for cervical cancer experience local recurrence at the vaginal stump or pelvic side wall without detectable distant metastases (Perez et al. 1983).

Conventional radiologic modalities, such as urography, barium enema X-ray examination, and endoscopic examinations, allow recurrence to be diagnosed only through indirect signs (Squillaci et al. 1988).

#### *7.5.1.1 Cytologic Study*

Cytologic examination is valuable, inexpensive, and easy to perform. It may provide an early diagnosis of local recurrence, before the onset of clinical signs and symptoms (SHIELD et al. 1991).

Cytologic abnormalities are detected with a correct diagnosis of tumor recurrence in 49% (SHIELD et al. 1991). However, the sensitivity of cytologic examination in the irradiated cervix is disappointingly low, ranging from 28% to 51% (HRICAK et al. 1993). The specificity of postradiation cytology is also low, because postradiation dysplasia, especially within 4 months after the treatment, makes it difficult to discriminate recurrent malignant cells (SHIELD et al. 1991). In addition, cytologic examination has definite limitations: tumor recurrence outside the central pelvis will not be detected, and sampling difficulties may lead to relatively high false-negative rates. A negative result should not, therefore, be considered a reliable indicator of absence of recurrence.

#### 7.5.1.2 Serum Assay for Squamous Cell Carcinoma Antigen

Squamous cell carcinoma antigen (SCC) level in serum has been associated with disease extent and has aided in the detection of recurrent disease (ROSE et al. 1992). SCC levels decline substantially after treatment, as primary tumor regresses.

#### 7.5.1.3 Ultrasonography

Ultrasonography allows the diagnosis only of large-volume recurrences. Therefore, US is not helpful in patients with a small recurrence or an extension to the rectal wall.

Transrectal US has been reported to allow accurate determination of the extent of recurrence and its infiltration into adjacent connective tissues. Transrectal US demonstrates tumor recurrence with a sensitivity of 100%, a specificity of 83.3%, and an overall accuracy of 90.5% (SQUILLACI et al. 1988). Furthermore, it can be used to guide fine-needle biopsy in cases with findings suggestive of recurrence.

The diagnosis can be made when the vaginal cuff is larger than 2.2 cm in anteroposterior diameter, when structural irregularities are found in a normal-sized vaginal cuff, when a hypoechoic mass is seen inside the vaginal cuff, and when there is infiltration of the bladder wall, rectovaginal septum, or parametrium (SQUILLACI et al. 1988). Additionally, transrectal US may show an accumulation of endometrial fluid secondary to stenosis from the recurrent tumor.

#### 7.5.1.4 Computed Tomography

Computed tomography has a sensitivity of 93% and an accuracy of 82% in the diagnosis of recurrent cervical carcinoma (HERON et al. 1988).

The most common CT feature of recurrent tumor is an irregular central pelvic mass between the bladder and the rectum (Figs. 7.13a, 7.14a). Such a tumor may be of homogeneous soft tissue density or may have central low-attenuation areas due to necrosis. Sometimes, enlargement of the cervix is the only criterion used for diagnosing recurrence (WILLIAMS et al. 1989).

The major difficulties encountered with CT are its inability to characterize parametrial change after irradiation. CT suggests radiation fibrosis if the parametria alone are abnormal. CT findings of masses at multiple sites and pelvic side wall extension associated with a parametrial mass are required to make a definitive diagnosis of parametrial recurrence (VICK et al. 1984).

Pelvic side wall extension most commonly occurs in the parametria next to the uterine corpus. Additional lateral extension occurs at the level of the cervix and at the level of the vagina. It is manifested by linear soft tissue strands extending to the obturator internus muscle or confluent solid tumor obliterating fat planes (Fig. 7.13a). However, it may be difficult to distinguish between true invasion and simple contiguity of tumor with the muscle.

In patients treated with radiation therapy, local recurrence of tumor or radiation fibrosis may cause obstruction of the cervical os with subsequent hydrometra, hematometra, or pyometra. The cause of obstruction can be recurrent tumor or radiation fibrosis. The obstruction will appear as a symmetrically enlarged uterus with a low attenuation, nonenhancing central mass on CT scan. The central low attenuation and lack of contrast enhancement help differentiate an obstructed uterus from other causes of uterine enlargement.

Computed tomography has difficulty in confirming a diagnosis of bladder or rectal invasion unless the tumor has penetrated through the serosa and muscularis. The diagnosis of bladder or rectal invasion can only be made with certainty when intraluminal tumor contiguous with extraluminal disease is identified (WALSH et al. 1981).

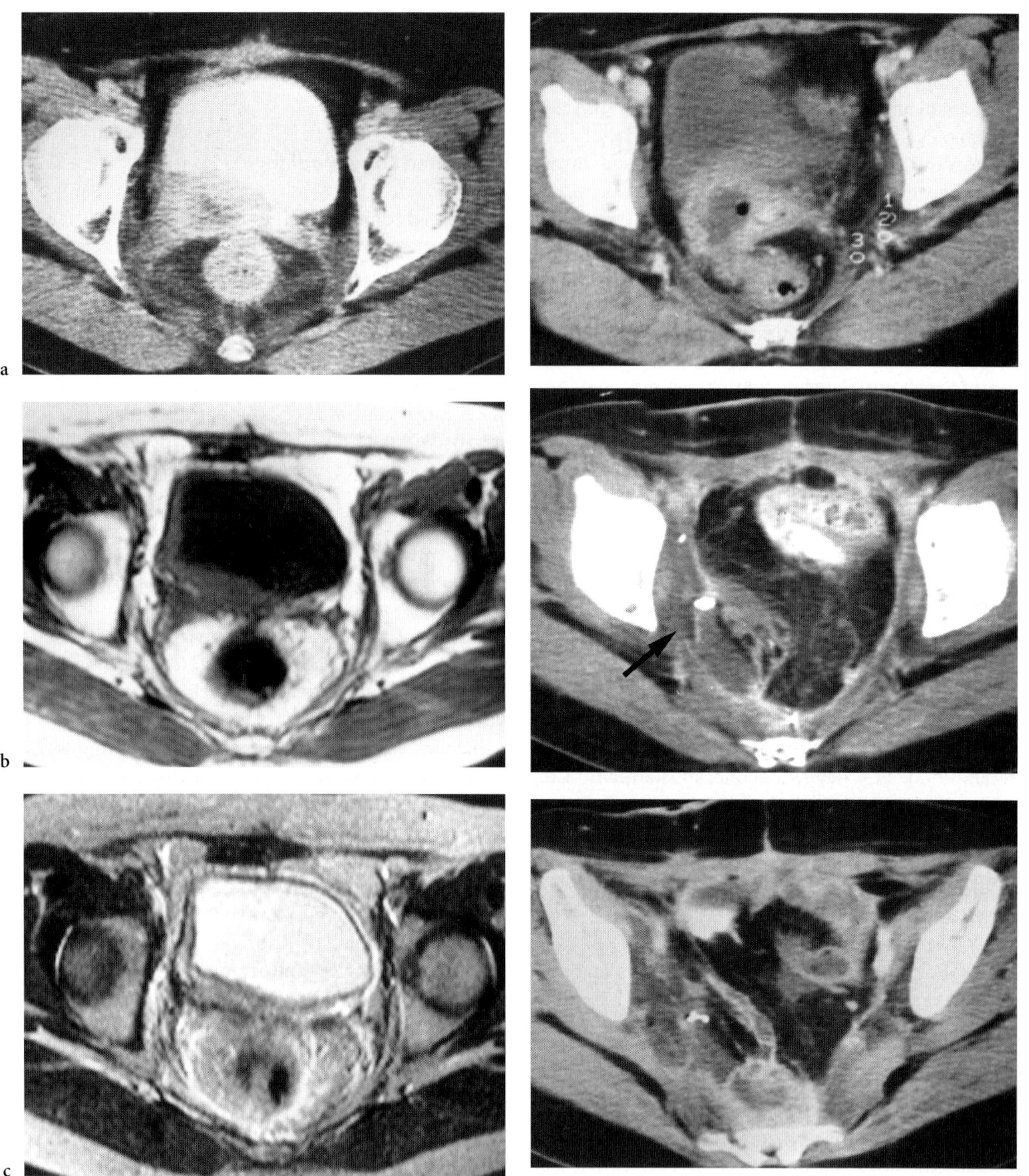

**Fig. 7.13 a–c.** A 56-year-old patient with cervical carcinoma, stage Ib, who underwent radical hysterectomy with additional radiation therapy. **a** Three years after treatment, CT shows an irregular centrally necrotic mass in the vaginal stump. Invasion of the posterior bladder wall and the right pelvic side wall is suggested, **b, c** Axial T1- and T2-weighted images show definite invasion of the bladder and right pelvic side wall. Combined operation and radiotherapeutic treatment (CORT) was performed including total pelvic exenteration, colostomy, ureterostomy with ileal conduit, omentectomy, and gracilis muscle flap, which proved extension to the pelvic side wall. bladder wall, and perirectal adipose tissue

**Fig. 7.14 a–c.** A 37-year-old patient with cervical carcinoma, stage IIb, who underwent radiation therapy. **a** One year after radiation therapy, CT shows a large residual mass in the cervix invading the posterior wall of the bladder, the rectum and the right pelvic side wall, as confirmed by subsequent CT-guided biopsy. CORT was performed with curative intent. **b** One month after CORT, CT shows no evidence of residual mass. The gracilis muscle flap and omental fat cover the surface of the right pelvic side wall (*arrow*). **c** Six months after CORT, CT shows a recurrent presacral mass with peripheral enhancement, confirmed by immediate CT-guided biopsy

Another contribution of CT is the detection of hydronephrosis and the determination of its etiology, that is, whether it is due to ureteral obstruction by a tumor mass. Often ureteral obstruction may result in rupture of the lymphatics of the fornix and decompression of the collecting system via this pathway.

Computed tomography can recognize direct bone invasion or bone metastases and lymph node metastasis. Nearly half of the patients with central pelvic recurrence also have pelvic adenopathy (WALSH et al. 1981). In more than one-sixth of patients with recurrent disease, para-aortic lymph nodes are the only site of disease.

#### *7.5.1.5*
#### *Magnetic Resonance Imaging*

Magnetic resonance imaging has been reported to show recurrent carcinoma with an accuracy of 80%, a sensitivity of 82%, and a specificity of 78% (WILLIAMS et al. 1989).

Recurrent tumor manifests as a discrete measurable region with a usually heterogeneous signal intensity that is generally higher than that of fibrosis on T2-weighted images (EBNER et al. 1988). T1-weighted images will generally fail to depict smaller lesions. Focal abnormal high signal intensity confined to the cervix, which is more intense on T2-weighted images than the adjacent pelvic muscle, is interpreted as recurrent tumor (Fig. 7.13b,c) (WEBER et al. 1995). By contrast, in patients without recurrent tumor, the cervix regains its normal morphologic features and characteristic low signal intensity (SUGIMURA et al. 1990).

Recurrent tumor is also diagnosed when an irregular or widened endocervical canal is depicted, or the cervical stroma is of high signal intensity. These findings, however, are nonspecific and in such cases differentiation between recurrent tumor and radiation changes cannot be made.

Secondary changes within the uterus, such as hematometra or pyometra due to obstruction caused by carcinoma or fibrosis, are readily shown by MRI.

The vaginal cuff and pelvic side wall are common sites of recurrence after hysterectomy; the incidence varies with the type of additional radiation given (WILLIAMS et al. 1989). Infiltrative recurrences without a definable mass are not common (EBNER et al. 1988).

Parametrial recurrence as a soft tissue mass lateral to the cervix can be assessed by MRI, such assessment including the size and possible extension to the pelvic side wall. Sagittal MRI can detect recurrent tumor around the uterovesical ligament anteriorly (HRICAK 1994). A soft tissue mass may, however, represent focal scarring and fibrosis rather than active tumor.

Recurrent tumor extending to the pelvic side wall is diagnosed when MRI shows a mass extending to the side wall with loss of the normal intervening fat planes on T1-weighted images. Associated abnormally high signal intensity within the mass on T2-weighted images is considered a confirmatory finding (WEBER et al. 1995). However, inflammatory changes or edema of the musculature of the pelvic side wall can lead to false-positive findings.

Bladder or rectal invasion is diagnosed when the low signal intensity of the bladder wall is focally disrupted and is replaced by a higher signal intensity tumor on T2-weighted images (Fig. 7.13b,c) (COBBY et al. 1990; HRICAK et al. 1988; KIM et al. 1990). However, edema and inflammatory change also show an increase in signal on T2-weighted images, and can consequently be confused with such invasion.

Magnetic resonance imaging is superior to CT in the assessment of bone metastases, and shows more extensive involvement by metastatic bone disease. MRI is a useful study to delineate bone marrow involvement of the pelvis and lumbar spine in patients who have low back pain and an equivocal CT study.

#### *7.5.1.6*
#### *Contrast-Enhanced MRI*

Although the use of contrast media has yielded encouraging results in cervical carcinoma preoperatively, it has limited value in the evaluation of the irradiated pelvis. It causes tumor enhancement, but similar enhancement of the parametrium, bladder, and vagina may be observed because of radiation-induced tissue injury. An enhancement study is only useful in selected patients with parametrial or pelvic side wall recurrence, or radiation-induced fistula (HRICAK 1994).

Differentiation of neoplastic and cicatricial contrast enhancement is difficult in patients with pelvic lesions after treatment of cervical carcinoma. Recently quantitative analysis with color-coded pharmacokinetic mapping has been used to distinguish between malignant and benign conditions, with good results (HAWIGHORST et al. 1995).

## 7.5.2 Recurrent Endometrial Carcinoma

The most important prognostic factor in patients with endometrial carcinoma is the extent of tumor. Among patients treated with surgery alone, recurrence occurs in 10%–15% of patients with stage I disease, 25% with stage II disease, and 75% with stage III disease (Reddy et al. 1979).

Both the degree of differentiation of the tumor and the depth of myometrial invasion increase the risk for the development of recurrence (Reddy et al. 1979). If all stages are considered, patients with well-differentiated tumors have an 81% 5-year survival rate. The 5-year survival rate decreases to 50% among patients with poorly differentiated tumors. Similarly, patients with superficial myometrial invasion have an 85% 5-year survival rate, while those with deep myometrial invasion have a 5-year survival rate of 50% (Heiken and Lee 1985).

The interval from treatment of the primary tumor to the diagnosis of recurrence has been reported to vary from 7 to 78 months, and about 80% of recurrences appear during the first 2 years (Reddy et al. 1979) and 90% occur within 3 years (Heiken and Lee 1985).

The sites of recurrence depend on the treatment used. When treatment consists of surgery alone, more than half of recurrences occur within the pelvis. Among patients treated with preoperative irradiation, only one-third of recurrences occur in the pelvis and vagina. The incidence of vaginal vault recurrence is 7.4% with surgery and 1.2% with surgery and adjunctive radiotherapy (Reddy et al. 1979).

Although therapeutic results for recurrent disease are not as good as for initial treatment, a cure can be achieved with aggressive treatment. One-third of patients with a recurrence localized to the pelvis after initial surgery can be salvaged by further radiation therapy. The 5-year disease-free survival rate is 33% and the local control rate is 44.4% (Reddy et al. 1979).

Nodal metastases primarily involve the external iliac and para-aortic lymph nodes, and they generally develop before hematogenous spread. About two-thirds recur as distant metastases in the peritoneum, mesentery, para-aortic nodes, lungs, liver, and spine (Reddy et al. 1979).

### *7.5.2.1 Ultrasonography*

Duplex and color Doppler US may be helpful in differentiating benign endometrial conditions from recurrent endometrial carcinoma (Bourne et al. 1991). However, in patients who have been treated with hysterectomy, recurrence is difficult to evaluate with US.

### *7.5.2.2 Computed Tomography*

Computed tomography has been the imaging modality of choice in detecting persistent and recurrent endometrial carcinoma and screening for lymphatic or peritoneal metastases (Dore et al. 1987). The most common CT findings in patients with recurrent tumor are a central pelvic mass and pelvic or para-aortic lymphadenopathy. A surprisingly high percentage of patients show peritoneal involvement manifested by ascites with or without omental thickening. About 16% have liver metastases (Balfe et al. 1983).

In patients treated with irradiation alone, recurrent tumor may appear as an enlarged uterus with a distended endometrial cavity. As in the initial CT staging of patients with endometrial carcinoma, intravenous contrast administration may be able to differentiate tumor from contrast-enhanced myometrium. Endometrial tumor enhances less than the normal uterine wall and thus appears as a hypodense lesion. Some endometrial tumors contain a central focus of enhancement within the hypodense lesion, representing an area of less necrotic tumor (Heiken and Lee 1985).

Uterine fluid collections in adult women are usually the result of occlusion of the internal cervical os from recurrent carcinoma (Walsh 1992). CT demonstrates an enlarged uterus with a distended and fluid-filled endometrial cavity surrounded by contrast-enhanced myometrium of varying thickness. Postradiation fibrosis can be differentiated from a large central tumor because the fluid within the uterus does not enhance, whereas tumor shows enhancement, although to a lesser degree than normal uterine tissue.

In patients with extrapelvic metastases, CT demonstrates diffuse omental thickening with ascites and metastases to the mesentery, peritoneum, and liver (Balfe et al. 1983). Discrete solid masses seen in the pelvis are thought to be localized recurrence in the surgical bed. Most false-positive examinations are due to misinterpretation of radiation fibrosis as recurrent tumor. False-negative results are most often due to small tumor deposits in the lymph nodes, vagina, peritoneum, or omentum (WALSH 1992).

Despite these limitations, CT can play a major role in the appropriate selection of patients for surgical or radiation treatment following local tumor recurrence.

#### 7.5.2.3 Magnetic Resonance Imaging

Magnetic resonance imaging may be the technique of choice in endometrial carcinomas in evaluating precise depth of invasion or extrauterine spread (HRICAK et al. 1987; LIEN et al. 1991; SIRONI et al. 1992; YAMASHITA et al. 1993). Most endometrial carcinomas are isointense to the uterus on T1-weighted images, and have intermediate signal intensity between normal endometrium and myometrium on T2-weighted images (WORTHINGTON et al. 1986; HRICAK et al. 1987; POSNIAK et al. 1990). Large tumors may exhibit considerable signal heterogeneity due to necrosis and hemorrhage. The endometrial cavity may become wide due to the recurrent tumor or an associated fluid collection (WORTHINGTON et al. 1986; HRICAK et al. 1987; POSNIAK et al. 1990).

In the pretreatment assessment of endometrial carcinoma, the use of contrast media is advocated. Contrast-enhanced study permits better tumor detection and improves differentiation between viable tumor and retained debris within the endometrial cavity (HRICAK et al. 1991; SIRONI et al. 1992; THURNHER 1992). In the postradiation uterus, however, the myometrium enhances remarkably well, so no clear outline of recurrent or residual tumor can be demonstrated.

Cervical invasion can be diagnosed on MRI when high signal intensity tumor expands the cervical canal or, more reliably, when the low signal intensity of stroma is disrupted (HRICAK et al. 1987; BELLONI et al. 1990).

Determination of extension beyond the serosa of the uterus requires MR findings of transmural interruption of the myometrium and serosal irregularity. Invasion of rectum and bladder is indicated by intramural areas of contrast uptake or increased signal intensity and disruption of the low-signal muscle layer (HRICAK et al. 1987; CHEN et al. 1990). Disappearance of the interposed fatty layer is highly suggestive of infiltration. However, the accuracy of MR is not well established because of the small number of patients reported.

### 7.5.3 Müllerian Mixed Mesodermal Tumor

Müllerian (or malignant) mixed mesodermal tumors (MMMTs) are rare tumors derived from the multipotential cells of müllerian mesenchyme, and exhibit differentiation toward endometrial and mesodermall cells. The latter may form muscle, cartilage, or bone within the tumor (SHAW et al. 1983).

Most of these tumors occur spontaneously in elderly women, but 7%–46% of patients have a history of pelvic irradiation for unrelated disease (KING and KRAMER 1980). The latent interval between the initial irradiation and the diagnosis of MMMT ranges from 5 to 40 years with a median of 16–21 years. If the latent interval is relatively short, special attention is needed to differentiate between an MMMT and a recurrent pelvic malignancy, usually from cervical carcinoma.

Prognosis is extremely poor because these tumors are aggressive and show lymphatic and myometrial invasion at initial presentation (NIELSEN et al. 1989). In evaluating the depth of myometrial invasion, MRI is superior to CT scan. MMMT shows diffuse low signal intensity with focal hemorrhagic foci on T1-weighted images and heterogeneous enhancement on contrast studies. On T2-weighted images, the tumor displays a heterogeneous, intermediate or high signal intensity (Fig.7.15) (SHAPEERO and HRICAK 1988).

Appearances on MRI are nonspecific and should be differentiated from recurrent cervical carcinoma or endometrial carcinoma. The relatively massive size and invasive nature of MMMT may help in this diagnosis (SHAPEERO and HRICAK 1988). A fluid collection in the endometrial cavity associated with a polypoid mass has been described as one of the findings of MMMT and endometrial carcinoma (HRICAK et al. 1987).

### 7.5.4 Persistent Gestational Trophoblastic Neoplasm

Gestational trophoblastic disease represents a spectrum of gynecologic pathology from hydatidiform mole to choriocarcinoma. Gestational trophoblastic neoplasia (GTN), a subset of this group, implies persistence of disease and consists of choriocarcinoma,

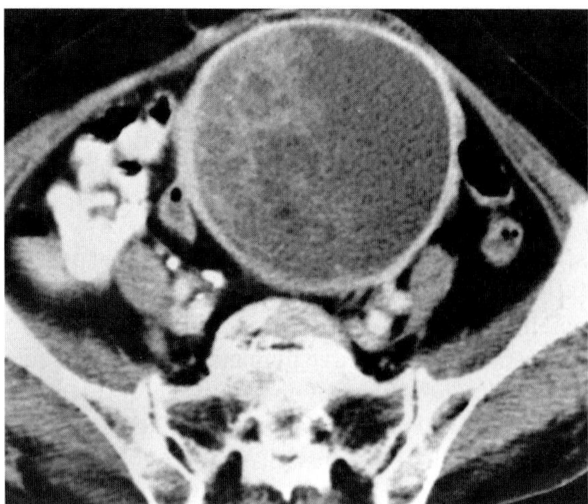

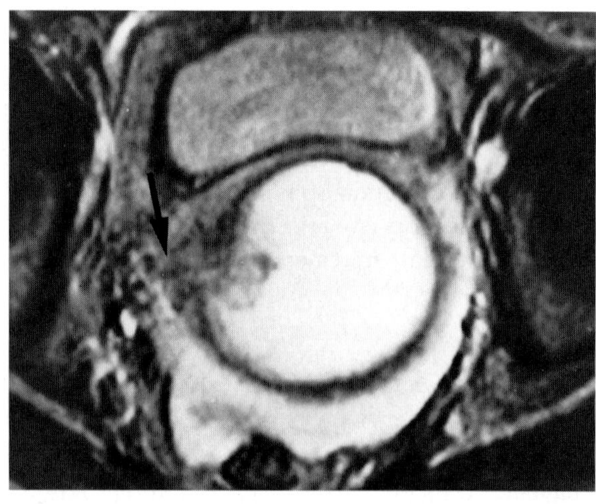

**Fig. 7.15 a,b.** A 72-year-old patient with an MMMT and a history of radiation therapy 15 years previously for stage IIIb cervical carcinoma. **a** Enhanced CT scan reveals distended endometrial cavity with fluid retention. Heterogeneously enhancing solid mass is attached to the right myometrial wall. The myometrium is remarkably effected. **b** A 54-year-old woman with an MMMT and a history of pelvic irradiation for stage IIb cervical carcinoma 8 years previously. Axial T2-weighted image shows endometrial fluid and ascites posterior to the uterus. An endometrial solid mass deeply invaded the myometrium and extended to the right parametrium (*arrow*), as was confirmed pathologically.

metastatic molar disease, and nonmetastatic molar disease with persistently elevated human chorionic gonadotropin (hCG).

The serum measurement of hCG is the most accurate test to detect persistent or recurrent GTN. After surgical evacuation of the uterus, serum hCG is followed. If titers rise or reach a plateau over 2 weeks, the patient is considered to have persistent trophoblastic disease and must be treated. At this point, risk category is assigned to determine the appropriate type of chemotherapy. The criteria for the high-risk category are: (a) brain or liver metastases; (b) metastatic disease with hCG greater than 40 000 mIU/ml at the begining of therapy; (c) failure of single-agent therapy; and (d) metastatic disease with therapy initiated greater than 4 months post-termination of the responsible pregnancy. Reported survival rates are 100% in low-risk and 72% in high-risk patients due to effective chemotherapy (Davis et al. 1984). High-risk status requires immediate aggressive therapy with combination chemotherapy, whereas low-risk patients are treated with a single agent (Davis et al. 1984). The levels of hCG do not correlate with uterine size, probably because nonuterine foci of trophoblastic tissue also are capable of producing hCG. Therefore, uterine size does not necessarily reflect total tumor burden.

Imaging studies may have a problem-solving role by serving to identify metastases in patients with recurrent GTN. Among the multiple radiologic modalities, CT is often used because it can readily evaluate all critical organs, as well as provide ancillary information, such as the presence of hemorrhage from a metastasis (Davis et al. 1984; Sanders and Rubin 1987).

#### 7.5.4.1 Ultrasonography

Ultrasonography, which is effective in the initial diagnosis of molar disease, is not useful in determining the risk of development of persistent disease (Davis et al. 1984).

The multiloculated, often bilateral theca lutein cysts secondary to elevated serum levels of hCG usually resolve after treatment of the intrauterine process; however, they can become quite large, producing pain from torsion.

Doppler US may be useful in the evaluation of GTN. These vascular tumors tend to show very high blood flow. More specifically, high diastolic flow, presumably the result of decreased peripheral resistance in the proliferating vessels of the neoplasm, has been identified in patients with persistent GTN (Desai and Desberg 1991; Carter et al. 1993). Sequential sonograms have shown regression of the neoplasm and normalization of its waveform with reduction in vascular pooling and arteriovenous shunting.

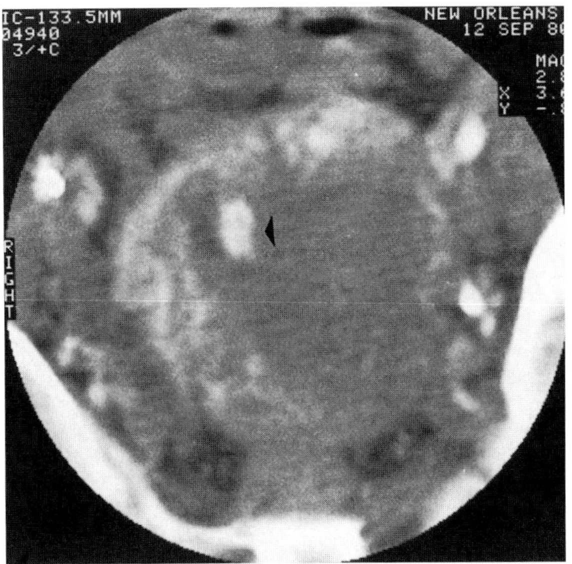


**Fig. 7.16.** Note the prominent vascularity and puddling of contrast medium in the muscularis of the uterus on dynamic CT during the vascular capillary phase. This is characteristic of choriocarcinoma destrunes. (From Lang 1989)

#### 7.5.4.2
#### *Computed Tomography*

The most common CT features of GTN are uterine enlargement (80%) and bilateral theca lutein cysts (54%) (Davis et al. 1984). Irregular, eccentric hypodense foci in the myometrium or endometrial cavity with central ringlike enhancement is seen, representing local tumor. The hypodense area of tumor probably corresponds to foci of hemorrhage or necrosis (Sanders and Rubin 1987).

During the capillary phase the rich neovascularity of choriocarcinoma is readily appreciated. On delayed phase CT, puddling of contrast medium is particularly well shown in cases of choriocarcinoma destruens (Fig. 7.16) (Lang 1989).

Direct extrauterine spread of GTN is represented by soft tissue density in the broad ligament contiguous with the uterus and obliterating the pelvic fat or muscle planes. When trophic tissue involves the broad ligaments or pelvic side walls, hysterectomy is not indicated. Dynamic CT can detect the vascular component of the tumor and can also detect the characteristic hypervascular liver metastases.

Computed tomography can detect unsuspected pulmonary metastatic nodules not detected by plain film. For brain involvement, CT is the unequivocal choice. These CT findings are predictive of a high-risk group of patients who fail initial chemotherapy.

#### 7.5.4.3
#### *Magnetic Resonance Imaging*

Usually MRI is performed to demonstrate intrapelvic spread in patients with a known persistent mole (Hricak et al. 1986). The impact of MRI findings on management decisions is minimal. Therefore, rather than being a routine examination, MRI is useful as a problem-solving tool in selected cases (Kohorn 1993).

Many tumors show heterogeneous, hypervascular masses that distort the normal zonal anatomy. Some tumors show areas of high signal intensity on T1-weighted images consistent with hemorrhagic foci. On serial MRI obtained following chemotherapy in patients with persistent GTN, there is a progressive decrease in uterine size, tumor size, and tumor vascularity, and progressively improved visualization of zonal anatomy (Hricak et al. 1986).

### 7.5.5
### Uterine Lymphoma

The uterus is rarely the primary site of lymphoma. Secondary involvement of the uterus, however, may occur in the later stages; therefore uterine lymphomas are usually discovered in patients with generalized disease. About 70% of uterine lymphomas originate in the cervix, and about 60% of them are diffuse large cell or histiocytic lymphoma (Harris and Scully 1984).

On US, lymphoma appears as a well-defined mass of low-level echogenicity in an enlarged uterus. Surrounding hyperechoic myometrium is compressed. On CT, a well-circumscribed lobular lesion shows homogeneous low density in the uterine cervix or body. A peripherally enhancing rim is noted. Characteristically no central necrosis is found even in a bulky mass.

Magnetic resonance imaging is useful for diagnosing uterine lymphoma. Uterine lymphoma shows a lesion of low signal intensity on T1-weighted images and inhomogeneous signal intensity with areas of high and low signal intensity on T2-weighted images (Fig. 7.17a). Contrast-enhanced study shows areas of inhomogeneous enhancement in the thickened myometrium (Kawakami et al. 1995). The junctional zone and cervical stromal ring are not disrupted (Fig. 7.17b). This finding is unique because endometrial carcinoma may disrupt the junctional zone, and cervical carcinoma may disrupt the cervical stromal ring of low signal intensity (Yamada and

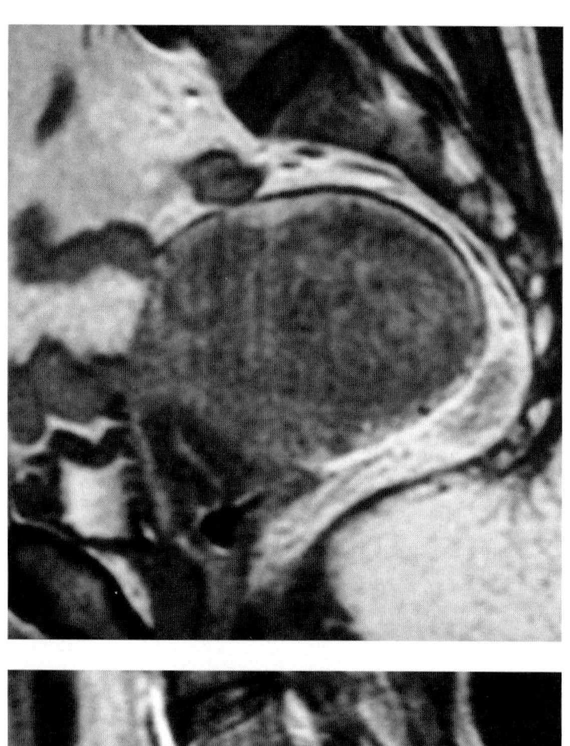

a

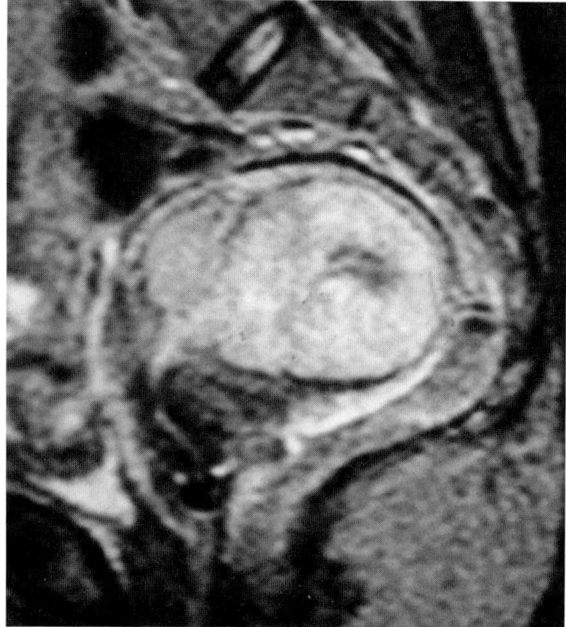

b

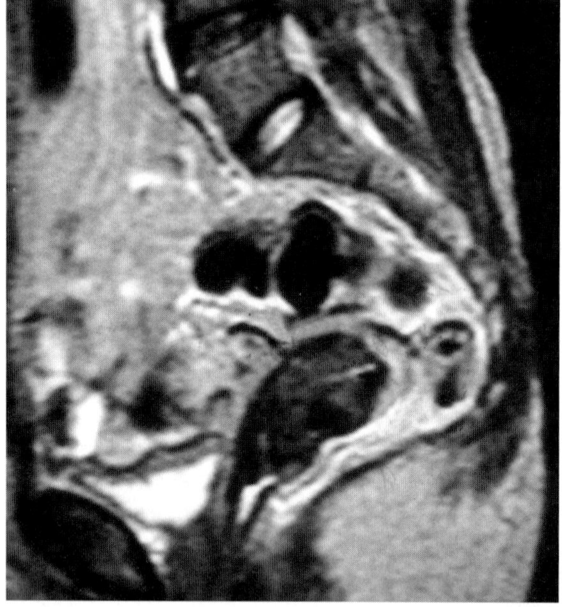

c

**Fig. 7.17 a–c.** A 62-year-old woman with diffuse large cell, histiocytic lymphoma. **a** Sagittal contrast-enhanced T1-weighted image shows a lobular enlarged uterus and an irregularly enhancing mass in the fundus and body. **b** Sagittal T2-weighted image shows a mass of high signal intensity in the myometrial wall. The junctional zone of low signal intensity is well preserved. **c** Four months after systemic chemotherapy there is no evidence of residual mass in the uterus, this being indicative of complete remission

Suzuki 1993). Uterine lymphomas show an excellent response to chemotherapy. The uterus shows a decrease in size and reconstitution of zonal anatomy (Fig. 7.17c).

### 7.5.6 Recurrent Ovarian Carcinoma

In contrast to endometrial and cervical carcinomas, ovarian carcinoma is often found to be advanced at the time of diagnosis and only about 30% of cases are surgically resectable. Although the initial response to therapy is good, 5-year survival for advanced disease is only 17% (Richardson et al. 1985).

When ovarian carcinoma is suspected, surgery is considered the staging procedure of choice. Surgery is both diagnostic and therapeutic by identifying the tumor stage, and allowing maximum cytoreduction (Meyer et al. 1995). Optimal cytoreduction is considered to have been achieved when no tumor of 2 cm or larger is left behind; this enhances the response to chemotherapy and improves long-term survival (HAND et al. 1993). However, surgery is often extensive and prolonged in clinically fragile patients and is associated with significant morbidity; incomplete cytoreduction is also common, occurring in as many as 40% of patients (YOUNG et al. 1993). Furthermore patients with bulky, nonresectable disease will not benefit from primary surgery, because surgical resection does not improve survival if the diameter of the residual lesion is greater than 2 cm (HOSKINS et al. 1994). In this group of patients, neoadjuvant chemotherapy followed by surgical debulking is a better approach (NIH 1995).

For residual or recurrent ovarian carcinoma, current treatment involves surgery and a variety of chemotherapeutic regimens with curative intent. Second-look laparotomy (SLL) with peritoneal washings has been performed to assess remission or microscopic relapse since the 1970s (GOLDHIRSCH et al. 1984; SILVERMAN et al. 1988). However, the justification for SLL in recurrent ovarian cancer has been questioned, because SLL does not improve overall survival, and about 30%–50% of cases will ultimately recur despite negative surgical findings (MILLER et al. 1992). Debulking at the time of SLL has also been questioned because secondary cytoreduction does not fulfill its goal in 70%–80% of patients (FRASCI et al. 1994). The routine use of SLL is no longer recommended in the presence of lesions greater than 2 cm, multiple retroperitoneal or pelvic lymph node metastases, or pulmonary and pleural metastases (NIH 1995). Various noninvasive modalities are applied to prove tumor recurrence and to spare these patients the morbidity of exploratory surgery (FORSTNER et al. 1995b).

Physical examination and laboratory analyses, such as determination of the CA-125 level, have not proved sufficiently accurate. Though pelvic tumor recurrences as small as 1.5 cm are detected by vaginal palpation, even large tumors can be missed by physical examination when they are located elsewhere (PRAYER et al. 1993).

Both CT and MRI may be used to predict successful cytoreduction, although they are too insensitive in detecting small metastatic foci. Optimal cytoreduction has not been achieved (a) when the tumor is larger than 2 cm at the root of the mesentery, porta hepatis, omentum of the lesser sac, intersegmental fissure of the liver, gastrosplenic ligament, diaphragm, or dome of the liver; (b) when lymph nodes at the celiac axis are enlarged (>1.0 cm); or (c) when presacral extraperitoneal disease is detected (NELSON et al. 1993). Tumor resectability depends predominantly on tumor location, with a sensitivity of 92% for CT and 97% for MRI (NELSON et al. 1993). Frequently missed nonresectable lesions include plaquelike diaphragmatic implants and lesions at the attachment of the spleen.

#### 7.5.6.1 Radioimmunoassay

The serial cancer antigen (CA) 125 assay is widely used to assess results of treatment and to detect recurrent ovarian carcinoma because of its reliability, ready availability, and low cost. Serum tumor markers decrease as the tumor regresses due to surgical resection or effective chemotherapy. If serum CA-125 levels are elevated at the completion of chemotherapy, there will be persistent disease at SLL (EINHORN et al. 1986). CA-125 level is elevated in 54% of patients with recurrence and seems to correlate with the extent of tumor, although a threshold level differentiating between microscopic and macroscopic disease cannot be established (PATSNER et al. 1990; BUIST et al. 1994).

Other conditions may cause false-positive results, e.g., benign ovarian neoplasms; thus the specificity of the test is somewhat limited. The false-negative rate can be as high as 59%; however, the maximum tumor diameter never exceeds 1 cm in these patients (BEREK et al. 1986). Despite these problems, the postoperative measurement of CA-125 may serve as a baseline from which to monitor disease recurrence. CT and MRI are important adjuncts to CA-125 assays rather than primary screening methods for detecting persistent or recurrent disease.

#### 7.5.6.2 Ultrasonography

While US is important in the detection and characterization of ovarian masses, its use in detecting recurrent ovarian carcinoma is limited. Recurrent ovarian carcinoma can present as either a localized pelvic mass or disseminated throughout the peritoneal cavity. In the case of a pelvic mass, color Doppler and pulsed Doppler flow imaging may be useful in differentiating between a benign and a malignant mass (BOURNE et al. 1989; KURJAK et al. 1991). The presence of color flow in the echogenic portion indicates the hypervascular nature of malignancy; absence of color flow in the echogenic portion indicates a cystic or hypovascular nature and hence a benign lesion (Jain 1994). In a case of disseminated recurrence, however, these techniques are not helpful in detecting peritoneal tumor implants.

### 7.5.6.3 Computed Tomography

Computed tomography is usually performed to document regression of disease, before SLL after chemotherapy in most patients with stage III or IV disease. If there is no radiologic evidence of recurrent disease, the patient must be surgically evaluated for confirmation because of the high false-negative rate for the detection of peritoneal disease. If CT shows residual disease or hepatic or retroperitoneal metastases, however, the morbidity of exploratory surgery can be obviated (Wagner et al. 1994). CT results accurately predict the residual tumor size, which is more predictive of prognosis than the number of lesions (Megibow et al. 1988).

The overall sensitivity of CT is 32%–84%, and the specificity is 77%–88% with a false-negative rate of 37%–41% (Silverman et al. 1988; Reuter et al. 1989; Walsh 1992). False-positive rates of 17%–19% are usually caused by misdiagnosis of adherent bowel loops as a tumor mass. A bowel "pseudotumor" may be due to adhesions or the effects of radiation therapy (Goldhirsch et al. 1984).

Detection of peritoneal implants depends mainly on their location in the peritoneal cavity rather than on lesion size. In the detection of lesions measuring 5 mm or larger, the sensitivity of CT is 100% in the subphrenic spaces, 80% in the pouch of Douglas, 67% in the greater omentum and the gastrocolic ligament, and 52% in the other regions of the peritoneum (Buy et al. 1988). While peritoneal implants greater than 2 cm are readily depicted with similar sensitivity by MRI and CT, diseases in the mesentery or implants on the small and large bowel are better evaluated with CT (Figs. 7.18, 7.19). When the greater omentum is involved, omental cake or a smudged infiltrative pattern is seen. If the metastases are implanted on the diaphragmatic surface of the liver, a thorough examination of the diaphragmatic surface is needed by means of peritoneoscopy. Surgically it is difficult to visualize the diaphragm through the standard midline incision.

Detection of peritoneal implants also depends on the presence of adjacent ascites. The presence of ascites alone is neither sensitive nor specific for the diagnosis of peritoneal disease, because small amounts of ascites can be seen in a wide variety of benign conditions. While CT does not depict small metastases to the bowel serosa and omentum in recurrent ovarian carcinoma, implants less than 5 mm in diameter are readily detected when a considerable amount of ascites is present. Ascites is present next to the lesion in 73% of true-positive CT scans and absent in 78% of false-negative CT scans (Buy et al. 1988).

Enhanced CT does not significantly improve detection of recurrent ovarian cancer, but the presence of enhanced peritoneum or small nodules on the peritoneum should be viewed with suspicion (Semelka et al. 1993).

The major limitation of CT in detecting recurrent ovarian cancer is its inability to detect miliary peritoneal seeding and small omental and mesenteric tumor nodules, especially in the absence of ascites. High-resolution CT scanners can be used to detect 50% of peritoneal implants as small as 5 mm (Buy et al. 1988). CT may be able to detect psammomatous calcification in plaquelike peritoneal metastases, even when a mass is not present (Mitchel et al. 1986).

### 7.5.6.4 Intraperitoneal Contrast-Enhanced CT

Intraperitoneal contrast-enhanced CT (IPC-CT) may increase the accuracy of detecting tumor implants

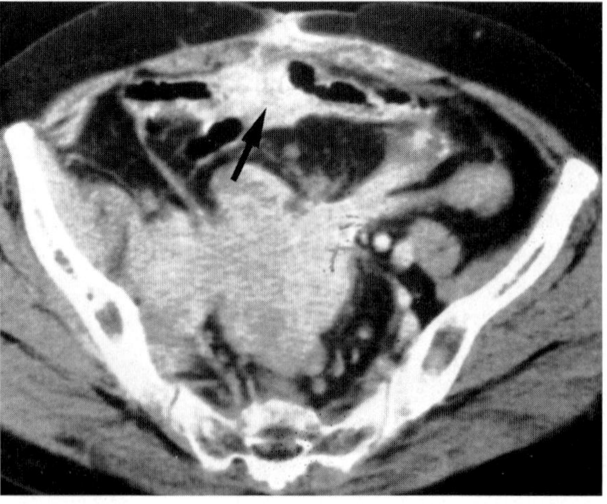

**Fig. 7.18.** A 39-year-old patient with ovarian carcinoma who underwent staging laparotomy and cytoreductive surgery. Follow-up CT shows a heterogeneous lobulated solid mass in the right pelvic cavity, and diffusely thickened wall of the small bowel representing serosal tumor implants (*arrow*), confirmed at subsequent second-look laparotomy.

two- to fourfold over conventional CT (HALVORSEN et al. 1991; FRASCI et al. 1994). IPC-CT detects small nodules less than 2 cm in diameter and misses macroscopic disease in only 12% of cases (HALVORSEN et al. 1991). IPC-CT varies in its accuracy depending on the location of the recurrent disease; the highest sensitivity is in the subphrenic and paracolic regions, and the lowest in the mesentery. IPC-CT has an overall sensitivity of 88% (FRASCI et al. 1994).

Second-look laparotomy demonstrates persistent disease where diffusion defects are noted. Nevertheless, diffusion defects represent only indirect evidence of persistent disease, as opposed to the direct evidence of imaging a tumor nodule. Along with persistent carcinoma, adhesions can be due to prior surgery, prior intraperitoneal chemotherapy, or radiation therapy. There are no details as to the type and extent of tumor involvement in these adhesions (FRASCI et al. 1994).

Although one report (NELSON et al. 1992) failed to show superiority of ICP-CT over conventional CT, IPC-CT alone may be considered more accurate in the detection of persistent disease than the combination of CT and CA-125. When IPC-CT results are combined with CA-125 data, sensitivity increases from 78% to 87% (FRASCI et al. 1994).

### 7.5.6.5
### Magnetic Resonance Imaging

Magnetic resonance imaging has no additional value in assessing the extent of the ovarian carcinoma, or in detecting abdominal or pelvic tumor implants (GHOSSAIN et al. 1991; BUIST et al. 1994). However, in patients with markedly elevated CA-125 levels and negative CT, MRI may provide additional diagnostic criteria for the evaluation of recurrent disease (STEVENS et al. 1991; HATA et al. 1992).

When MRI findings are combined with the CA-125 level, detection of recurrent disease rises from 53% to 75%. However, the negative predictive value of the combination of CA-125 assay and MRI remains low, which raises the need for SLL as a diag-

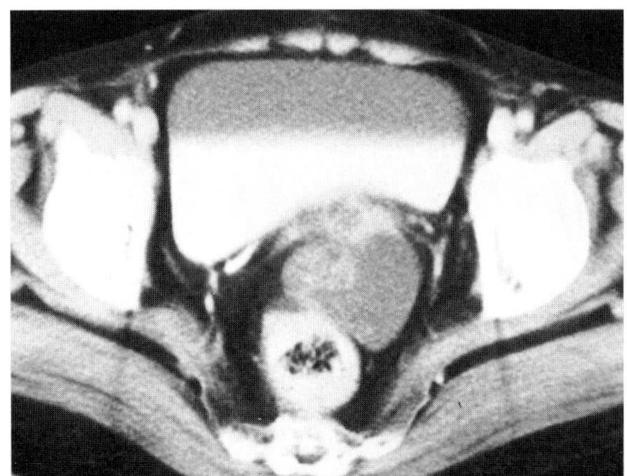
a

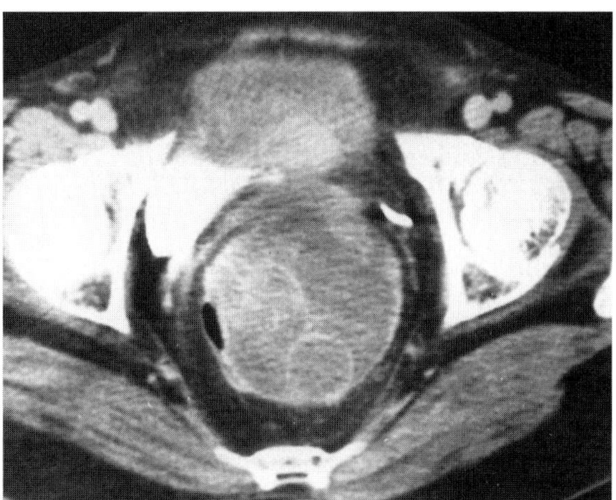
b

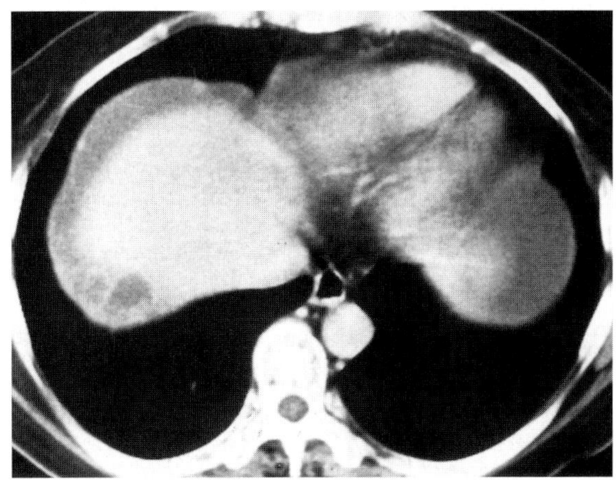
c

**Fig. 7.19 a–c.** A 49-year-old patient with mucinous cystadenocarcinoma of the ovary who underwent staging laparotomy and cytoreductive surgery. **a** One year after surgery, CT shows a large heterogeneous mass between the rectum and the bladder without separation from the adjacent vaginal stump. The patient received additional chemotherapy. **b** Six months later the serum CA-125 level was elevated to 119 U/ml. CT shows enlargement of the pelvic mass, which is invading the rectum. **c** Near the diaphragmatic surface, multiple enhancing tumor implants are noted, surrounded by ascites. Secondary debulking laparotomy was performed (pelvic mass debulking, total cystectomy with ileal conduit, resection and reanastomosis of the sigmoid colon, total omentectomy) and invasion of the bladder and rectum was confirmed. This patient received additional intraperitoneal radioisotope (holmium) treatment

nostic tool when laboratory and radiologic tests do not show an abnormality (Patsner et al. 1990).

While diagnoses of recurrence in CT are based only on morphologic criteria such as irregular configuration with signs of invasive growth, the signal intensities of pathologic changes provide essential information. A small tumor infiltrating the apex of the vagina can be inhomogeneously hyperintense on T2-weighted images but not on CT (Prayer et al. 1993).

Uterine invasion is diagnosed by means of localized distortion of the uterine contour, irregular interface between tumor and myometrium, and high signal intensity in the involved myometrium on T2-weighted images (Forstner et al. 1995a).

Invasion of the sigmoid colon or urinary bladder is diagnosed when there is loss of the tissue plane between the tumor and the wall of the colon or bladder, when the colon is encased, or when direct tumor extension is observed (Fig. 7.20). While the positive predictive value of MRI for the detection of colon invasion is excellent (91%), the negative predictive value (69%) is only moderate (Forstner et al. 1995a).

Pelvic side wall invasion is diagnosed with similar sensitivity and specificity by either CT or MRI when the tumor approaches to within 3 mm of the pelvic wall or when iliac vessels are surrounded or distorted by the tumor (Fig. 7.13b,c). The sensitivity for pelvic side wall invasion is low for both CT and MRI

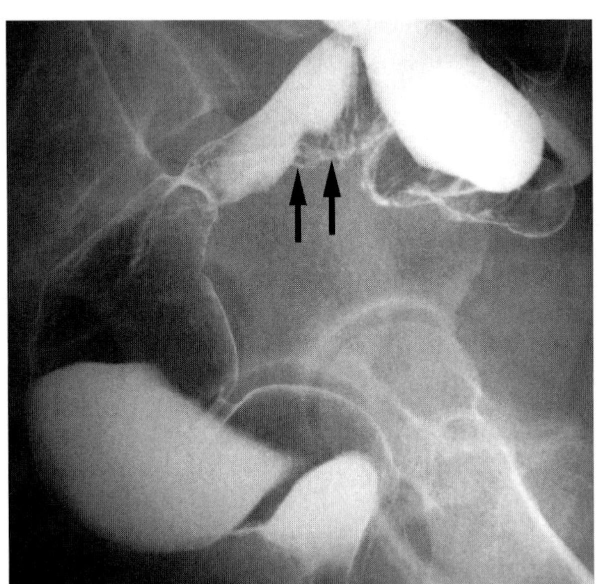
a

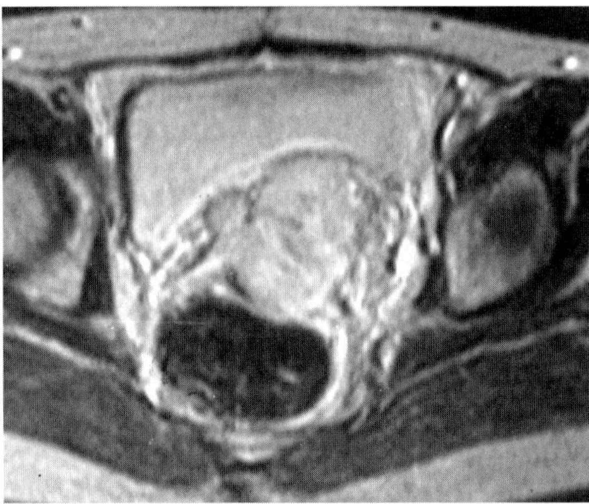
c

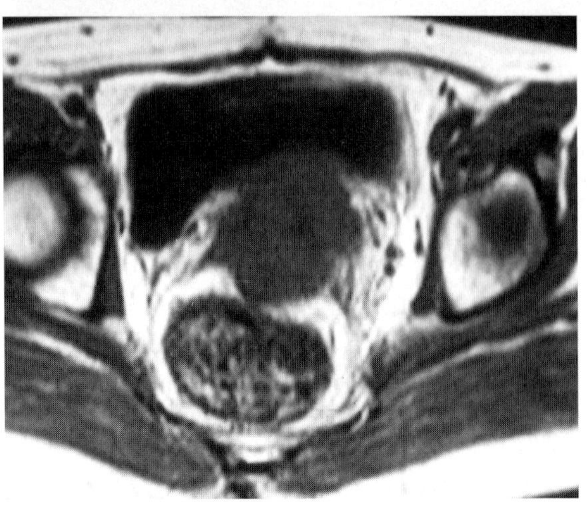
b

**Fig. 7.20 a–c.** A 40-year-old patient with poorly differentiated papillary serous cystadenocarcinoma of the ovary with a history of hysterectomy, bilateral salpingo-oophorectomy, and omentectomy 1 year previously. **a** The barium enema x-ray examination shows irregular luminal narrowing of the rectosigmoid and shaggy mucosal surface (*arrows*). **b, c** Axial T1- and T2-weighted images show a lobulated mass between the bladder and the rectum with an irregular lateral margin. The posterior wall of the urinary bladder is focally thickened, but true invasion cannot be ascertained due to the chemical shift artefact. On subsequent total exenteration, invasion of the rectosigmoid and posterior wall of the urinary bladder was confirmed

(Forstner et al. 1995a). This may be explained by the surgical findings of dense adhesions.

The characteristic appearance of omental cake can be identified by its infiltrative, nodular appearance and can be distinguished from bowel by enhancement.

Contrast-enhanced MRI can achieve 83% accuracy for the detection of recurrent disease (Stevens et al. 1991). Tiny peritoneal implants in the paracolic gutters and omentum are reliably diagnosed with the use of oral and intravenous contrast media when small amounts of surrounding ascites are present (Semelka et al. 1993). Serosal implants cannot be seen even on contrast-enhanced MRI, suggesting underestimation of peritoneal spread with relapse. Observations based on contrast-enhanced CT suggest that malignant lesions enhance more rapidly than benign lesions and to a greater extent (Buy et al. 1991), suggesting a role for dynamic MRI.

The accuracy of various procedures in the detection of tumor recurrence has been evaluated. Palpation with CA-125 has been reported to have a sensitivity of 100%, as compared with 66.6% for CT and 77.7% for MRI. A specificity of 93.3% has been found for all methods, with reported accuracy rates of 95.8% for palpation with CA-125, 83.3% for CT, and 87.5% for MRI (Prayer et al. 1993).

## 7.6 Assessment of Lymph Node Metastases

Cervical and endometrial carcinomas spread out of the pelvis along the three lymphatic routes: through the parametrial lymphatics to the external iliac and common iliac nodes, along the round ligament to the inguinal nodes, and along the gonadal vessels directly to the para-aortic nodes (Mezrich 1994).

The lymphatic drainage from the right ovary is to precaval and laterocaval nodes between the aortic bifurcation and the renal hilus. The left ovary drains to nodes above and below the left renal vein. An accessory pathway drains into the middle chain of the external iliac group of nodes. Pelvic and retroperitoneal lymph node involvement is common in ovarian carcinoma at all stages of the disease. Sometimes the only manifestation of recurrent ovarian carcinoma is lymph node metastases, which has an incidence of 11%–17% (Heiken and Lee 1985). The presence of para-aortic metastatic adenopathy is itself a poor prognostic indicator.

Lymph node metastases usually are not palpable on physical examination and are difficult to predict by clinical data. The modalities for the detection of metastatic lymph nodes are CT, MRI, lymphoscintigraphy, and lymphangiography with or without percutaneous needle biopsy.

Computed tomography may play an important role in patients whose recurrent disease manifests as lymph node metastases. CT or MRI criteria other than nodal size are not sufficiently specific or sensitive. The size criterion of pelvic lymph node metastases varies between 1.0 and 2.0 cm in diameter (Waggenspack et al. 1988), but recently lymph nodes have been considered malignant when the diameter of the short axis exceeds 1 cm irrespective of the location (Hricak et al. 1988; Kim et al. 1993). If this minimal axial diameter of a node is used as a criterion, higher accuracy (90.4%) results (Kim et al. 1994).

The accuracy of MRI and CT in detecting pelvic lymph node metastases is similar: 73%–83% for CT and 76%–100% for MRI (Hricak et al. 1988; Togashi et al. 1989; Kim et al. 1993). MRI has a sensitivity of 75% and a specificity of 88% in predicting lymph node metastases (Hawnaur et al. 1994). Higher accuracy can be achieved in detecting para-aortic lymph node metastases: the sensitivity of CT in respect of such metastases has been reported to be 67%–77%, its specificity 86%–100%, and its overall accuracy 80%–98% (Villasanta et al. 1983; Bandy et al. 1985; Camilien et al. 1988).

Theoretically, replacement of lymph nodes by low signal intensity tumor should render them more visible than benign or normal-sized nodes on MRI (Hawnaur et al. 1994). However, the MR signal characteristics of enlarged nodes are not useful in determining the presence or absence of metastatic disease. Enlarged lymph nodes without tumor involvement are not identifiable, probably due to fatty infiltration or sinus histiocytosis which renders the nodes isointense to surrounding pelvic fat.

Although on MRI enlarged lymph nodes are normally distinguishable from pelvic vessels containing fast-flowing blood, there is a difficulty with slow-flowing pelvic veins causing increases signal intensity. The external iliac vein frequently has an intermediate signal intensity similar to lymphadenopathy on T1-weighted images. Recent biopsy, pelvic inflammatory disease, or pregnancy can result in prominent pelvic veins due to increased vascularity.

There are no significant differences in the degree of contrast enhancement between metastatic and nonmetastatic lymph nodes (Kim et al. 1994). The presence of central necrosis is not helpful in differentiating metastatic from nonmetastatic nodes.

One of the limitations of CT or MRI is that it is impossible to delineate intranodal architecture, so small nodes harboring microscopic tumor may go undetected, and enlarged nodes with inflammatory changes may be interpreted as malignancy. Furthermore, unopacified bowel loops may mimic enlarged lymph nodes due to a similar signal intensity and thus lead to a false-positive diagnosis. Routine use of oral contrast media opacifying all bowel loops may mitigate this potential problem.

Lymphangiography can demonstrate disturbance of intranodal architecture and thereby adds an additional parameter in the diagnosis of metastatic disease in normal-sized lymph nodes.

The accuracy in assessing retroperitoneal lymph node metastases can be enhanced by CT-guided biopsy (MATSUKUMA et al. 1989; HELLER et al. 1990). CT localization of retroperitoneal lymph node metastases can be used to adjust radiation therapy ports to include the abdomen.

## 7.7 Treatment of Recurrences

### 7.7.1 Pelvic Exenteration

Pelvic exenteration offers the last chance for survival for patients with central recurrences who have failed radiation therapy or surgical treatment. Five-year survival rates have been reported to be up to 50% after pelvic exenteration (HOECKEL and KNAPSTEIN 1992). However, the survival rate is less than 2% at 2 years if the margins of surgical resection are involved or if surgery is not possible due to fixed or distant disease (SHINGLETON et al. 1989). Even if distant metastases develop, local control may be regarded as worthwhile palliation.

The morbidity and complication rates of pelvic exenteration are high, at up to 47%–52.5%, and most complications involve the gastrointestinal and urinary tracts. Therefore, in order to select patients who have a reasonable chance of long-term survival, it is important to confirm the recurrence histologically and ascertain the extent of disease (CRAWFORD et al. 1996).

Contraindications to pelvic exenteration include pelvic side wall extension, metastatic lymphadenopathy, leg edema indicating venous or lymphatic compromise, and sciatic nerve pain from neural invasion (POPOVICH et al. 1993).

Most oncologic surgeons still consider exploratory laparotomy with biopsy to be necessary to select patients for exenteration. With the operative procedure, 33% will have a laparotomy that does not continue to exenteration and a further 8% will have disease at the resection margins (SHINGLETON et al. 1989).

In the past, radiologic evaluation of candidates for pelvic exenteration was largely restricted to chest radiography, excretory urography, and barium enema x-ray examination. CT has improved the selection of candidates for exenteration. CT may predict inoperability based on extension to the pelvic side walls (Fig. 7.13a), encasement of adjacent vessels, ureteric dilatation, or lymph node enlargement. Ascites as the only abnormal finding other than a central pelvic mass is not a contraindication to exenteration. In a patient in whom CT shows the aforementioned relative contraindications to exenteration, noncurative surgery can be avoided (CRAWFORD et al. 1996). Microscopic disease at the resection margins cannot be predicted by CT and may only become evident on the histologic review.

Magnetic resonance imaging is also valuable in surgical planning in candidates for pelvic exenteration. The accuracy of MRI is 83% in selecting patients for pelvic exenteration (POPOVICH et al. 1993). It is to be noted, however, that the MRI appearance of tumor invasion of the pelvic side wall cannot be reliably distinguished from radiation changes within 6 months of radiation therapy (EBNER et al. 1988). Many of these patients will still require exploratory laparotomy for diagnosis, although percutaneous biopsy may provide the diagnosis in some cases.

Evaluation by MRI of tumor extension into the bladder and rectum is helpful in planning the appropriate surgical approach. Cystoscopy and proctosigmoidoscopy may be useful when MR findings are equivocal or when specific indications of bladder or rectal involvement are present. Evidence of tumor extension into the bladder and rectum necessitates total pelvic exenteration, whereas extension into only the bladder allows an anterior approach and invasion into only the rectum allows a posterior exenteration. The accuracy of MRI in identifying bladder and rectal invasion is lower than its accuracy in respect of the pretreatment carcinoma. The discrepancy in accuracy is attributed to tissue damage caused by radiation therapy (POPOVICH et al. 1993).

### 7.7.2 Combined Operative and Radiotherapeutic Treatment

Recently a combined operative and radiotherapeutic treatment (CORT) approach has been developed for recurrent pelvic malignancies. It is suggested that CORT combines synergistic surgical and radiation treatment factors to improve the therapeutic ratio between tumor control and tissue tolerance. Therefore local radiation doses higher than those of conventional methods can be applied in cases previously treated by surgery. Reirradiation with potentially curative doses seems to be possible after previous primary or adjuvant radiation (HOECKEL and KNAPSTEIN 1992).

The operative part consists in staging laparotomy, maximum tumor debulking at the pelvic side wall and exenteration of infiltrated central pelvic organs, implantation of guiding tubes into the residual tumor at the pelvic wall, pelvic wall plasty with muscle, musculocutaneous, and omentum flaps, and surgical reconstruction of bowel and bladder.

CORT may be undertaken in patients who are not candidates for pelvic exenteration, such as in patients with pelvic side wall extension of a recurrent tumor. Usually tumor bulk is located centrally with peripheral infiltration of the pelvic wall. Peripheral tumor also exhibits seromuscular infiltration of pelvic hollow organs such as the bladder, rectosigmoid colon, and small bowel.

Either CT or MRI permits identification of those who are candidates for exenteration and those who are candidates for CORT on the basis of the findings regarding pelvic side wall involvement (Figs. 7.13, 7.14). Although encouraging, the results of CORT for the treatment of pelvic wall recurrences are still preliminary.

## 7.8 Conclusion

Computed tomography or MRI is recommended for visualization of recurrent carcinomas of the cervix and endometrium, detection of persistent and metastatic gestational trophoblastic disease, and evaluation of recurrent ovarian cancers. In spite of its limited tissue contrast resolution, CT remains the primary and the most practical imaging modality because of easy accessibility, lower cost, the fast examination time, and a superior sensitivity for the detection of macroscopic abdominal metastasis. CT is particularly advantageous in screening for lymph node metastases and in guided biopsy of metastases and recurrent tumor. These data are used to supplement clinical assessment in recommending suitable candidates for exenteration, CORT, additional radiation therapy, or chemotherapy.

After treatment of malignancies, MRI is useful in the assessment of the pelvis owing to its potential for differentiating radiation-induced change from recurrent tumor. MRI is reserved as a problem-solving modality in patients with a contraindication to iodinated contrast media, who are pregnant, or in whom CT findings are inconclusive.

*Acknowledgments.* I am grateful for the help and support of Du Hwan Choe, MD, Jung Hoon Lee, MD, Byung Hee Lee, MD, and Soo Yil Chin, MD at the Korea Cancer Center Hospital. I also thank Robert C. Kim, MD, at Nephrology Associates, Bridge Port, Connecticut, for his review of the manuscript.

## References

Arrive L, Chang YCF, Hricak H, et al. (1989) Radiation induced uterine changes: MR imaging. Radiology 170:55–58

Balfe DM, Van Dyke J, Lee JKT, Weyman PJ, McClennan BL (1983) Computed tomography in malignant endometrial enoplasms. J Comput Assist Tomogr 7:677–681

Bandy LC, Clarke-Pearson DL, Silverman PM, Creasman WT (1985) Computed tomography in evaluation of extrapelvic lymphadenopathy in carcinoma of the cervix. Obstet Gynecol 65:73–76

Belloni C, Del Maschio A, Sironi S (1990) Magnetic resonance imaging in endometrial carcinoma staging. Gynecol Oncol 37:172–177

Berek JS, Knapp RC, Malkasian GD, et al. (1986) CA 125 serum levels correlated with second-look operations among ovarian cancer patients. Obstet Gynecol 67:685–689

Bourne TH, Campbell S, Steer C, Whitehead MI, Collins WP (1989) Transvaginal color flow imaging: a possible new screening technique for ovarian cancer. BMJ 299:1367–1371

Bourne TH, Campbell S, Steer CV, Royston P, Whitehead MI, Collins WP (1991) Detection of endometrial cancer by transvaginal ultrasonography with color flow imaging and blood flow analysis: a preliminary report. Gynecol Oncol 40:253–259

Buist MR, Golding RP, Burger CW, et al. (1994) Comparative evaluation of diagnostic methods in ovarian carcinoma with emphasis of CT and MRI. Gynecol Oncol 52:191–198

Buy JN, Moss AA, Ghossain MA, et al. (1988) Peritoneal implants from ovarian tumors: CT findings. Radiology 169:691–694

Buy JN, Ghossain MA, Sciot C, et al. (1991) Epithelial tumors of the ovary: CT findings and correlation with US. Radiology 178:811–818

Camilien L, Gordon D, Fruchter RG, Maiman M, Boyce JG (1988) Predictive value of computerized tomography in the presurgical evaluation of primary carcinoma of the cervix. Gynecol Oncol 30:209–215

Carter J, Fowler J, Carlson J, et al. (1993) Transvaginal color flow Doppler sonography in the assessment of gestational trophoblastic disease. J Ultrasound Med 12:595–599

Chen SS, Rumancik WM, Spiegel G (1990) Magnetic resonance imaging in stage I endometrial carcinoma. Obstet Gynecol 75:274–277

Cobby M, Browning J, Jones A, Whipp E, Goddard P (1990) Magnetic resonance imaging, computed tomography, and endosonography in the local staging of carcinoma of the cervix. Br J Radiol 63:673–679

Crawford RAF, Richards PJ, Reznek RH, Ngan HYS, Shepherd JH (1996) The role of CT in predicting the surgical feasibility of exenteration in recurrent carcinoma of the cervix. Int J Gynecol Cancer 6:231–234

Davis WK, McCarthy S, Moss AA, Braga C (1984) Computed tomography of gestational trophoblastic disease. J Comput Assist Tomogr 8:1136–1139

DeLange EE, Fechner RE, Wanebo HJ (1989) Suspected recurrent rectosigmoid carcinoma after abdominoperineal resection: MR imaging and histopathologic findings. Radiology 170:323–328

Desai RK, Desberg AL (1991) Diagnosis of gestational trophoblastic disease: value of endovaginal color flow Doppler sonography. AJR 157:787–788

Dore R, Moro G, D'Andrea F, LaFianza A, Franchi M, Bolis PF (1987) CT evaluation of myometrium invasion in endometrial carcinoma. J Comput Assist Tomogr 11:282–289

Doubleday LC, Bernardino ME (1980) CT findings in the perirectal area following radiation therapy. J Comput Assist Tomogr 4:634–638

Ebner F, Kressel HY, Mintz MC, et al. (1988) Tumor recurrence versus fibrosis in the female pelvis: differentiation with MR imaging at 1.5 T. Radiology 166:333–340

Einhorn N, Bast RC, Knapp RC, Tjerngerg B, Zurawski VR (1986) Presoperative evaluation of serum CA 125 levels in patients with primary epithelial ovarian cancer. Obstet Gynecol 67:414–416

Flueckiger F, Ebner F, Poschauko H, Tamussino K, Einspieler R, Ranner G (1992) Cervical cancer: serial MR imaging before and after primary radiation therapy- a 2-year follow-up study. Radiology 184:89–93

Forstner R, Hricak H, Occhipinti KA, Powell CB, Frankel SD, Stern JL (1995a) Ovarian cancer: staging with CT and MR imaging. Radiology 197:619–626

Forstner R, Hricak H, Powell CB, Azizi L, Frankel SB, Stern JL (1995b) Ovarian cancer recurrence: value of MR imaging. Radiology 196:715–720

Frasci G, Contino A, Iaffaioli RV, Mastrantonio P, Conforti S, Persico G (1994) Computerized tomography of the abdomen and pelvis with peritoneal administration of soluble contrast (IPC-CT) in detection of residual disease for patients with ovarian cancer. Gynecol Oncol 52:154–160

Ghossain MA, Buy JN, Ligneres C, Bazot M, Hassen K, Malbec L, Hugol D (1991) Epithelial tumors of the ovary: comparison of MR and CT findings. Radiology 181:863–870

Goldhirsch A, Triller JK, Greiner R, Dreher E, Davis BW (1984) Computed tomography prior to second-look operation in advanced ovarian cancer. Radiology 152:861–867

Halvorsen RA, Panushka C, Oakley GJ, Letourneau JG, Adcock LL (1991) Intraperitoneal contrast material improves the CT detection of peritoneal metastases. AJR 157:37–40

Hand R, Fremgen A, Chmiel JS, et al. (1993) Staging procedures, clinical management, and survival outcome for ovarian carcinoma. JAMA 269:1119–1122

Harris NL, Scully RE (1984) Malignant lymphoma and granulocytic sarcoma of the uterus and vagina: a clinicopathologic analysis of 27 cases. Cancer 53:2530–2545

Hata K, Hata T, Manabe A, Sugimura K, Kitao M (1992) A critical evaluation of transvaginal Doppler studies, transvaginal sonography, magnetic resonance imaging, and CA 125 in detecting ovarian cancer. Obstet Gynecol 80:922–926

Hawighorst H, Knapstein PG, Schaeffer U, et al. (1995) Pelvic lesions in patients with treated cervical carcinoma: efficacy of pharmacokinetic analysis of dynamic MR images in distinguishing recurrent tumors from benign conditions. AJR 166:401–408

Hawnaur JM, Johnson RJ, Buckley CH, Tindall V, Isherwood I (1994) Staging, volume estimation and assessment of nodal status in carcinoma of the cervix: comparison of magnetic resonance imaging with surgical findings. Clin Radiol 49:443–452

Heiken JP, Lee JKT (1985) Recurrent pelvic malignancy. In: Walsh JW (ed) Computed tomography of the pelvis. Churchill Livingstone, New York, pp 185–209

Heller PB, Malfetano JH, Bundy BN, Barnhill DR, Okagaki T (1990) Clinical-pathologic study of stage IIB, III, and IVA carcinoma of the cervix: extended diagnostic evaluation for paraaortic node metastasis – a gynecologic oncology group study. Gynecol Oncol 38:425–430

Heron CW, Husband JE, Williams MP, Dobbs HJ, Cosgrove DO (1988) The value of CT in the diagnosis of recurrent carcinoma of the cervix. Clinical Radiology 39:496–501

Hoeckel M, Knapstein PG (1992) The combined operative and radiotherapeutic treatment (CORT) of recurrent tumors infiltrating the pelvic wall: first experience with 18 patients. Gynecol Oncol 46:20–28

Hoskins WJ (1993) Surgical staging and cytoreductive surgery of epithelial ovarian cancer. Cancer 71:1534–1540

Hoskins WJ, McGuire WP, Brady MF, et al. (1994) The effect of diameter of largest residual disease on survival after primary cytoreductive surgery in patients with suboptimal residual epithelial ovarian carcinoma. Am J Obstet Gynecol 170:974–980

Hricak H (1994) Magnetic resonance imaging evaluation of the irradiated female pelvis. Semin Roentgenol 29:70–80

Hricak H, Demas BE, Braga CA, Fisher MR, Winkler ML (1986) Gestational trophoblastic neoplasm of the uterus: MR assessment. Radiology 161:11–16

Hricak H, Stern JL, Fisher MR, Shapeero LG, Winkler ML, Lacey CG (1987) Endometrial carcinoma staging by MR imaging. Radiology 162:297–305

Hricak H, Lacey CG, Sandles LG, Chang YCF, Winkler ML, Stern JL (1988) Invasive cervical carcinoma: comparison of MR imaging and surgical findings. Radiology 166:623–631

Hricak H, Hamm B, Semelka RC, et al. (1991) Carcinoma of the uterus: use of gadopentetate dimeglumine in MR imaging. Radiology 181:95–106

Hricak H, Swift PS, Campos Z, Quivey JM, Gildengorin V, Goeranson H (1993) Irradiation of the cervix uteri: value of unenhanced and contrast-enhanced MR imaging. Radiology 189:381–388

Jain KA (1994) Prospective evaluation of adnexal masses with endovaginal gray-scale and duplex and color Doppler US: correlation with pathologic findings. Radiology 191:63–67

Johnson RJ (1993) Radiology in the management of ovarian cancer. Clin Radiol 48:75–82

Kawakami S, Togashi K, Kojima N, Norikawa K, Nori T, Konishi J (1995) MR appearance of malignant lymphoma of the uterus. J Comput Assist Tomogr 19:238–242

Kim KH, Lee BH, Do YS, et al. (1994) Stage IIb cervical carcinoma: MR evaluation of effect of intraarterial chemotherapy. Radiology 192:61–65

Kim SH, Choi BI, Lee HP, Kang SB, Choi YM, Han MC, Kim CW (1990) Uterine cervical carcinoma: comparison of CT and MR findings. Radiology 175:45–51

Kim SH, Choi BI, Han JK, et al. (1993) Preoperative staging of uterine cervical carcinoma: comparison of CT and MRI in 99 patients. J Comput Assist Tomogr 17:633–640

Kim SH, Kim SC, Choi BI, Han MC (1994) Uterine cervical carcinoma: evaluation of pelvic lymph node metastasis with MR imaging. Radiology 190:807–811

King ME, Kramer EE (1980) Malignant müllerian mixed tumors of the uterus. A study of 21 cases. Cancer 45:188–190

Kohorn EI (1993) Evaluation of the criteria used to make the diagnosis of nonmetastatic gestational trophoblastic neoplasia. Gynecol Oncol 48:139–147

Krestin GP, Steinbrich W, Friedmann G (1988) Recurrent rectal cancer: diagnosis with MR imaging versus CT. Radiology 168:307–311

Kuhlman JE, Fishman EK (1990) CT evaluation of enterovaginal and vesicovaginal fistulas. J Comput Assist Tomogr 14:390–394

Kurjak A, Azlud I, Alfirevic Z (1991) Evaluation of adnexal masses with transvaginal color ultrasound. J Ultrasound Med 10:295–297

Lang EK (1989) Management of hemorrhagic pelvis neoplasms by transcatheter embolization. J Intervent Radiol 4:113–117

Libshitz HI (1994) Radiation changes in bone. Semin Roentgenol 29:15–37

Lien HH, Blomlie V, Trope C, Kaern J, Abeler VM (1991) Cancer of the endometrium: value of MR imaging in determining depth of invasion into the myometrium. AJR 175:1221–1223

Matsukuma K, Tsukamoto N, Matsuyama T, Ono M, Nakano H (1989) Preoperative CT study of lymph nodes in cervical cancer: its correlation with histological findings. Gynecol Oncol 33:168–171

Megibow AJ, Bosniak MA, Ho AG, Beller U, Hulnick DH, Beckman EM (1988) Accuracy of CT in detection of persistent or recurrent ovarian carcinoma: correlation with second-look laparotomy. Radiology 166:341–345

Meyer JI, Kennedy AW, Friedman R, Ayoub A, Zepp RC (1995) Ovarian carcinoma: vlaue of CT in predicting success of debulking surgery. AJR 875–878

Mezrich R (1994) Magnetic resonance imaging: applications in uterine cervical cancer. MRI Clin North Am 2:211–243

Miller DS, Spirtos NM, Ballon SC, et al. (1992) Critical reassessment of second look laparotomy for epithelial ovarian cancer. Cancer 69:502–510

Mitchel DG, Hill MC, Hill S, et al. (1986) Serous carcinoma of the ovary: CT identification of metastatic calcified implants. Radiology 158:649–652

Nelson BE, Rosenfield AT, Schwartz PE (1993) Preoperative abdominopelvic computed tomographic prediction of optimal cytoreduction in epithelial ovarian carcinoma. J Clin Oncol 11:166–172

Nelson RC, Chezmar JL, Hoel MJ, Buck DR, Sugarbaker PH (1992) Peritoneal carcinomatosis: preoperative CT with intraperitoneal contrast material. Radiology 182:133–138

Ng HT, Shyu SK, Chen YK, Yuan CC, Chao KC, Kan YY (1992) A scoring system for predicting recurrence of cervical cancer. Cancer 2:75–78

Nielsen SN, Podratz KC, Scheithauer BW, O'Brien PC (1989) Clinicopathologic analysis of uterine malignant mixed müllerian tumors. Gynecol Oncol 34:372–378

NIH Consensus Development Panel on Ovarian Cancer (1995) Ovarian cancer: screening, treatment and follow-up. JAMA 273:491–496

Park SY, Kim BG, Kim KH, et al. (1995) Phase I/II study of neoadjuvant intraarterial chemotherapy with mitomycin-C, vincristine, and cisplatin in patients with stage IIb bulky cervical carcinoma. Cancer 76:814–823

Patsner B, Orr JW, Mann WJ, Taylor PT, Partridge E, Allmen T (1990) Does serum CA-125 level prior to second-look laparotomy for invasive ovarian adenocarcinoma predict size of residual disease? Gynecol Oncol 37:319–322

Perez CA, Breaux S, Madoc-Jones H, et al. (1983) Radiation therapy alone in the treatment of carcinoma of uterine cervix. 1. Analysis of tumor recurrence. Cancer 51:1393–1402

Popovich MJ, Hricak H, Sugimura K, Stern JL (1993) The role of MR imaging in determining surgical eligibility for pelvic exenteration. AJR 160:525–531

Posniak HV, Olson MC, Dudiak CM, et al. (1990) MR imaging of uterine carcinoma: correlation with clinical and pathologic findings. Radiographics 10:15–17

Prayer L, Kainz C, Kramer J, et al. (1993) CT and MR accuracy in the detection of tumor recurrence in patients treated for ovarian cancer. J Comput Assist Tomogr 17:626–632

Ramsey RG, Zacharias CE (1985) MR imaging of the spine after radiation therapy: easily recognizable effects. AJR 144:1131–1135

Reddy S, Lee MS, Hendrickson FR (1979) Pattern of recurreneces in endometrial carcinoma and their management. Radiology 133:737–740

Reuter K, Griffin T, Hunter RE (1989) Comparison of abdominopelvic computed tomography results and find ings at second-look laparotomy in ovarian carcinoma patients. Cancer 63:1123–1128

Richardson GS, Scully RE, Nikrui N, Nelson JH (1985) Common epithelial cancer of the ovary (part I). N Engl J Med 312:415–424

Rose PG, Nelson BE, Fournier L, Junter RE (1992) Serum squamous cell carcinoma antigen levels in invasive squamous vulvar cancer. J Surg Oncol 50:183–186

Sanders C, Rubin E (1987) Malignant gestational trophoblastic disease: CT findings. AJR 148:165–168

Semelka RC, Lawrence PH, Shoenut JP, Heywood M, Kroeker MA, Lotocki R (1993) Primary ovarian cancer: prospective comparison of contrast-enhanced CT and pre-and postcontrast, fat-suppressed MR imaging, with histologic correlation. J Magn Reson Imaging 3:99–106

Shapeero LG, Hricak H (1988) Mixed müllerian sarcoma of the uterus: MR imaging findings. AJR 153:317–319

Shaw RW, Lynch PF, Wade-Evans T (1983) Müllerian mixed tumor of the uterine corpus: a clinical histopathological review of 28 patients. Br J Obstet Gynecol 90:562–569

Shield PW, Wright RG, Free K, Daunter B (1991) The accuracy of cervicovaginal cytology in the detection of recurrent cervical carcinoma following radiotherapy. Gynecol Oncol 41:223–229

Shingleton HM, Soong SJ, Gelder MS, Hatch KD, Baker VV, Austin JM (1989) Clinical and histopathologic factors predicting recurrence and survival after pelvic exenteration for cancer of the cervix. Obstet Gynecol 73:1027–1034

Silverman PM, Osborne M, Dunnick NR, Bandy LC (1988) CT prior to second-look operation in ovarian cancer. AJR 150:829–832

Sironi S, Belloni C, Taccagni G, Del Maschio A (1991) Invasive cervical carcinoma: MR imaging after preoperative chemotherapy. Radiology 180:719–722

Sironi S, Colombo E, Villa G, Taccagni G, Belloni C, Garancini P, Del Maschio A (1992) Myometrial invasion by endometrial carcinoma: assessment with plain and gadolinium-enhanced MR imaging. Radiology 185:207–212

Squillaci E, Salzani MC, Grandinetti ML, Auffermann W, Marsella A, Maresca G, Colagrande C (1988) Recurrence of ovarian and uterine neoplasms: diagnosis with transrectal US. Radiology 169:355–358

Stevens SK, Moore SG, Kaplan ID (1990) Early and late bone-marrow changes after irradiation: MR evaluation. AJR 154:745–750

Stevens SK, Hricak H, Stern JL (1991) Ovarian lesions: detection and characterization with gadolinium-enhanced MR imaging at 1.5 T. Radiology 181:481–488

Sugimura K, Carrington BM, Quivey JM, Hricak H (1990) Postirradiation changes in the pelvis: assessment with MR imaging. Radiology 175:805–813

Tavares NJ, Arrive L, Demas BE, Quivey J, Hricak H (1988) Bladder morphology following radiation therapy: assessment with MR imaging (abstr). Radiology 169:169

Taylor PM, Johnson RJ, Eddleston BE, Hunter RD (1990) Radiological changes in the gastrointestinal and genitourinary tract following radiotherapy for carcinoma of the cervix. Clin Radiol 41:165–169

Thorvinger B, Horvath G, Samuelsson L (1990) CT demonstration of fistulae in patients with gynecologic neoplasms. Acta Radiologica 31:357–360

Thurnher SA (1992) MR imaging of pelvic masses in women: contrast enhanced vs unenhanced images. AJR 159:1243–1250

Togashi K, Nishimura K, Sagoh T, et al. (1989) Carcinoma of the cervix: staging with MR imaging. Radiology 171:245–251

Vick CW, Walsh JW, Wheelock JB, et al. (1984) CT of the normal and abnormal parametria in cervical cancer. AJR 143:597–603

Villasanta U, Whitley NO, Haney PJ, Brenner D (1983) Computed tomography in invasive carcinoma of the cervix: an appraisal. Obstet Gynecol 62:218–224

Waggenspack GA, Amparo EG, Hannigan EV (1988) MR imaging of uterine cervical carcinoma. J Comput Assist Tomogr 12:409–414

Wagner BJ, Buck JL, Seidman JD, McCabe KM (1994) Ovarian epithelial neoplasms: radiologic pathologic correlation. Radiographics 14:1351–1374

Walsh JW (1992) Computed tomography of gynecologic neoplasms. Radiol Clin North Am 30:817–830

Walsh JW, Amendola MA, Hall DJ, Tisnado J, Goplerud DR (1981) Recurrent carcinoma of the cervix: CT diagnosis. AJR 136:117–122

Weber TM, Sostman HD, Spritzer CE, Ballard RL, Meyer GA, Clarke-Pearson DL, Soper JT (1995) Cervical carcinoma: determination of recurrent tumor extent versus radiation changes with MR imaging. Radiology 194:135–139

Williams MP, Husband JE, Heron CW, Cherryman GR, Koslin DB (1989) Magnetic resonance imaging in recurrent carcinoma of the cervix. Br J Radiol 62:544–550

Worthington JL, Balfe DM, Lee JKT, et al. (1986) Uterine neoplasms: MR imaging. Radiology 159:725–830

Yamada I, Suzuki S (1993) Primary uterine lymphoma: MR imaging. AJR 160:662–663

Yamashita Y, Mizutani H, Torshima M, et al. (1993) Assessment of myometrial invasion by endometrial carcinoma: transvaginal sonography vs contrast-enhanced MR imaging. AJR 161:595–599

Yong RC, Perez CA, Hoskins W (1993) Cancer of the ovary. In: De Vita VT, Hellman S, Rosenberg SA (eds) Cancer: principles and practice of oncology, 4th edn, vol 1. Lippincott, Philadelphia, pp 1226–1263

# 8 Magnetic Resonance Imaging of Invasive Mole

Y. Yamashita and M. Takahashi

CONTENTS



## 8.1 Introduction

Gestational trophoblastic disease (GTD) comprises a spectrum of proliferative abnormalities of trophoblasts ranging from partial and complete hydatidiform mole to postmolar GTD and choriocarcinoma. The biologic behavior varies from the rarely invasive hydatidiform mole to the highly aggressive choriocarcinoma. Although the division of these diseases is useful in understanding the various manifestations and progression of disease, it should be recognized that since the advent of an accurate immunologic biologic marker for this disease (beta-human chorionic gonadotropin, β-hCG), this division has had less clinical utility.

## 8.2 Hydatidiform Mole

Complete hydatidiform mole develops when an empty ovum is fertilized by two sperm or by one diploid sperm. It is classically described as a mass of grape-like vesicles. Histologically, a complete mole is characterized by swelling of chorionic villi, which are enveloped by atypical, hyperplastic trophoblasts. Ultrasound (US) excludes the presence of a normal intrauterine gestation. The typical US appearance is distention of the uterine cavity by a soft tissue mass containing numerous small cystic spaces. These lesions are rarely imaged on magnetic resonance (MR) imaging.

Y. Yamashita, MD, Associate Professor, Department of Radiology, Kumamoto University School of Medicine, 1-1-1 Honjo, Kumamoto, 860, Japan
M. Takahashi, MD, Professor and Chairman Department of Radiology, Kumamoto University School of Medicine, 1-1-1 Honjo, Kumamoto, 860, Japan

## 8.3 Invasive Mole and Choriocarcinoma

Postmolar GTD refers to both locally invasive disease (invasive mole) and distant metastases. Invasive mole forms an irregular hemorrhagic mass that raggedly penetrates the myometrium; an extrauterine site may also be identified (Salafia and Popek 1996). Postmolar GTD most commonly follows a complete hydatidiform mole but may occur subsequent to any gestational event, including abortion, ectopic pregnancy, or term pregnancy. "Invasive" implies that molar villi and trophoblasts have extended more deeply and widely than the normal uterine implantation. Approximately 20% of patients undergoing an evacuation of a complete hydatidiform mole develop postmolar GTD. Approximately 70%–90% of these cases consist of a histologically defined invasive mole while the remainder are choriocarcinoma. Postmolar GTD is clinically assessed by monitoring of the β-hCG level (Soper et al. 1992; Hilgers and Lewis 1982).

Treatment of postmolar GTD varies according to the degree of invasion and the presence of metastases. Evacuation of a molar pregnancy is curative in most patients. Patients are usually followed by measurement of the serum β-hCG level, which is a sensitive indicator of the presence of disease. A rise or plateau in the serum β-hCG level following evacuation is diagnostic of invasive or postmolar GTD. Postmolar GTD is extremely sensitive to chemotherapy, and even patients with distant metastases have a cure rate approaching 100%.

Metastases occur most frequently to the lungs (80%), vagina (30%), pelvis (20%), liver, and brain.

Therefore, the diagnosis of postmolar GTD requires assessment of local and distant disease for optimal therapy (Soper et al. 1992; Hilgers and Lewis 1982). Computed tomographic (CT) scanning of the chest, abdomen, and pelvis is used to detect both local extension of disease and distant metastases in patients with GTD. Although GTD is usually sensitive to chemotherapy, tumors involving the uterine wall are frequently resistant (Hertz 1971). Delayed hysterectomy is often necessary to control residual tumor foci in the pelvis when resistance to chemotherapy develops. Therefore, identification of tumor nodules in the myometrium or parametrium may have therapeutic implications (Sanders and Rubin 1987). The diagnosis of myometrial involvement by invasive trophoblasts is difficult to make by means of uterine curettage.

Although the diagnosis of hydatidiform mole and persistent GTD is made clinically on the basis of the serum β-hCG level, diagnostic imaging can play a useful role in certain clinical settings. Various imaging techniques have been used to demonstrate the focus of myometrial involvement (Soper et al. 1992). In patients with persistently elevated serum β-hCG level following molar evacuation, US is useful to exclude intrauterine pregnancy and may demonstrate focal areas of increased echogenicity within the uterus. Color Doppler imaging may assist in the detection of myometrial involvement. However, evaluation of myometrial disease is often difficult with US. Formerly, angiography and CT were applied for evaluation of uterine disease. The recently introduced MR imaging provides advantages over these modalities in staging of the disease. The role of MR imaging in the diagnosis of GTD has not been defined, but it is considered to be superior to other imaging techniques in tumor detection and follow-up (Hricak et al. 1986).

In postmolar GTD, MR imaging detects tumors deeply invading the myometrium without extension to the endometrial surface. Recognition of invasive trophoblastic disease on conventional T2-weighted images depends on the presence of hyperintense areas in the myometrium (Figs. 8.1, 8.2). The findings

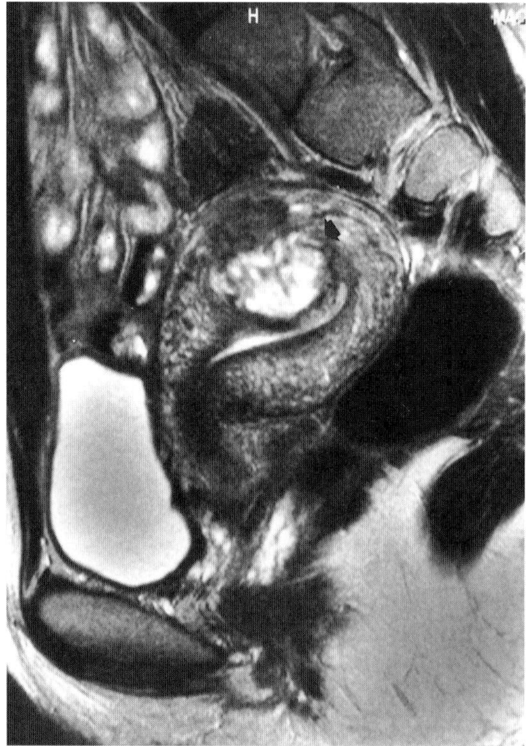


a

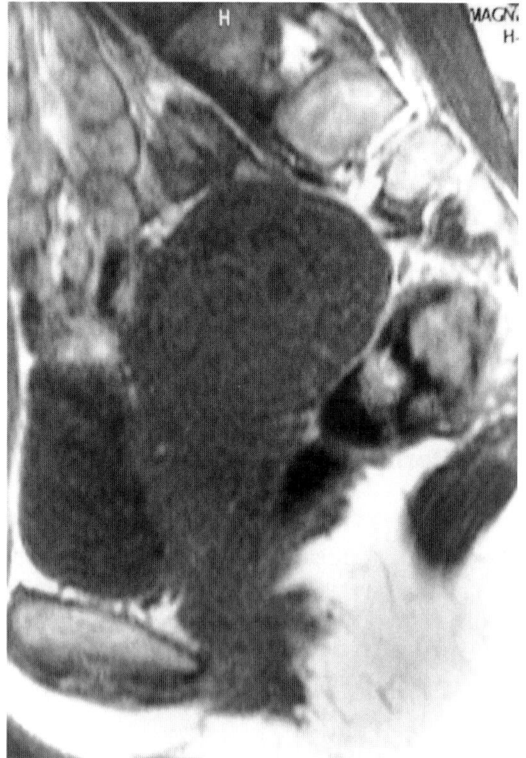


b

**Fig. 8.1 a,b.** A 37-year-old female with invasive GTD. **a** Sagittal T2-weighted image before chemotherapy shows a heterogeneously hyperintense mass in the anterior wall of the uterus (*arrow*). The zonal anatomy is preserved. **b–d** Dynamic MR images (**b** precontrast, **c** early phase, **d** delayed phase) demonstrate markedly enhancing spots within the mass, indicating viable trophoblastic tissue in the early phase. The remaining tissue shows little enhancement, indicating necrotic tissue. **e** After seven courses of chemotherapy, when the serum β-hCG level had decreased to the normal range, the myometrial mass had decreased in size, although hypointense lesions remain on this T2-weighted image

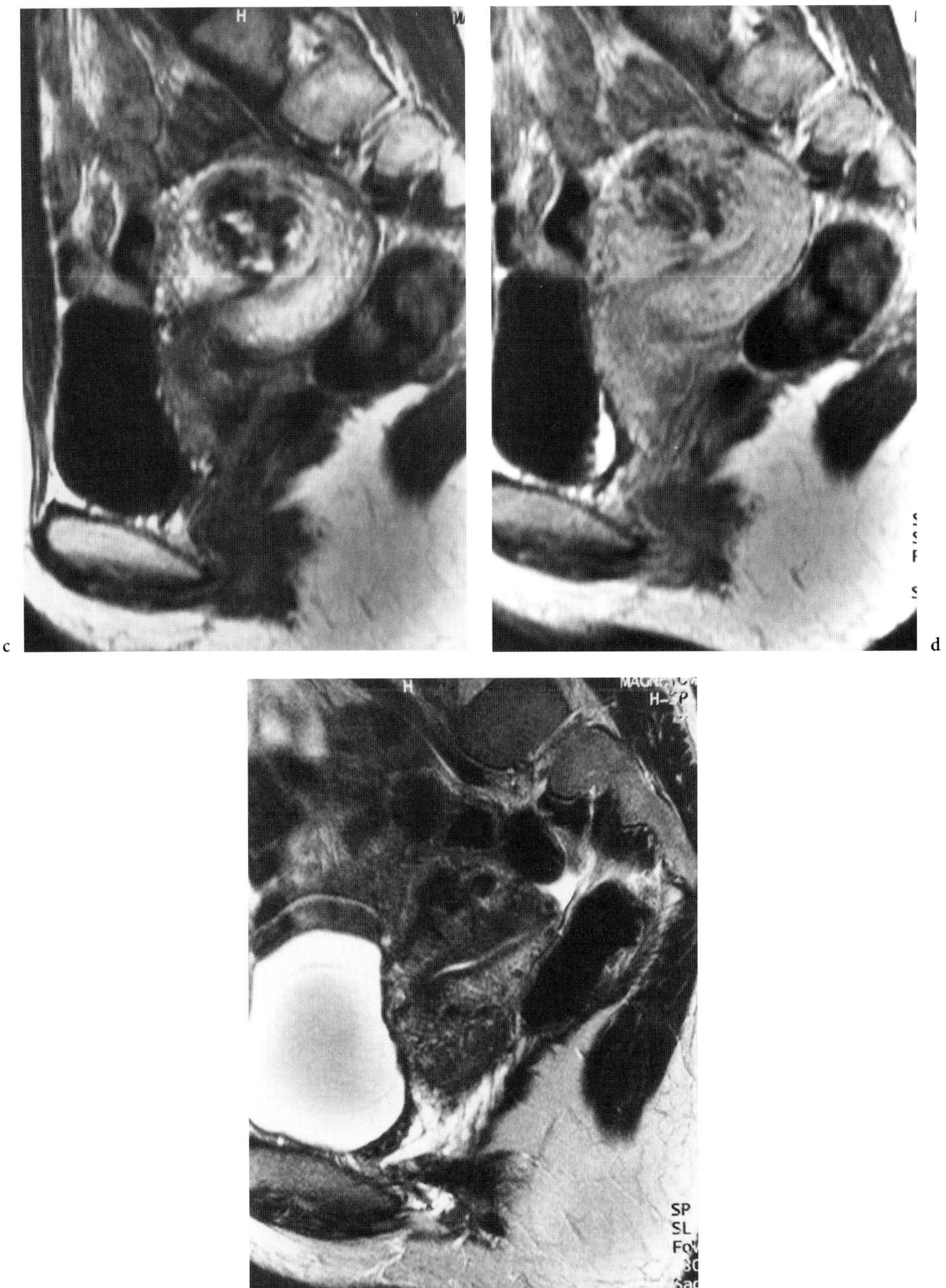


Fig. 8.1 a,b. *Continued*

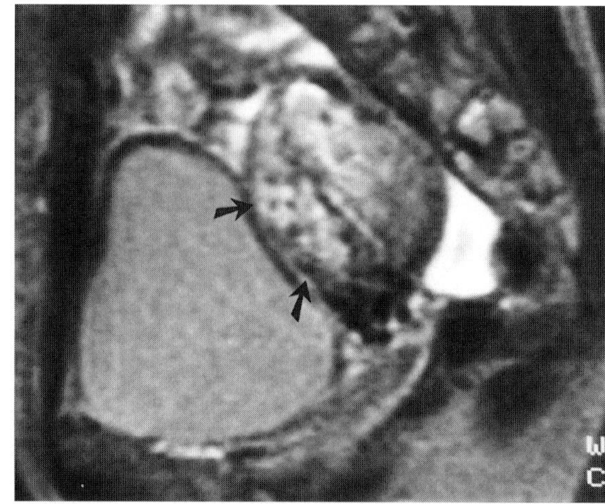


a

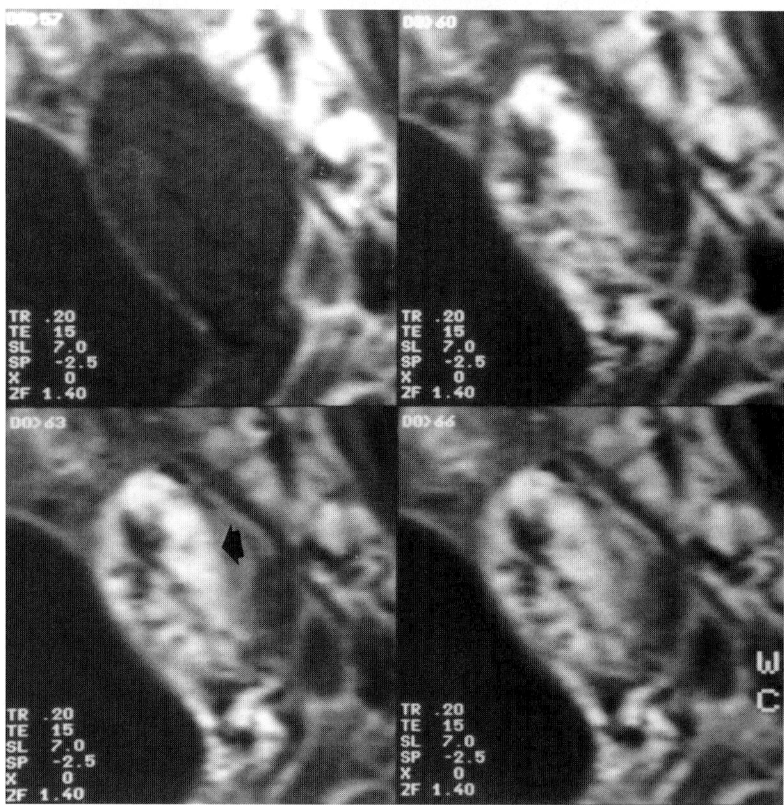


b

**Fig. 8.2 a–d.** A 24-year-old female with invasive GTD. **a** Sagittal T2-weighted image before chemotherapy shows a markedly large hyperintense mass with engorged spotty vessels in the uterine cervix (*arrows*). The zonal anatomy is obscured. **b** Dynamic MR images (*upper left*, precontrast; *upper right*, 30 s; *lower left*, 120 s; *lower right*, 180 s) demonstrate a markedly enhancing mass in the cervix (*arrowheads*). **c** After three courses of chemotherapy, when the serum β-hCG level had decreased to the normal range, the cervical mass appears slightly decreased in size. **d** On dynamic images, the abnormal enhancement is remarkably reduced (*arrow*) (from Yamashita et al., Acta Radiol 36:188–192)

of postmolar GTD may vary; however, marked heterogeneity is seen in the myometrium on T2-weighted images due to tumor necrosis, hemorrhage, and cyst formation (Sanders and Rubin 1987; Barton et al. 1993). Tumors as well as these associated myometrial findings appear hyperintense or hypointense on T2-weighted images (Figs. 8.1, 8.2). In addition, these abnormalities are nonspecific and may also be present in patients with missed abortions or ectopic pregnancy (Salafia and Popek 1996).

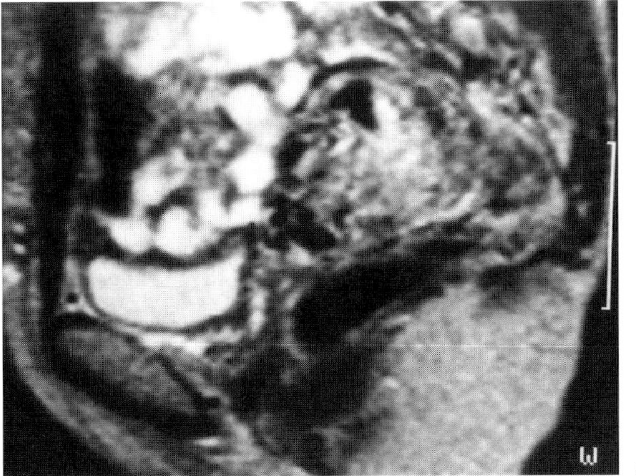

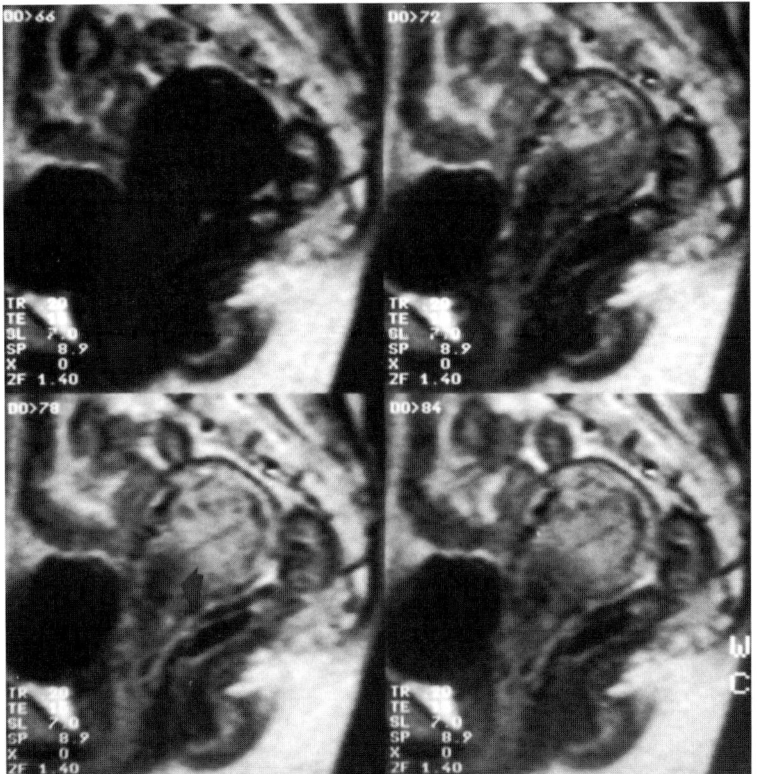

Fig. 8.2 a–d. *Continued*

As patients respond to chemotherapy, the tumor vascularity decreases, intralesional hemorrhage develops, and the normal uterine zonal anatomy reappears on T2-weighted images (Fig. 8.3) (HRICAK et al. 1986). MR imaging also reveals a decrease in uterine volume, and disappearance of the theca luteal cysts. However, myometrial abnormalities remain after several courses of chemotherapy, when the serum β-hCG level has been normalized (Figs. 8.1, 8.3). Research is ongoing to determine whether a MR imaging can be used to predict patients who will develop persistent GTD or who will respond to chemotherapy.

Contrast-enhanced dynamic MR imaging after rapid injection of Gd-DTPA has proved a useful technique in the evaluation of uterine neoplasms (HIRANO et al. 1992; YAMASHITA et al. 1993). Because invasive GTD is usually extremely hypervascular, (COCKSHOTT et al. 1964; BORELL et al. 1955), we perform both conventional T2-weighted and contrast-enhanced dynamic MR imaging in patients with postmolar GTD for the

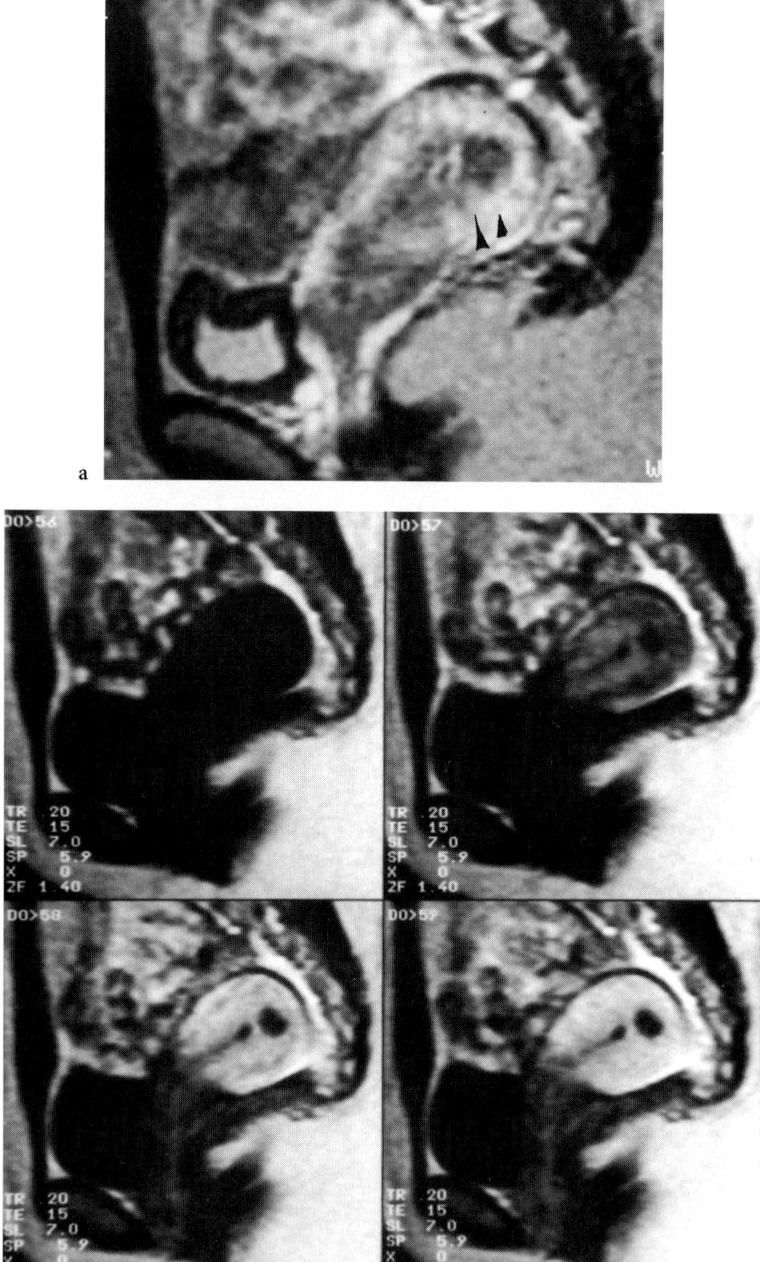


**Fig. 8.3 a,b.** A 21-year-old female with postmolar persistently elevated hCG. The serum β-hCG level was 4 mIU/ml at the time of MR study. **a** Sagittal T2-weighted image shows a hypointense mass in the myometrium (*arrowheads*). The zonal anatomy is partially obscured. **b** On dynamic MR images (*upper left*, pre; *upper right*, 30 s; *lower left*, 120 s; *lower right*, 180 s), the fundal lesion seen on the T2-weighted image displays no contrast enhancement, probably indicating necrosis, cyst, or hemorrhage. The rest of the myometrium shows a normal enhancement pattern (from YAMASHITA et al., Acta Radiol 36:188–192)

assessment of myometrial lesions (BORELL et al. 1955).

The area of focal enhancement on contrast-enhanced dynamic MR images correlates with changes in the serum β-hCG level indicating the amount of active trophoblastic tissue present (Fig. 8.4) (MORROW and TOWNSEND 1987). Areas of marked enhancement in the early dynamic phase indicate viable trophoblastic cells accompanied by villous stroma and inflammatory reactions of the surrounding myometrium. Extensive enhancement was seen in patients with a markedly elevated β-hCG

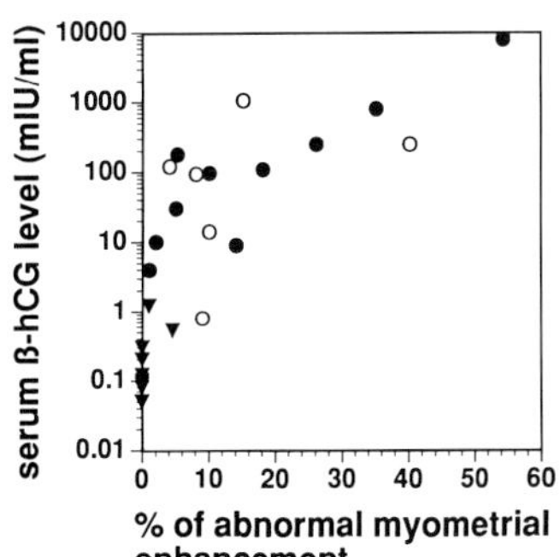


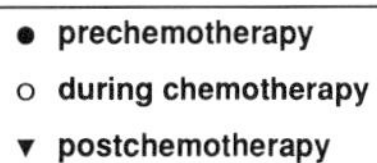


**Fig. 8.4.** Correlation of area of abnormal enhancement on dynamic MR imaging with serum β-hCG level. *Solid circles*, prechemotherapy; *open circles*, during chemotherapy; *triangles*, often chemotherapy. The degree of contrast enhancement correlated with the serum β-hCG level obtained before, during, and after chemotherapy (r = 0.72, $P$ = 0.003) (from YAMASHITA et al., Acta Radiol 36:188–192)

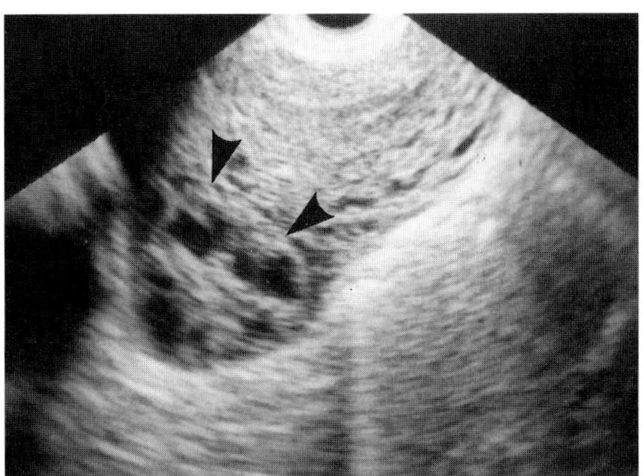

a

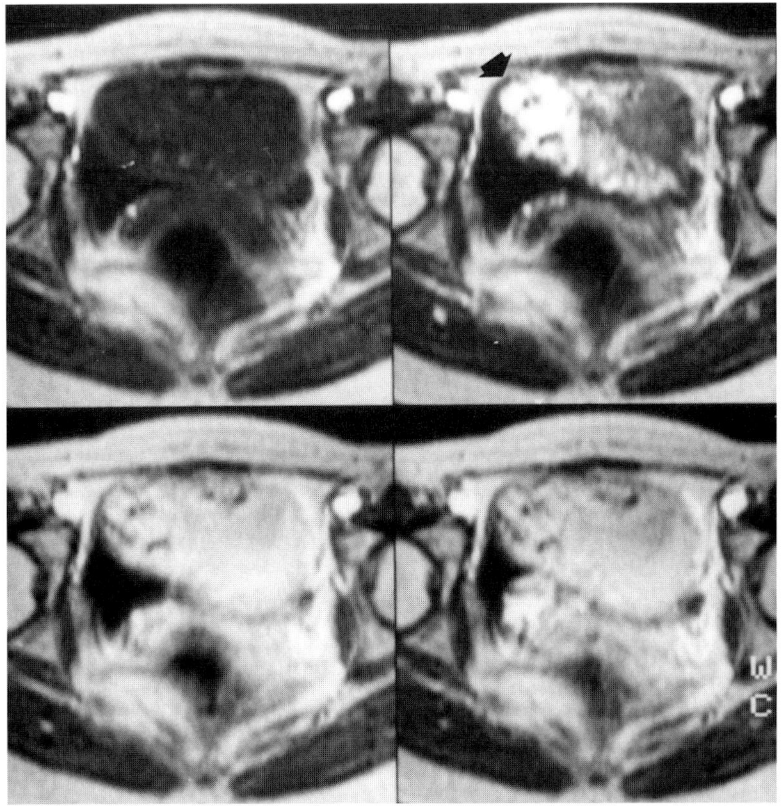

b

**Fig. 8.5 a,b.** A 22-year-old female with ectopic (interstitial) pregnancy simulating invasive GTD. The patient had been amenorrhea for the last 2 months and the urine β-hCG level was elevated (8000 IU/dl). **a** Transvaginal ultrasound shows an irregular echoic mass (*arrows*) at the right cornu of the uterus. **b** Dynamic MR imaging shows remarkable contrast enhancement (*arrow*), suggesting the lesion is very vascular. Histologic examination revealed the mass to be composed of normal villi, consistent with ectopic pregnancy in the right cornu of the uterus (Permission from YAMASHITA et al., Comp Med Imag & Graphics 19:211–246)

level, and the enhancement decreased with reduction in the serum β-hCG level after repeated courses of chemotherapy. Therefore, contrast-enhanced dynamic MR imaging might be useful for the follow-up of myometrial diseases in postmolar GTD (Yamashita et al. 1995a). Postcontrast T1-weighted images are of limited value compared with dynamic MR images because the tumor–myometrial contrast decreases on delayed images, on which enhancement of the normal myometrium occurs (Fig. 8.1d).

Choriocarcinoma in preceded by complete hydatidiform mole in 50% of cases, by miscarriage in 25%, by normal pregnancy in 24%, and by an ectopic pregnancy in 1.5%. Grossly the tumor is hemorrhagic and friable. The tumor widely invades maternal vessels, with extensive hemorrhage and necrosis. We have not experienced a case of this rare disease.

## 8.4 Differential Diagnosis

Similar MR findings can be seen in missed abortions or ectopic pregnancy (Barton et al. 1993; Yamashita et al. 1995b). Although the differential diagnosis of invasive mole and ectopic pregnancy in a previously pregnant woman should be made clinically or by measurement of the β-hCG level, diagnostic imaging can play a useful role. In patients with an elevated β-hCG level but negative histology on D&C, MR imaging can accurately demonstrate persistent uterine disease. However, the radiologic findings of both entities can be similar, probably because (a) a fetus or gestational sac is not usually seen in ectopic pregnancy and (b) both ectopic pregnancy and GTD have abundant vascular spaces between trophoblasts. Among these diseases, interstitial pregnancy is particularly difficult to diagnose not only on clinical examination but also on imaging studies (Yamashita et al. 1995) (Fig. 8.5). When the fertilized ovum implants within the interstitial segment of the tube, interstitial pregnancy results; such cases account for about 2.5% of all tubal gestations. Because of the greater distensibility of the myometrium covering the interstitial portion compared to the other segments of the tube, rupture of an interstitial pregnancy is likely to occur later, but may be fatal due to the abundant blood supply from branches of both uterine and ovarian arteries immediately adjacent to the implantation site (Pritchard et al. 1985).

## 8.5 Conclusion

In conclusion, the role of MR imaging in cases of invasive mole lies in the detection of myometrial abnormalities and in follow-up. The appearance on T2-weighted images is usually nonspecific. Contrast-enhanced dynamic MR imaging seems to have potential for the demonstration of myometrial involvement is postmolar GTD and may be useful in monitoring treatment effect.

## References

Barton JW, McCarthy SM, Kohorn EI, Scoutt LM, Lange RC (1993) Pelvic MR imaging findings in gestational trophoblastic disease, incomplete abortion, and ectopic pregnancy: are they specific? Radiology 186:163–168

Borell U, Fernstrom I, Westman A (1955) Value of pelvic arteriography in diagnosis of mole and chorioepithelima. Acta Radiol 44:378–383

Cockshott WP, Evans KT, deV Hendrickse JP (1964) Arteriography of trophoblastic tumors. Clin Radiol 15:1–8

Hertz R (1971) Biological aspects of gestational neoplasms derived from trophoblast. Ann NY Acad Sci 172:279–287

Hilgers RD, Lewis JL (1982) Gestational trophoblastic disease. In: Danforth DN (ed) Obstetrics and gynecology. Harper & Row, Philadelphia, pp 393–406

Hirano Y, Kubo K, Hirai Y, et al. (1992) Preliminary experience with gadolinium-enhanced dynamic MR imaging for uterine neoplasms. Radiographics 12:243–256

Hricak H, Demas BE, Braga CA, Fisher MR, Winkler ML (1986) Gestational trophoblastic neoplasm of the uterus: MR assessment. Radiology 161:11–16

Morrow CP, Townsend DE (1987) Tumors of the ovary: general considerations, classification, the adnexal mass. In: Morrow CP, Townsend DE (eds) Synopsis of gynecologic oncology. Wiley, New York, pp 231–255

Pritchard JA, MacDonald PC, Gant NF (1985) Ectopic pregnancy. In: Williams' obstetrics, 17 edn. Appleton-Century-Crofts, Norwalk, pp 423–439

Salafia CM, Popek EJ (1996) Placenta. In: Damjanov I, Linder J (eds) Anderson's pathology, 7 edn. vol 2. Mosby, St. Louis, pp 2310–2353

Sanders C, Rubin E (1987) Malignant gestational trophoblastic disease: CT findings. AJR 148:165–168

Soper JT, Hammond CB, Lewis JLJ (1992) Gestational trophoblastic disease. In: Hoskins WJ, Peterz CA, Young RC (ed) Principles and practice of gynecologic oncology. Lippincott, Philadelphia, pp 795–825

Yamashita Y, Torashima M, Takahashi M, et al. (1995) Contrast-enhanced dynamic MR imaging of postmolar gestational trophoblastic disease. Acta Radiol 36:188–192

Yamashita Y, Harada M, Torashima M, et al. (1995) Unruptured interstitial pregnancy: a pitfall of MR Imaging. Comp Med Imag & Graphics 19:241–246

# 9 Magnetic Resonance Imaging of the Ovary: Correlation with Ultrasound

Y. YAMASHITA and M. TAKAHASHI

CONTENTS



## 9.1 Introduction

The detection and characterization of an ovarian mass represent a continuing clinical and radiological challenge. Characterization is of utmost importance in the preoperative evaluation of an ovarian neoplasm, as it enables the surgeon to anticipate carcinoma of the ovary before the operation so that adequate procedures are planned. However, the imaging characteristics of ovarian masses do not always permit differentiation of malignant from benign lesions. Numerous investigators have tried to solve this problem, but thus far no clear-cut answers have been obtained.

Although ultrasonography (US) remains the foremost imaging modality for screening patients with adnexal lesions, magnetic resonance (MR) imaging has demonstrated potential in the evaluation of pathologic adnexal conditions and has been used in the diagnosis of various types of adnexal masses (OSMERS et al. 1990; NYBERG, et al. 1987; NISHIMURA et al. 1987; TOGASHI et al. 1987, 1991). Indeed, MR imaging and transvaginal or transabdominal US have been reported to show a similar sensitivity in the characterization of adnexal masses (BROWN et al. 1990; GRANBERG et al. 1991), although in one recent prospective study transvaginal US (TVUS) did emerge as the better modality (JAIN et al. 1993).

A number of studies have evaluated the sensitivity and specificity of MR imaging in distinguishing benign from malignant ovarian masses. With conventional MR imaging, the fine internal architectural details are not visualized, and this is considered to preclude specific diagnosis. Contrast-enhanced MR imaging allows better depiction of the internal architecture and differentiation of cystic from solid lesions, and is therefore particularly useful in differentiation between malignant and benign lesions (STEVENS et al. 1991; THURNHER et al. 1990). It has been shown that contrast enhancement with Gd-DTPA considerably improves the sensitivity and specificity of MR imaging (STEVENS et al. 1991; OUTWATER and KRESSEL 1992; YAMASHITA et al. 1995). Because of its high cost its use should be limited to assisting in the characterization of a mass, particularly when a sonogram is suboptimal or indeterminate (RICCIO et al. 1990; TAYLOR and SCHWARTZ 1994).

Characterization of some epithelial or stromal ovarian lesions is occasionally difficult. In order to differentiate such diagnostically indeterminate lesions, various trials have utilized morphologic characteristics (LERNER et al. 1994; SASSONE et al. 1991) or flow analysis using color Doppler (KURJAK et al. 1991; FLEISCHER et al. 1991; WEINER et al. 1992). However, whichever criteria are employed, there is still considerable overlap between benign and malignant lesions (BROWN et al. 1994).

## 9.2 US and MR Finding in Respect of the Normal Ovary

The ovaries are paired pelvic organs that lie on either side of the uterus close to the lateral pelvic wall,

Y. YAMASHITA, MD, Associate Professor, Department of Radiology, Kumamoto University School of Medicine, 1-1-1 Honjo, Kumanoto, 860, Japan
M. TAKAHASHI, MD, Professor and Chairman Department of Radiology, Kumamoto University School of Medicine, 1-1-1 Honjo, Kumamoto, 860, Japan

behind the broad ligament and anterior to the rectum. The ovary is joined to the posterior aspect of the broad ligament by the mesovarium, to the ipsilateral uterine cornu by the ovarian ligament, and to the lateral pelvic wall by the suspensory ligament.

On both TVUS (Fig. 9.1) and high-resolution MR imaging (Fig. 9.2), small follicles are almost invariably identified in the ovaries of normal women of child-bearing age and may occasionally be found in postmenopausal women as well. Adult ovaries are ovoid, measuring approximately 3–5 cm in maximum diameter. The size varies considerably depending on age and content of follicular derivatives (Prat 1996). Normal ovarian size also fluctuates with the phase of the menstrual cycle, and the ovary containing the ovulatory follicle is usually larger. On MR imaging, ovarian stroma and the capsule are evident. Occasionally, hemorrhage is seen in the follicle.

## 9.3 Benign Lesions

Ovarian diseases of surgical importance can be broadly divided into nonneoplastic cysts, inflammation, and neoplasms. Benign lesions include nonneoplastic cysts (inclusion cysts, functional cysts, etc.), hyperplasia, inflammation, endometriosis, and benign ovarian neoplasms. Unfortunately, there is considerable overlap in the US and MR appearance of neoplastic and nonneoplastic diseases, and these imaging modalities cannot distinguish malignant from benign neoplasms with the accuracy necessary to avert surgery.

Lesions can be confidently diagnosed as benign when three of the following four criteria are met: (a) the lesion size is less than or equal to 4 cm in maximum diameter, (b) the lesion is entirely cystic, (c) the lesion wall is less than 3 mm thick, and (d) there is a lack of internal structure. In both solid and cystic lesions, absence of all of the following ancillary findings is indicative of a benign mass: adjacent pelvic organ involvement; extension to the pelvic side wall; peritoneal, mesenteric, or omental disease; ascites; and adenopathy (Stevens et al. 1991; Morrow and Townsend 1987).

Both US and MR imaging studies can distinguish solid from cystic adnexal masses with a high degree of reliability. However, some solid-appearing lesions may represent hemorrhagic or complex cysts. From a radiologic point of view, cystic masses can be categorized as simple, complex, or hemorrhagic. Differential diagnosis of cystic pelvic masses includes functional cyst, parovarian cyst, peritoneal inclusion cyst, cystadenoma or carcinoma, cystic teratoma, endometrioma, hydrosalpinx or tubo-ovarian abscess, and lymphocele.

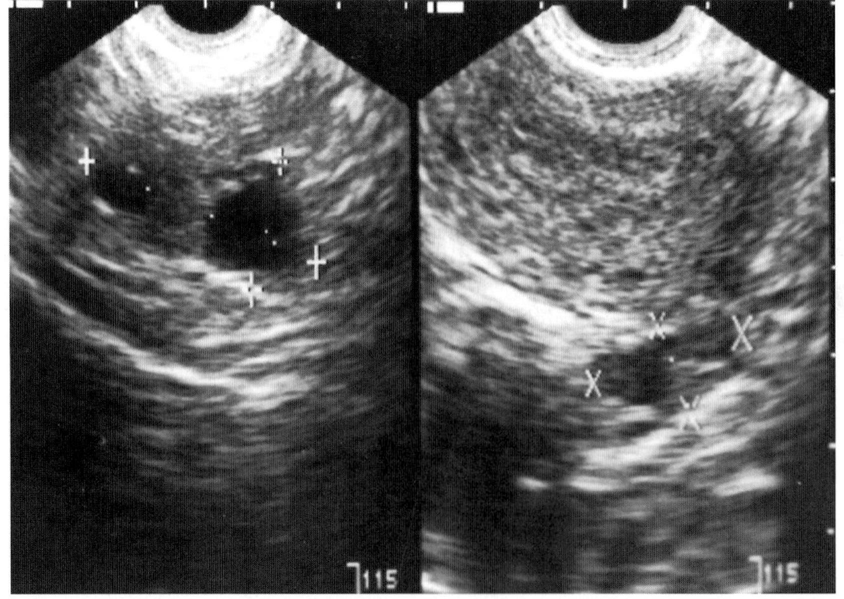


**Fig. 9.1 a,b.** US findings in respect of the normal ovary. Transverse (**a**) and longitudinal (**b**) TVUS views show a normal appearance of the ovary, which contains multiple small follicles. A small cyst is seen

### 9.3.1 Simple Cysts

Simple cysts carry a very low risk of malignancy. The diagnosis for a simple cyst includes functional cyst, parovarian or paratubal cyst, peritoneal inclusion cyst, and benign cystadenoma. Sonographic criteria for simple cysts include an anechoic cystic mass with a well-delineated wall and no internal echoes, septations, or mural nodules (Fig. 9.3). MR imaging characteristics include smooth, well-defined walls and a homogeneous signal intensity (Fig. 9.4). Simple fluid usually has a very long T1 and therefore has low signal intensity on T1-weighted images. The T2 of simple fluid is longer than that of any other soft tissue, causing high signal intensity on T2-weighted images. Administration of Gd-DTPA reveals a smooth thin wall. All these lesions can be considered benign.

### 9.3.2 Complex Cysts

Any mass causing a simple cyst can also produce a complex cystic appearance; in addition, ovarian hemorrhage (Fig. 9.5), endometrioma, abscess, or ovarian tumor (Fig. 9.6) can present such an appearance. On US the diagnosis is based on the presence of a cystic mass containing thin septations and/or internal echoes but not satisfying the strict criteria for simple cyst, hemorrhagic cyst, or endometrioma. In cases of hemorrhagic cyst the sonographic findings include a specific pattern of multiple fine interdigitating septations, giving a fishnet appear-

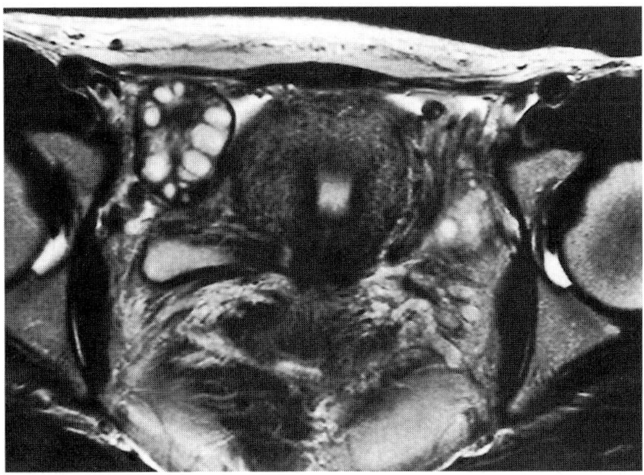

**Fig. 9.2.** MR findings of the normal ovary. The image of the right ovary shows multiple normal follicles, ovarian stroma, and the capsule

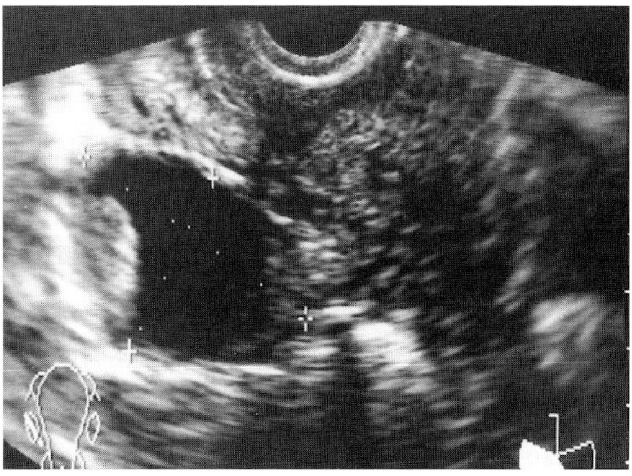

**Fig. 9.3.** US appearance of a simple cyst in a 24-year-old female. A unilocular cystic mass is seen in the right ovary. The nodule on the right side is normal ovary

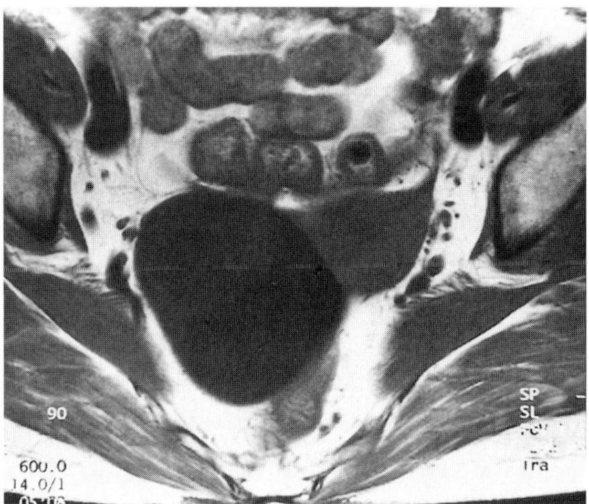


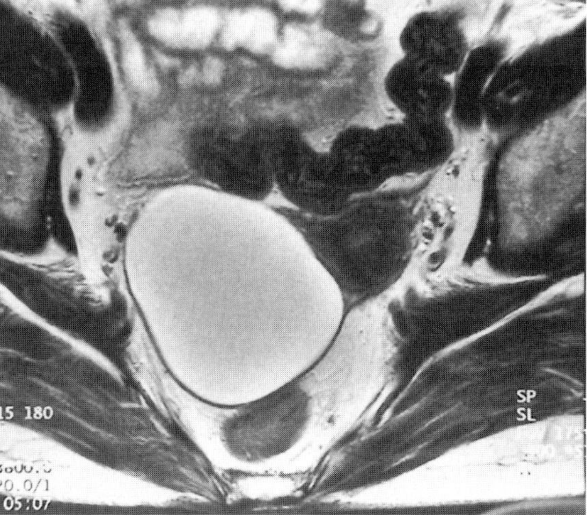


**Fig. 9.4 a,b.** Right ovarian simple cyst in a 28-year-old female. On the T1-weighted image (**a**), an ovarian cyst is seen as a hypointense mass adjacent to the uterus. On the T2-weighted image (**b**), the cyst is markedly hyperintense. The wall of the cyst is thin and smooth

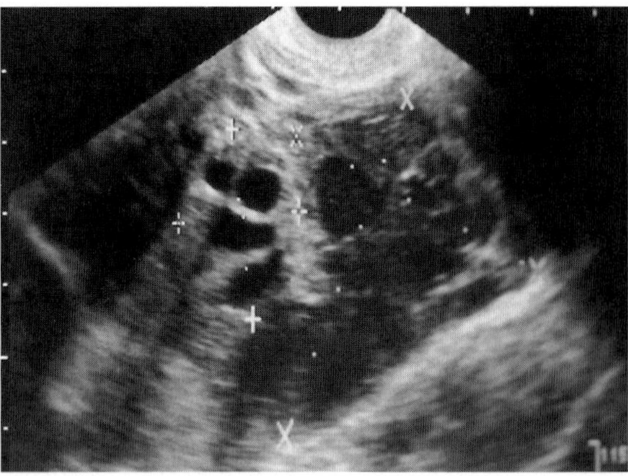

Fig. 9.5. Ovarian hemorrhage in a 23-year-old femals. TVUS shows an enlarged ovary with an irregular internal echo. The hypoechoic area represents hematoma (arrow)

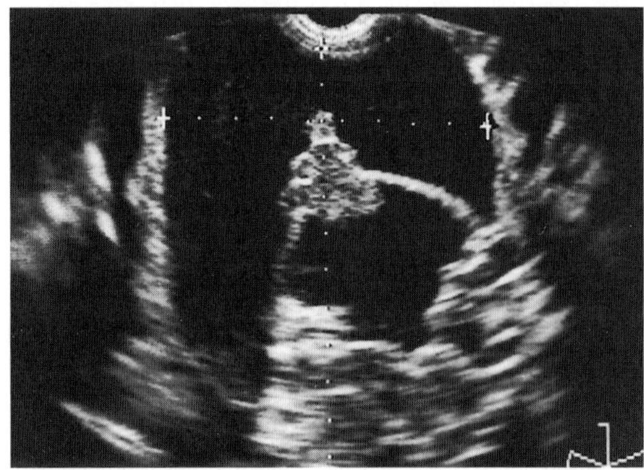

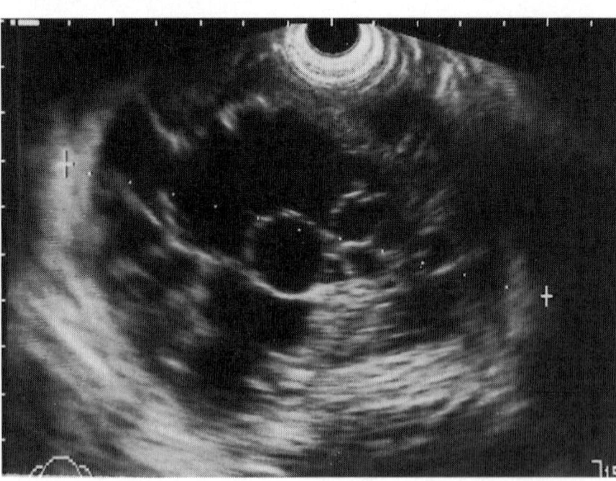

Fig. 9.6 a,b. Complex cystic appearance of benign and malignant ovarian masses on TVUS. a A cystic mass with septations and a large septal nodule in a 43-year-old female. Although these findings suggest carcinoma, this cystic mass turned out to be benign mucinous cystadenoma. b A large multiloculated cystic mass in a 23-year-old female. The wall of the cyst is irregular. This cystic lesion proved to be ovarian carcinoma (mucinous cystadenoma, borderline malignancy)

ance due to a whorled pattern of clotted blood associated with sharply marginated walls and enhanced through sound transmission.

On MR imaging, a diagnosis of complex cyst should be considered when mixed signal intensity is seen in a cystic mass on T1- and T2-weighted MR images. Administration of Gd-DTPA reveals a thickened wall with or without septations, mural nodules, or solid components (Fig. 9.7). A hemorrhagic mass usually appears homogeneous and isointense or hyperintense relative to fat on T1-weighted images and isointense or hyperintense to both fat and urine on T2-weighted images. In the acute stage hematoma (ovarian hemorrhage) may appear hyperintense on T1-weighted images and hypointense on T2-weighted images (Fig. 9.8).

## 9.3.3 Endometrioma and Dermoid Cyst

Endometrioma and dermoid cyst are very common cystic lesions which can present with a confusing imaging appearance on US. MR imaging can readily distinguish these lesions.

### *9.3.3.1 Endometrioma*

After repeated episodes of bleeding during menstruation, large deposits can produce a complex and predominantly cystic mass. Nevertheless, most of the endometrial implants cannot be detected on conventional MR studies because (a) they are usually too small, (b) peristasis may cause blurring, and (c) contrast between endometrial implants and adipose tissue is not sufficient for clear depiction of the small implants (Arrive et al. 1989).

The sonographic criteria include a specific pattern of diffuse, homogeneously dispersed low-level echoes within a well-marginated cystic mass (ground-glass pattern). However, the sonographic appearance may vary depending on the content of fluid (Fig. 9.9). On MR images, a definitive diagnosis of endometriosis may be made when a cyst that is hyperintense on T1-weighted images exhibits hypointense signal on T2-weighted images (shading) or when the lesion consists of multiple hyperintense cysts on T1- and T2-weighted images (Figs. 9.10, 9.11). Although very small endometrial implants cannot be detected on fat-saturated images, such images do seem superior to conventional T1- and

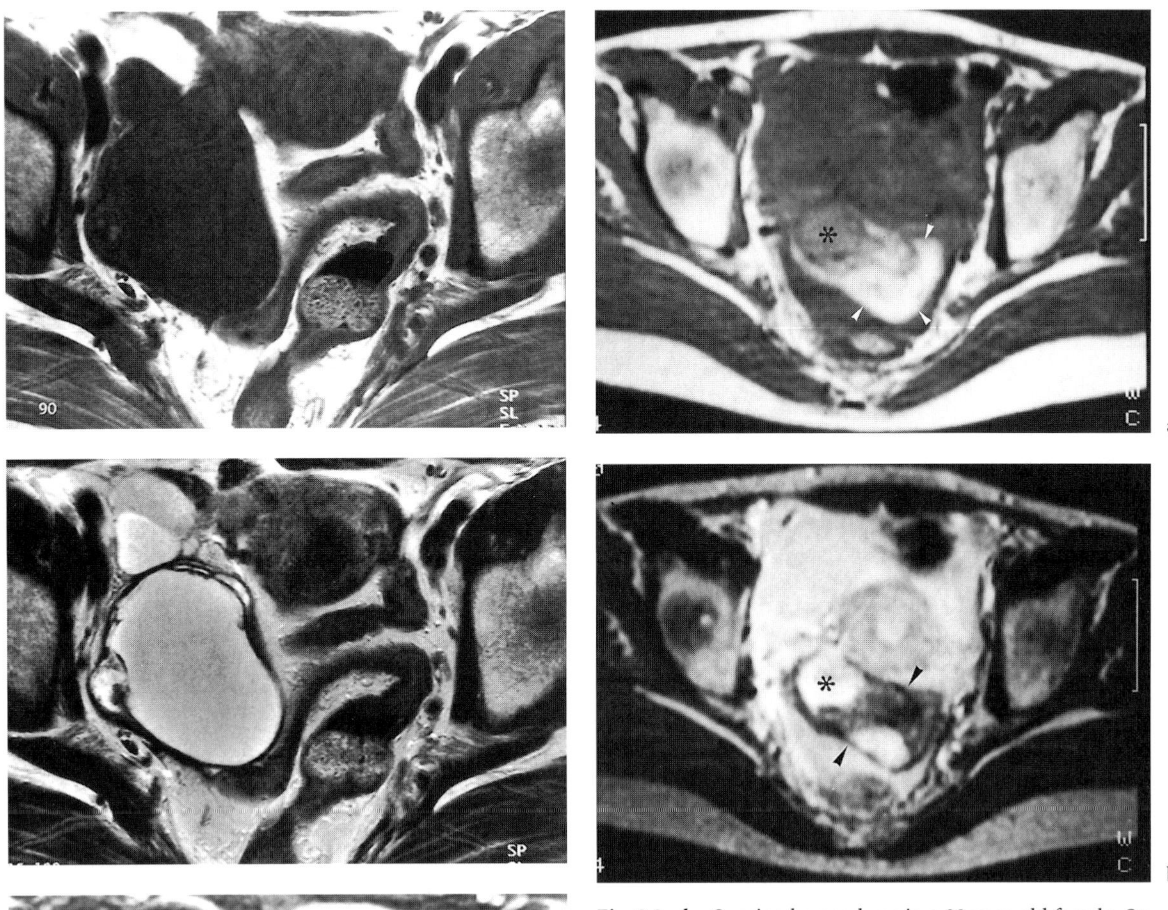

**Fig. 9.7a–c.** Complex cyst (serous cystadenoma) in a 23-year-old female. T1-weighted (**a**) and T2-weighted (**b**) images show a large complex cystic mass in the right ovary. On postcontrast T1-weighted images (**c**), the wall of the cyst is somewhat thick (Permission from YAMASHITA et al., Acta Radiol 38:572–577)

**Fig. 9.8 a,b.** Ovarian hemorrhage in a 28-year-old female. On the T1-weighted image (**a**), a hyperintense lesion is seen (*arrowheads*). On the T2-weighted image (**b**), the lesion is hypointense, indicating acute stage hematoma (presumably deoxyhemoglobin). Ruptured follicle (*) appears hypointense on T1-weighted images and hyperintense on T2-weighted images

T2-weighted spin-echo images owing to the better contrast that is obtained between the hemorrhagic lesion and peritoneal fat. In hemorrhagic tissues where a chemical shift effect does not occur, hyperintensity is seen due to the prolonged T1 effect. The signal decays in longer TEs are caused by the T2* effect (MITCHELL et al. 1991).

### 9.3.3.2
### Dermoid Cyst

Dermoid cyst (benign cystic teratoma) is probably the most common ovarian neoplasm in patients younger than 50 years. Such cysts are usually benign and inert but rarely they become malignant. Bilaterality occurs in 8%–15% of cases. Almost any component may become malignant, but squamous cell carcinoma accounts for 90% of the cases (PRAT 1996).

In mature cystic teratomas of the ovary, the contents of the cyst are usually greasy liquid composed

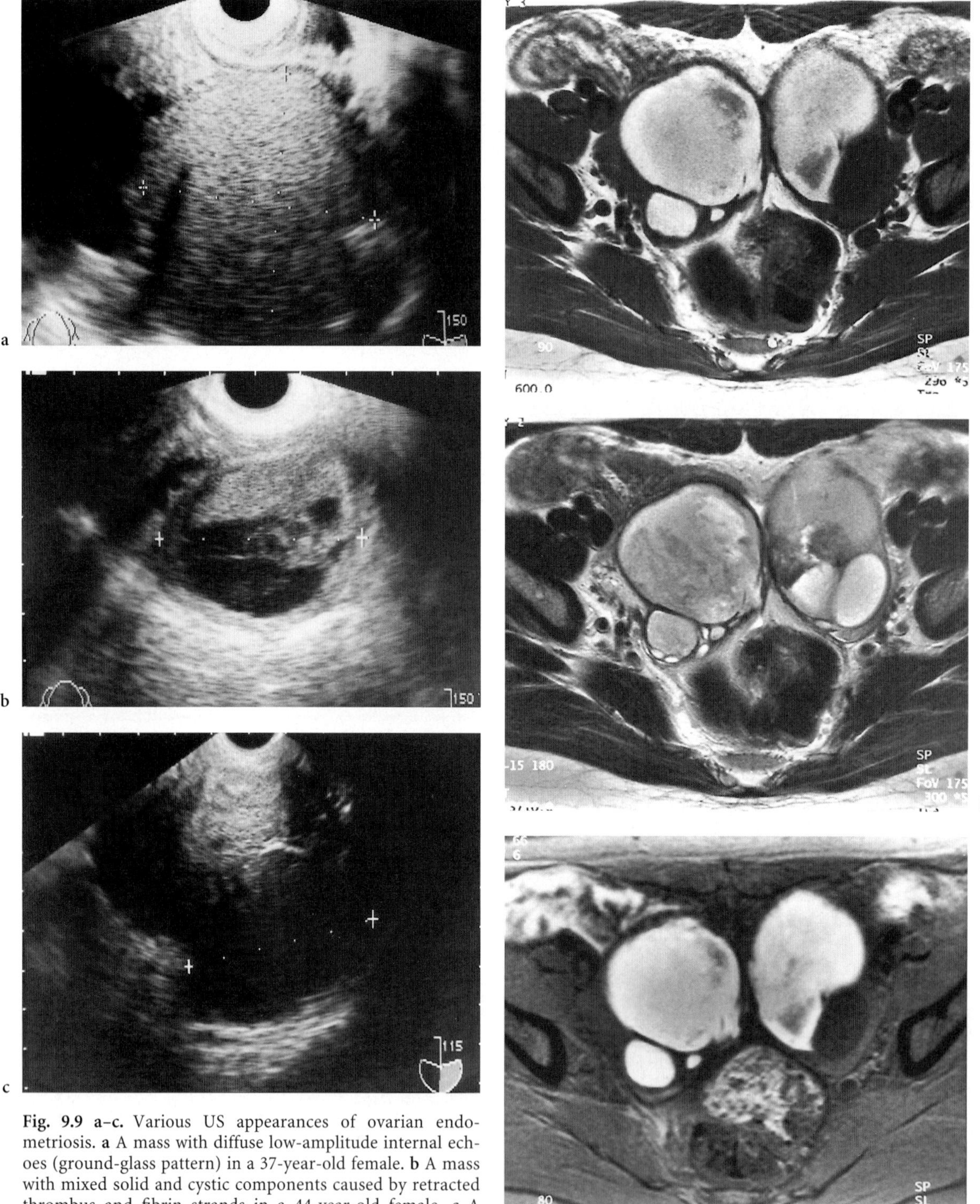

Fig. 9.9 a–c. Various US appearances of ovarian endometriosis. **a** A mass with diffuse low-amplitude internal echoes (ground-glass pattern) in a 37-year-old female. **b** A mass with mixed solid and cystic components caused by retracted thrombus and fibrin strands in a 44-year-old female. **c** A unilocular sonolucent cystic mass in a 33-year-old female

Fig. 9.10 a–c. Bilateral ovarian endometrioses in a 25-year-old female. T1-weighted (**a**) and T2-weighted (**b**) images show multiple hyperintense cystic masses in the bilateral ovaries. On the T2-weighted image, a small hypointense area is seen, indicating old clot or viscous fluid. Fat-saturated image (**c**) shows persistence of high signal intensity

of keratin, sebum, and hairs, with a surrounding firm capsule of varying thickness. Fatty components in the cystic lumen are present in 93%–96% of cases. Fat may be seen in the cyst cavity or as a round mass

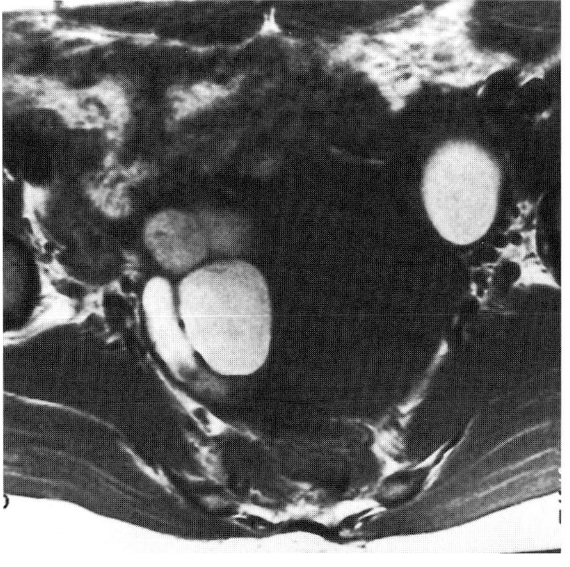

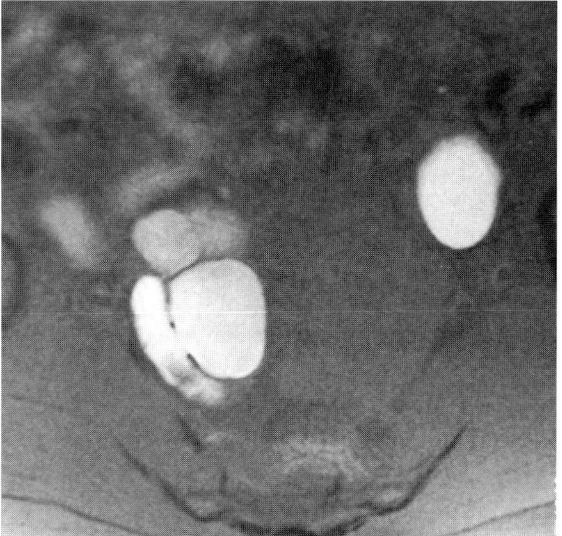

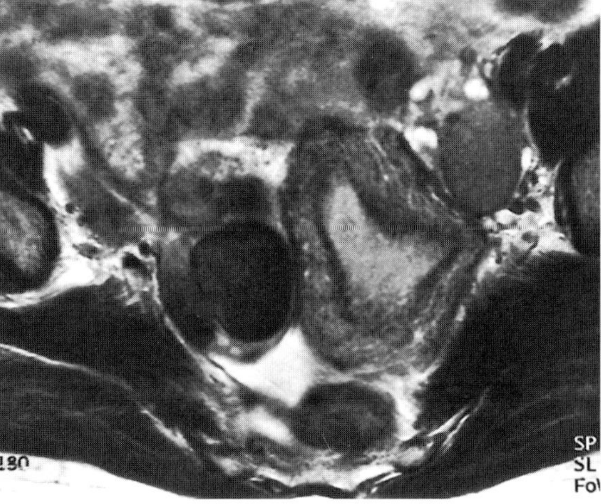

**Fig. 9.11 a–c.** Bilateral ovarian endometriosis in a 35-year-old female. T1-weighted (**a**) and fat-saturated T1-weighted (**b**) images show multiple hyperintense lesions in both ovaries. On the T2-weighted image (**c**) most of the lesions appear hypointense (*shading*)

floating in the interface between water and fatty fluid. The diagnosis may be overlooked in the small number of cases in which the cyst does not contain fat. Yellow fatty liquid in the dermoid consists predominantly of sebum and is usually liquid at temperatures above 34°C. The tumor is usually unilocular but may be multilocular, divided by septa into a number of compartments (Rosai 1989; Talerman 1987).

Mature cystic teratomas have a broad spectrum of appearance. Typical sonographic criteria include the presence of fat-fluid levels, a hyperechoic mural nodule (dermoid plug), and areas of calcification. An intensely hyperechoic mass within the ovary is also diagnostic for dermoid (Fig. 9.12). The most common error is to diagnose these lesions as solid

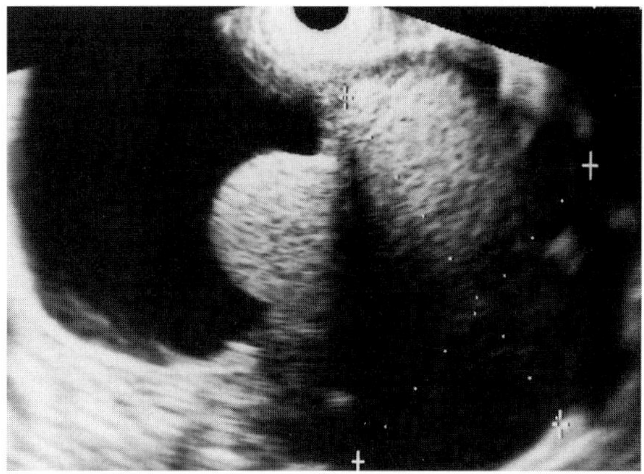

**Fig. 9.12.** Dermoid cyst with the typical US appearance in a 30-year-old female. Bright echoes and shadowing are seen

masses because they demonstrate numerous high-amplitude echoes and transmit sound poorly or not al all. Sometimes they may appear as a unilocular anechoic or hypoechoic cyst with a thin or somewhat thickened wall (Fig. 9.13). It should be noted that pure sebum tends to be anechoic or hypoechoic.

Mature cystic teratoma can be diagnosed with greater accuracy by MR imaging techniques because fat in the cystic cavity can be readily identified and causes characteristic imaging features such as chemical shift artifact, gravity-dependent debris, and protrusions (Togashi et al. 1987; Buy et al. 1989; Sheth et al. 1988). On MR imaging, the mass has signal intensity similar to fat on T1- and T2-weighted images (Fig. 9.14). An internal pattern of layering or floating of debris, as well as nodular or frondlike protrusions within the cystic mass, is also seen. The signal intensity is not equal to that of subcutaneous fat on T1- and T2-weighted images owing to either a small fatty component or a large amount of sebum or debris. Although the presence of fat inside the ovarian tumor is considered to be specific for mature cystic teratoma, fat can be present in other uncommon ovarian tumors such as immature teratoma, lipoma, liposarcoma, and lipid cell tumor (Buy et al. 1989; Scully 1979). Fat can develop within a solid mass as a result of hemorrhage and necrosis.

The diagnosis of mature cystic teratoma may be overlooked in the rare teratoma that does not contain fat in the cystic cavity (Yamashita et al. 1994); histologically, the fatty component is usually seen in the wall of the cyst (Fig. 9.15). Because such tumors lack the characteristic findings of mature cystic teratomas, a gradient-echo technique with both in-phase and opposed-phase images is useful to show a small amount of fat. Parenchymal signal loss from tissue containing a small amount of fat is greater on opposed-phase images than on fat-saturated images (Fig. 9.16) because lipid signal intensity is merely removed from the latter whereas it is actually used for negative contrast in the former technique. In subcutaneous fat, the oscillations of the signal occur as a result of the chemical shift between the vinyl CH protons and the $CH_2$ moiety of the long-chain fatty acid (Wehrli et al. 1987). In sebum or dermoid nipple containing both fat and nonfatty tissue, prominent periodic signal changes occur at a cycle of 4.4 ms. Summation of water and fat components in a voxel occurs in the in-phase image, while signal cancellation is seen in the opposed-phase image. In tissues containing predominantly lipid or water the effect of phase cycling is small. In teratomas seen in girls, the cystic cavity is usually filled with aqueous fluid and fat cannot be seen (Fig. 9.17).

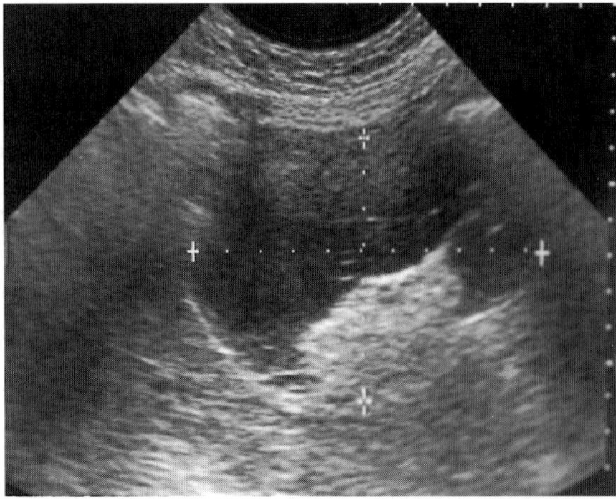

Fig. 9.13. Dermoid cyst in a 38-year-old female. TVUS shows a predominantly hypoechoic appearance due to pure sebum

### 9.3.3.3 Differentiation between Endometrioma and Dermoid Cyst on MR Imaging

Although differentiation of cystic teratomas from endometriomas and other hemorrhagic adnexal lesions is readily performed when typical MR findings are present, diagnosis may be difficult or sometimes impossible with conventional MR techniques (Nyberg et al. 1987; Togashi et al. 1987; Arrive et al. 1989; Dooms et al. 1986; Zawin et al. 1989). Lipid-containing lesions appear hyperintense on T1-weighted images because lipid has a short T1 relaxation time. Hemorrhagic lesions can display signal characteristics similar to those of lipid-containing lesions on both T1- and T2-weighted images if the lesion contains methemoglobin, which shortens both T1 and T2 relaxation times (Gomori and Grossman 1988). Endometriomas may appear isointense with fat on both T1- and T2-weighted images depending on the age of the blood within the lesion. In addition, useful diagnostic criteria such as the presence of chemical shift artifact or dermoid plug in teratomas (Togashi et al. 1987), shading, or a thick fibrous capsule or multilocularity in endometriomas (Nishimura et al. 1987; Togashi et al. 1991; Arrive et al. 1989; Zawin et al. 1989) may be absent.

Several fat-suppression MR imaging techniques can differentiate between fat and blood because the

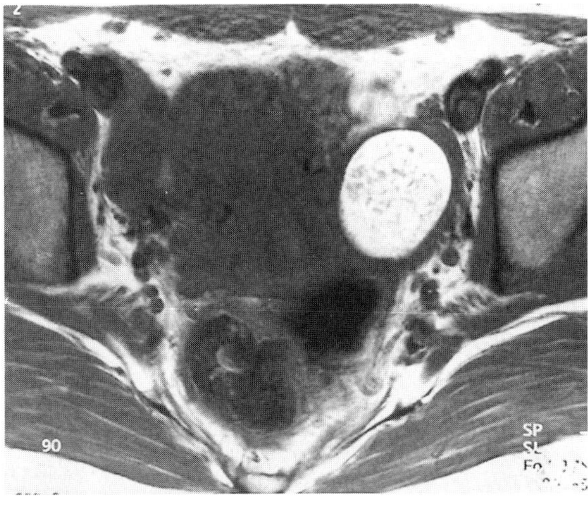
a

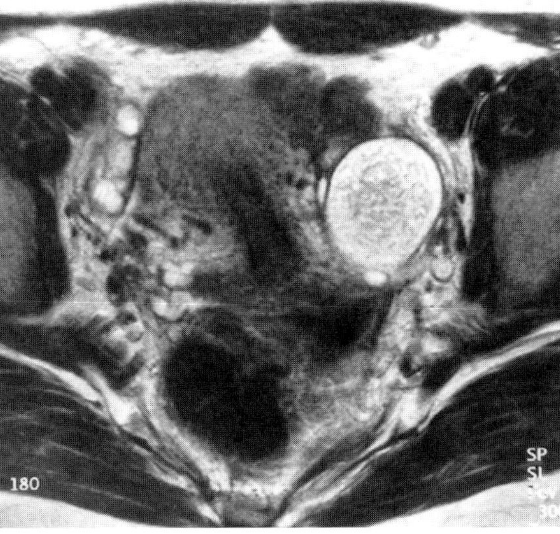
b

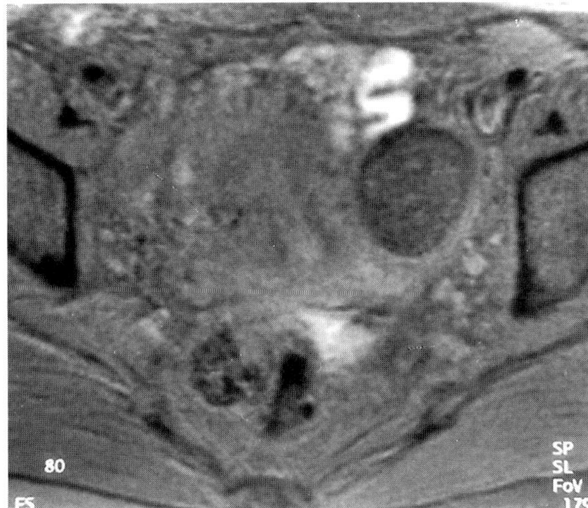
c

**Fig. 9.14 a–c.** Dermoid cyst with typical MR appearances in a 31-year-old female. On the T1-weighted SE MR image (**a**), a tumor is heterogeneously hyperintense. On the T2-weighted SE MR image (**b**), tumor is again heterogeneously hyperintense. Chemical shift artifact is seen within the cystic cavity. On the fat-saturated image (**c**), the hyperintense signal on the T1-weighted image is suppressed

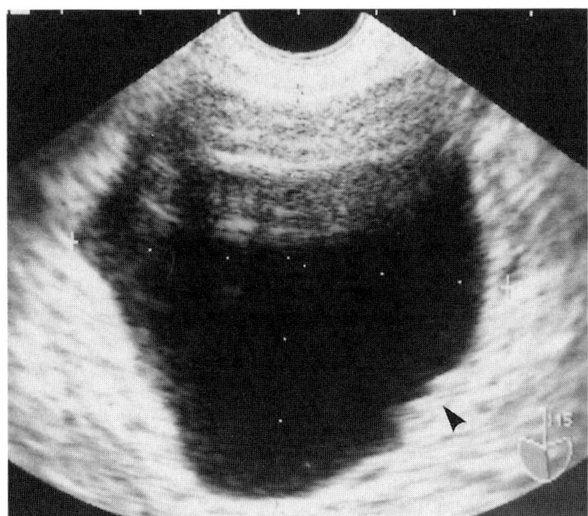
a

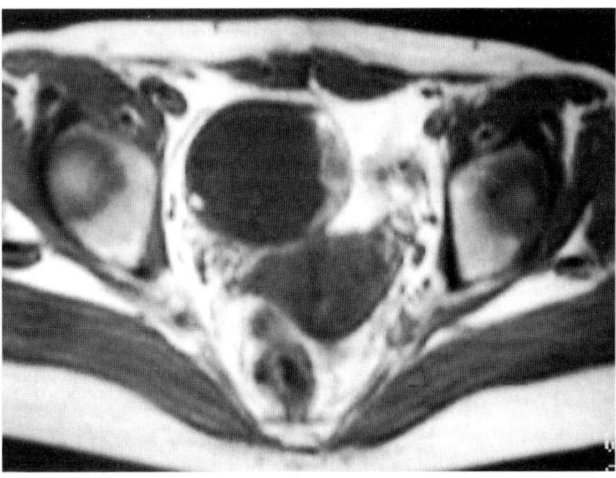
b

**Fig. 9.15 a,b.** Mature cystic teratoma appearing as a purely cystic mass in a 30-year-old female. TVUS (**a**) shows a cystic mass with an echogenic mural nodule (*arrowhead*). On the T1-weighted MR image, hyperintense areas are demonstrated in the cystic wall (**b**). Histologically the fatty component is usually seen in the wall of such cysts ((a) Permission of YAMASHITA et al., Radiology 194:557–565. (b) Permission of YAMASHITA et al., AJR 163:613–616)

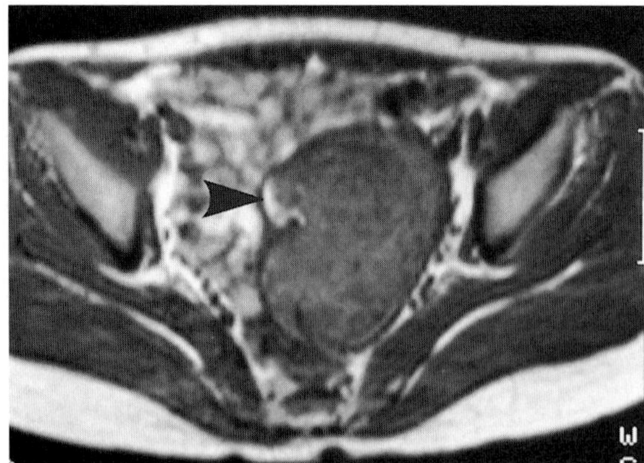

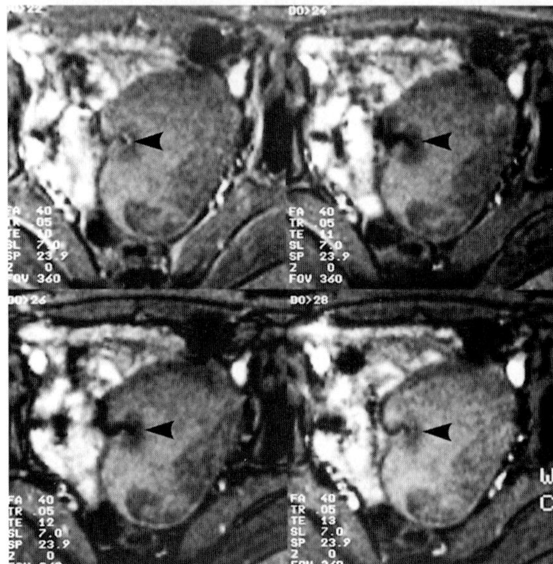

Fig. 9.16 a,b. Mature cystic teratoma of the right ovary with a slight amount of fat in a 30-year-old female. Histologic evaluation revealed the small amount of fat in the wall of the cyst. Most of the cyst cavity contained mucinous fluid with hair. On the T1-weighted SE MR image (**a**), the tumor is mostly hypointense. Hyperintense areas are seen in the cyst wall (*arrowhead*). On FLASH MR images (**b**), TE was varied from 10 to 13 ms: TE = 10 ms, in-phase (*upper left*); TE = 11 ms, opposed-phase (*upper right*); TE = 12 ms, opposed-phase (*lower right*); and TE = 13 ms, in-phase (*lower left*). The high-intensity signal on T1-weighted imaging is markedly suppressed (*arrowheads*) ((a) Permission of YAMASHITA et al., Radiology 194:557–565. (b) Permission of YAMASHITA et al., AJR 163:613–616)

source of high signals on T1-weighted images is the water proton for hemorrhage vs the lipid proton for fatty tissue (TIEN 1992). The proton-selective fat saturation technique has been shown to be useful for differentiating between hemorrhagic lesions and cystic teratomas (KIER et al. 1992; STEVENS et al. 1993; KELLER et al. 1987) and detecting small endometriomas (SUGIMURA et al. 1993).

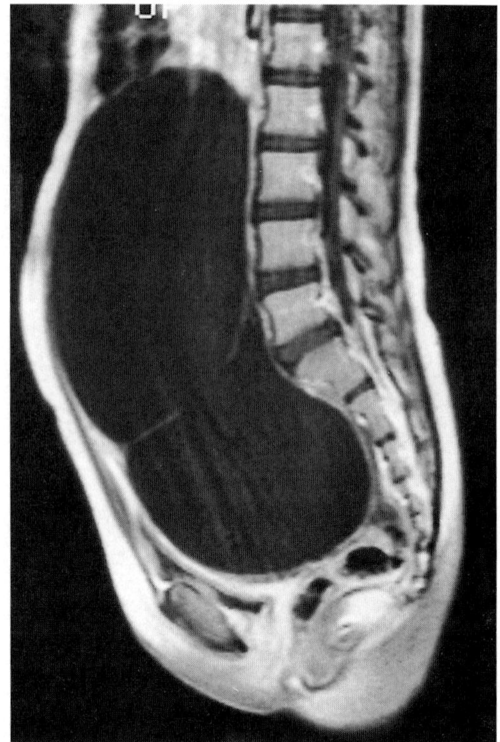

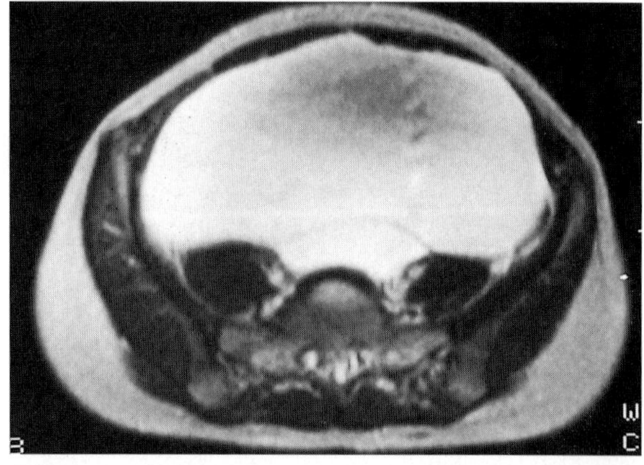

**Fig. 9.17 a,b.** Mature cystic teratoma of the right ovary with a minimal amount of fat in a 13-year-old girl. The small fatty component was demonstrated on histologic examination in the wall of the cyst. T1-weighted SE MR image (**a**) after administration of contrast material shows a hypointense multiloculated cystic mass without any fatty component. T2-weighted SE MR image (**b**) shows marked hyperintensity of the cyst cavity, indicating that the fluid is aqueous ((a) Permission of YAMASHITA et al., Radiology 194:557–565. (b) Permission of YAMASHITA et al., AJR 163:613–616)

## 9.3.4 Fibroma and Thecoma

Fibromas and thecomas are considered to arise from ovarian stromal cells specialized in steroid hormone production. Both tumors are usually solid and have

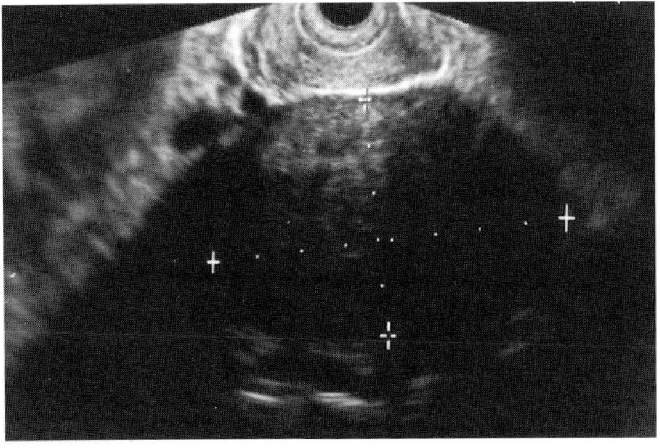

Fig. 9.18. Fibroma in a 45-year-old female. TVUS shows an echogenic mass with an anechoic component with acoustic enhancement

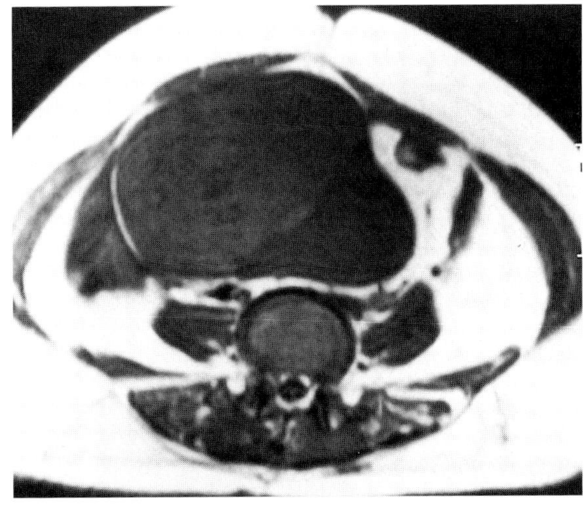

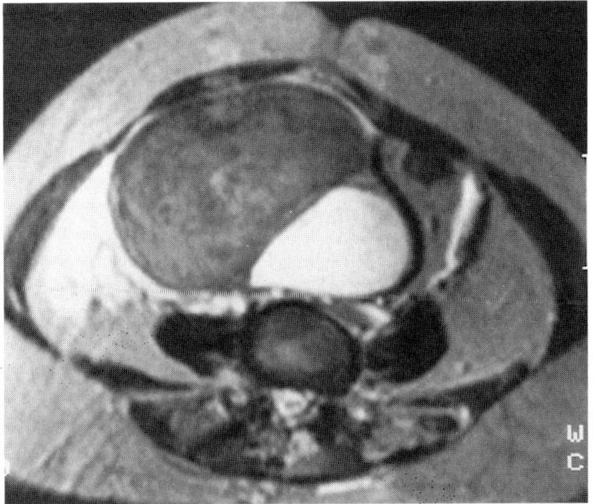

Fig. 9.19 a,b. Fibroma in a 41-year-old female. T1-weighted (a) and T2-weighted (b) images show a mass with two components. The mass is predominantly slightly hyperintense on the T1-weighted image and hypointense on the T2-weighted image. The cystic component is seen in the left side of the mass. The hypointensity of the solid component is a characteristic feature of this tumor (Permission from YAMASHITA et al., Acta Radiol 38:572–577)

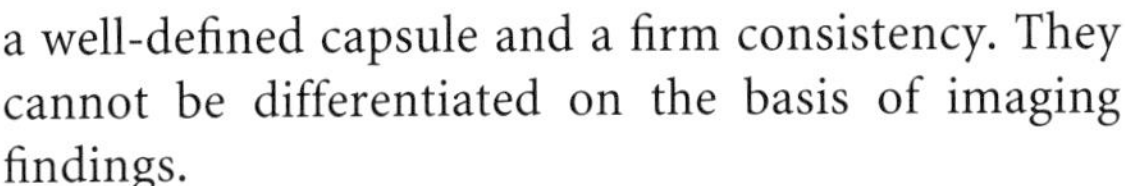

a well-defined capsule and a firm consistency. They cannot be differentiated on the basis of imaging findings.

On US fibromas and thecomas present as a solid mass of similar echogenicity to myometrium or an anechoic mass with acoustic enhancement or a complex mass with mixed echogenicity (Fig. 9.18). Identification of calcific foci within the mass is supportive of the diagnosis. At MR imaging, tumors that are isointense to or less intense than myometrium on T1-weighted images and of predominantly low signal intensity on T2-weighted images may be diagnosed as benign ovarian fibromas or thecomas (Fig. 9.19), though distinction from Brenner tumor and Krukenberg tumor, which present similar imaging findings, is necessary.

### 9.3.5 Tubo-ovarian Abscess

Tubo-ovarian abscess typically appears as a complex cystic mass. With US, identification of a tubular fluid-filled mass separate from the ovary is a useful criterion. Mucosal folds are helpful in establishing the tubal origin. Layering of echogenic debris is suggestive of blood or pus (Fig. 9.20). On MR imaging, an oblong fluid-filled tubular structure with high signal intensity on T1- and T2-weighted images is typically seen, but the tubular structure occasionally appears as a multiloculated cystic mass (Fig. 9.21). The exact appearance depends on the blood or protein content of the fluid, and its signal intensity may be complex. Enhancement of the tubal structure is seen.

## 9.4 Diagnosis of Malignant Lesions

The vast majority of ovarian malignancies arise from the surface epithelium, from either the germ cells or the stroma cells. On the basis of histologic features and clinical behavior, tumors can be classified into benign forms, borderline malignancies, and a higher grade malignant form. Borderline lesions have a better prognosis than higher grade malignancies but need to be treated like the malignant form. Borderline lesions usually present at an earlier age than the invasive form.

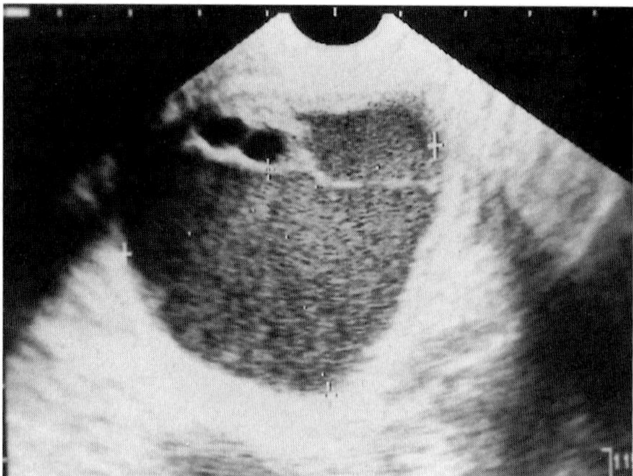

Fig. 9.20. Tubo-ovarian abscess in a 76-year-old female. TVUS shows a cystic mass with layering of echogenic debris, suggestive of pus

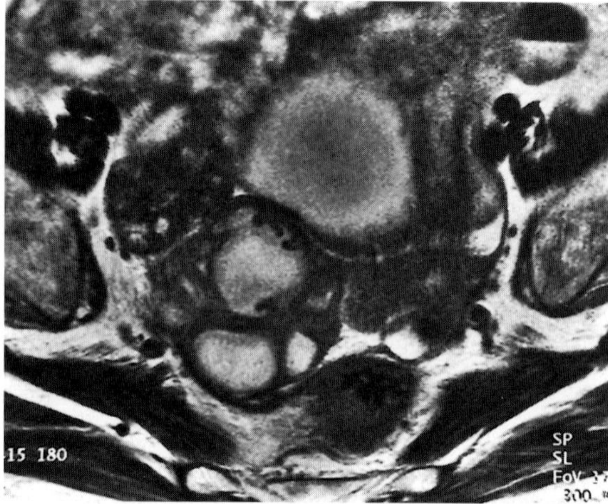

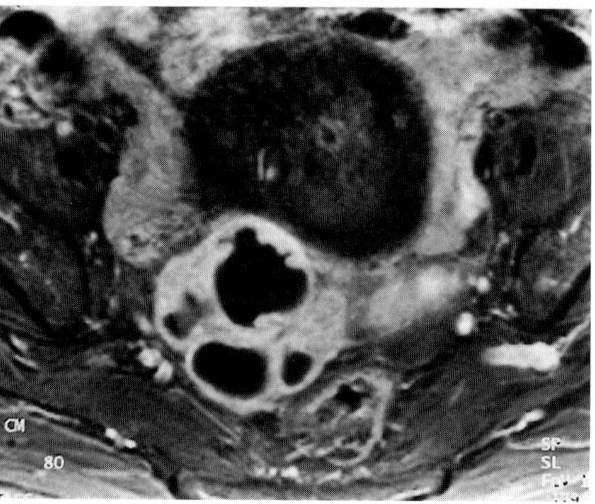

Fig. 9.21 a,b. Tubo-ovarian abscess in a 76-year-old female. On T2-weighted (a) and postcontrast fat-saturated T1-weighted (b) images a multiloculated cystic mass is seen in the right adnexa. The wall of the cystic lesion is somewhat thick. It would be difficult to distinguish such a presentation from a cystic ovarian neoplasm

A prospective diagnosis of malignancy can be made on either TVUS and MR imaging when lesion size exceeds 4 cm and either (a) the lesion is cystic but wall thickness exceeds 3 mm and/or nodularity, vegetations, or a large solid component is present; or (b) the lesion is completely or predominantly solid, with or without areas of necrosis or hemorrhage; or (c) any of the following findings are present: involvement of adjacent pelvic organs, extension to the pelvic side wall, or presence of peritoneal, mesenteric, or omental disease, ascites, or adenopathy (Stevens et al. 1991; Morrow and Townsend 1987). Distinction between primary tumor and metastasis may not be possible.

Small cystic or epithelial neoplasms are better characterized with TVUS due to its ability to resolve internal architectural details such as the focal mural wall thickness or a solid protruding component within a predominantly cystic mass (Fig. 9.22). Based on the morphologic characteristics of a mass, US is able to differentiate benign from malignant masses with reasonable accuracy (Lerner et al. 1994; Sassone et al. 1991). False-positive diagnoses are frequently made in cases of mature cystic teratoma and fibrothecoma and less frequently in cases of endometrioma because these diseases have variable sonographic appearances.

Although US remains the foremost imaging modality for screening patients with adnexal lesions, MR imaging may assist greatly in identifying the presence of malignancy before surgery (Osmers et al. 1990; Nyberg et al. 1987; Nishimura et al. 1987; Togashi et al. 1987, 1991). The MR appearance of ovarian malignancy includes both solid and mixed solid and cystic masses. These lesions are usually heterogeneous in signal intensity and internal architecture and often contain thick walls and thick, nodular septations. The administration of Gd-DTPA improves visualization of intratumoral architecture, septations, nodularity, wall thickness, and areas of necrosis (Figs. 9.23–9.25).

Ultrasonography, MR imaging, and CT all have a potential role in staging patients with ovarian malignancies. It has not been clarified which modality is the best for staging; their accuracy is being evaluated in a multicenter trial. Both CT and MR modalities can detect ascites, implants, and lymph nodes. Ascites is sometimes complex and often bloody; it has a heterogeneous signal intensity and may be loculated, containing thick septa. The detection of

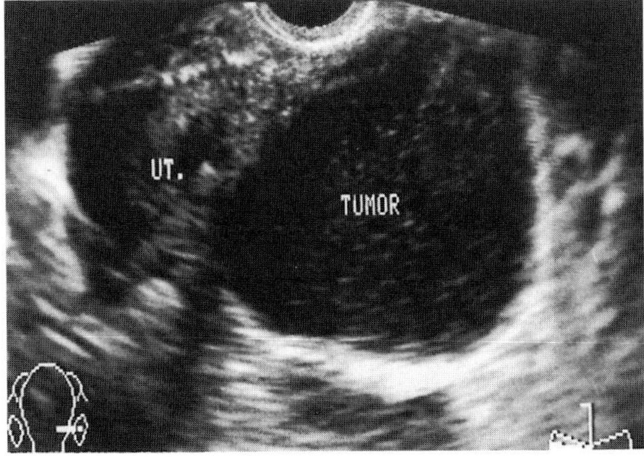


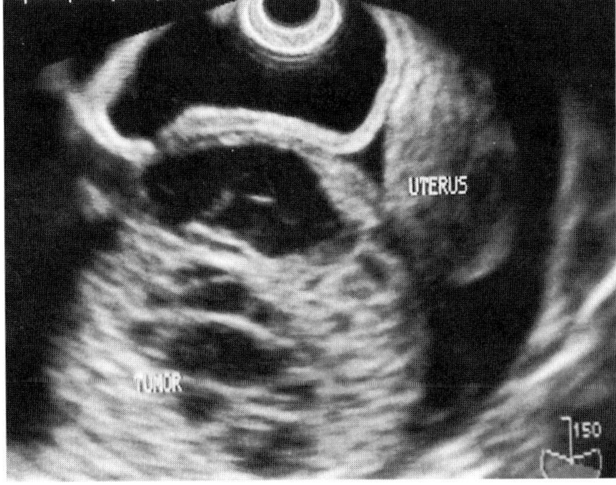


**Fig. 9.22 a,b.** Predominantly solid malignant ovarian solid masses. **a** A hypoechoic and predominantly solid mass in a 55-year-old female. **b** A mixed solid and cystic mass containing a cystic area, thick internal septations, and a soft tissue nodule in a 67-year-old female. A slight amount of ascites is seen b: Permission of YAMASHITA et al., Radiology 194:557–565

implants is critical but difficult, especially when they are small and microscopic. The presence of ascites may help in the detection of small metastatic foci. Implants are more conspicuous on fat-suppressed gadolinium-enhanced T1-weighted images (Fig. 9.25). The ability of MR imaging to detect lymph nodes is considered equal to that of CT. The signal void of flow allows for differentiation of vessels from internal iliac lymph nodes. All nodes larger than 1 cm are regarded as abnormal in the female pelvis.

Ultrasonography, MR imaging, and CT also can be used to distinguish between benign and malignant lesions using morphologic characteristics (LERNER et al. 1994; SASSONE et al. 1991) or flow analysis using color Doppler (KURJAK et al. 1991; WERNER et al. 1992). However, whichever criteria are employed there is still considerable overlap between benign and malignant lesions in the case of

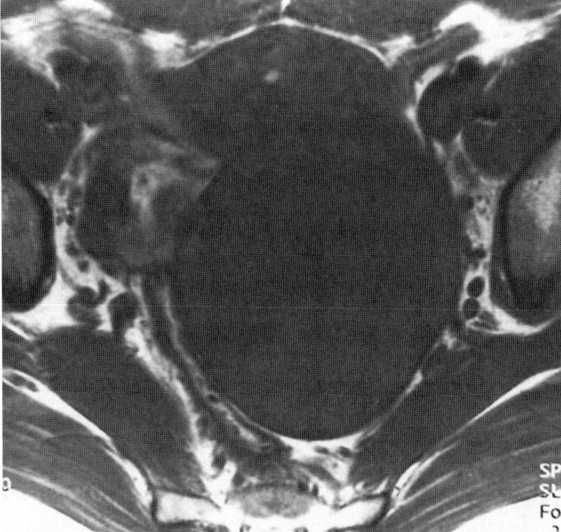

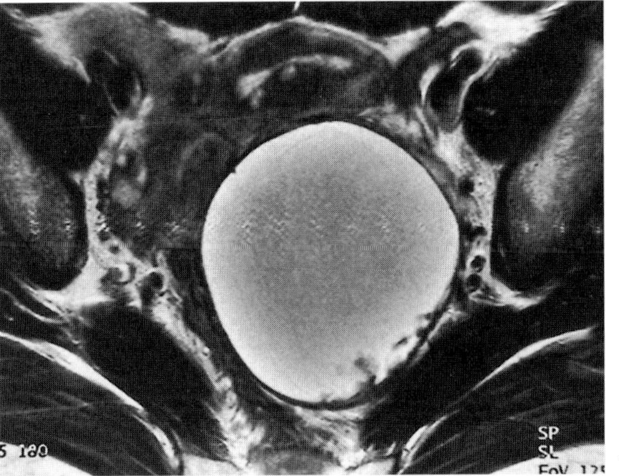

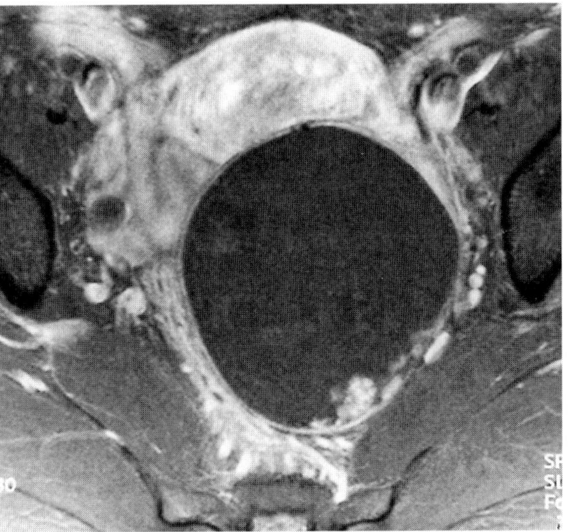

**Fig. 9.23 a–c.** Serous cystadenocarcinoma of low malignant potential in the left adnexa in a 44-year-old female. T1-weighted image (**a**) shows a hypointense tumor. On T2-weighted (**b**) and postcontrast (**c**) images, an irregular wall is evident

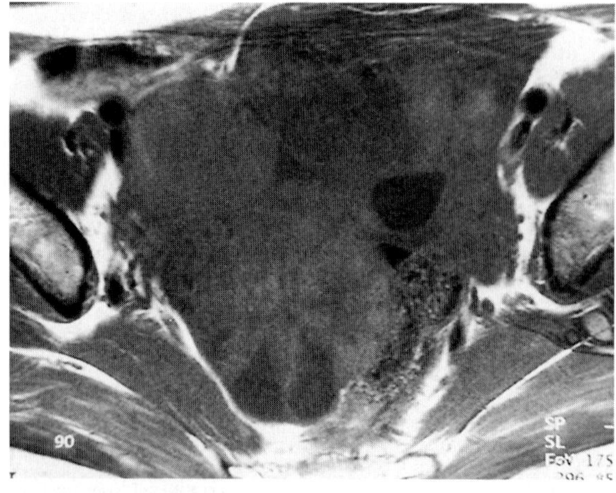

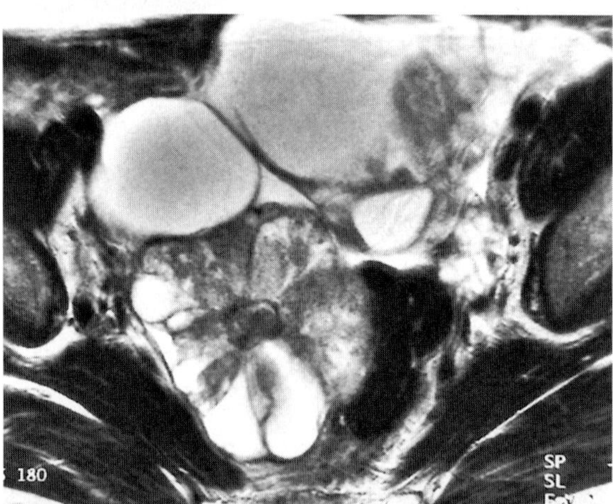

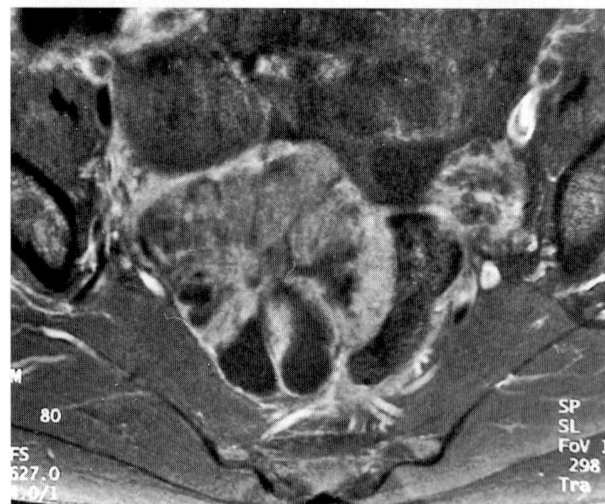

**Fig. 9.24 a–c.** Serous cystadenocarcinoma with tubal invasion in a 51-year-old female. T1-weighted image (**a**) shows an irregular hypointense tumor. On T2-weighed (**b**) and postcontrast (**c**) images, a predominantly solid mass with an irregular cyst is evident

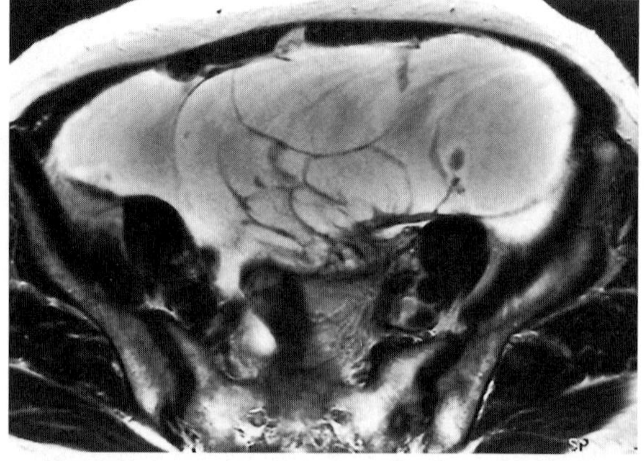

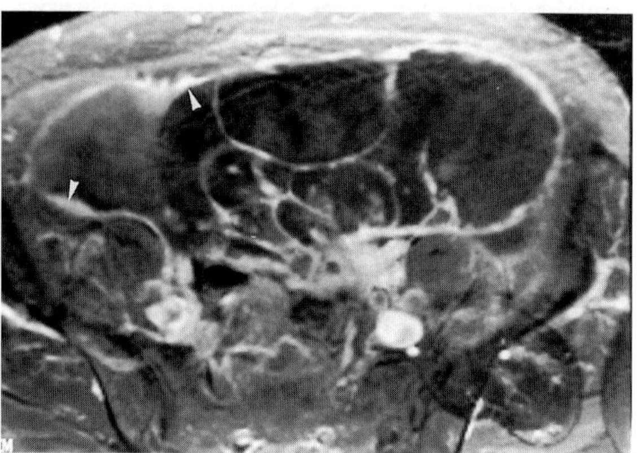

**Fig. 9.25 a,b.** Mucinous cystadenocarcinoma with peritoneal implantation in a 67-year-old female. On T2-weighted (**a**) and postcontrast (**b**) images, a multiloculated cystic mass with wall irregularity is demonstrated. Thick peritoneal enhancement is seen, indicating peritoneal implantation (*arrowheads*) on the postcontrast image

several epithelial or stromal ovarian lesions (Brown et al. 1994; Figs. 9.26, 9.27).

## 9.5 Comparison of MR Imaging and TVUS

Transvaginal US visualizes detailed internal architecture of the adnexal masses characteristic for various histologic types, thereby allowing a specific diagnosis. A number of studies have evaluated the sensitivity and specificity of pelvic US and MR imaging in distinguishing benign from malignant ovarian masses. The sensitivity of TVUS for discrimination between benign and malignant ovarian lesions was found to range from 82% to 100%, and its specificity from 83% to 95% (Sassone et al. 1991; Herrmann et al. 1987; Granberg et al. 1990; Finkler et al. 1988; Benacerraf et al. 1990).

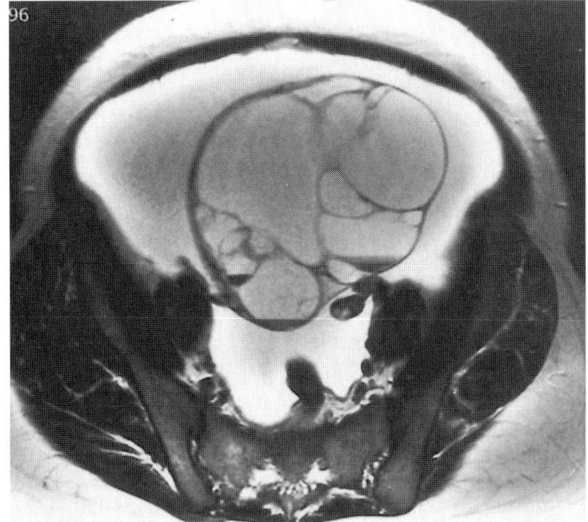

a

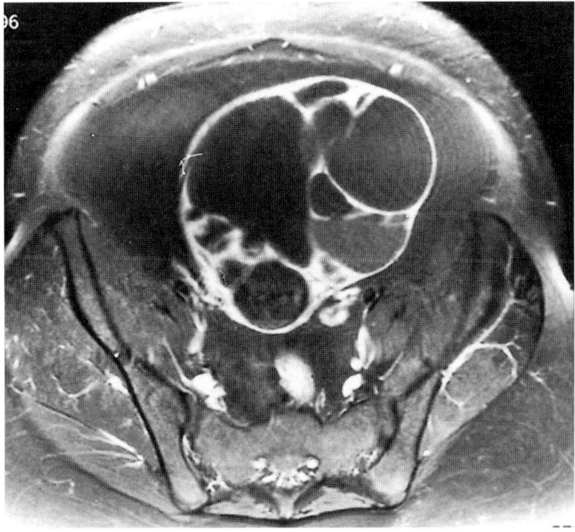

b

**Fig. 9.26 a,b.** Granulosa cell tumor in a 27-year-old female. On T2-weighted (**a**) and postcontrast (**b**) images, a multiloculated cystic mass with a thick but smooth wall is seen. Massive ascites is also demonstrated. Peritoneal enhancement is not evident

Conventional MR imaging does not visualize the fine internal architectural detail as well as does TVUS, which may preclude specific diagnosis. Contrast-enhanced MR imaging allows better depiction of the internal architecture and differentiation of cystic from solid lesions and has been found to be particularly useful in differentiation between malignant and benign lesions (STEVENS et al. 1991; THURNHER et al. 1990). According to STEVENS et al. (1991), the rate of correct characterization of malignant masses by MR imaging increased from 83% to 100% after administration of Gd-DTPA. Because internal details are as clearly depicted as with TVUS

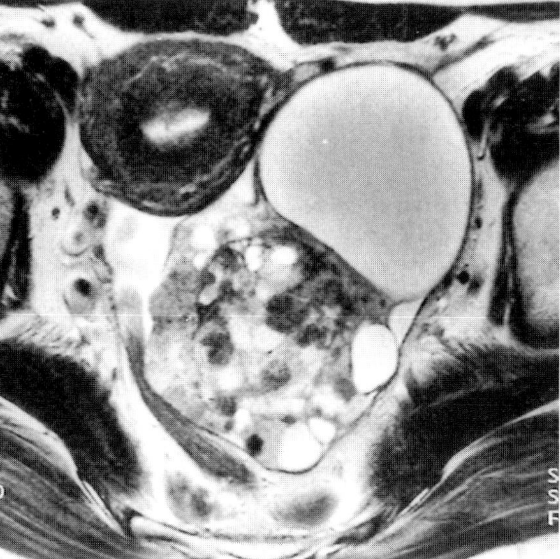

**Fig. 9.27.** Struma ovarii in a 33-year-old female. On T2-weighted images, a complex mass with multiple variously sized cysts and a solid component (Permission from YAMASHITA et al., Abdominal Imaging 22:100–102)

and the tissue contrast is superior, discrimination between malignant and benign lesions can be achieved with greater confidence on Gd-enhanced MR imaging.

The diagnostic capability of TVUS and MR imaging differs depending on the histology. TVUS and MR imaging are equally accurate in the diagnosis of large solid ovarian carcinomas. MR imaging can allow differentiation of the nature of the mass – simple fluid, atypical fluid, blood, solid tissue, fibrous tissue, fat, etc. – but these features frequently do not lead to a specific diagnosis. Small cystic epithelial neoplasms are better characterized with TVUS due to its ability to resolve internal architectural details such as the focal mural wall thickness or the presence of a solid protruding component within a predominantly cystic mass.

In cases of cystic lesions, TVUS and enhanced MR imaging are equally accurate in characterization of malignancy. MR imaging is significantly superior in the characterization of dermoid cysts and endometriomas. On TVUS, these tumors frequently lack previously reported typical findings such as a fishnet pattern for endometriomas and gravity-dependent layering or rounded nodules for dermoid cysts; in fact endometriomas may appear as solid or pure cystic, while some simple cysts have a fishnet appearance. Teratomas are frequently interpreted as malignant tumors.

In some rare instances, detection of malignant foci in benign masses is difficult on MR imaging. Although walls of cysts are usually thick, almost all endometriomas are benign; however, endometrial carcinoma may develop. Solid parts are dominant in benign mature cystic teratomas with malignant transformation or immature teratoma; such a presentation does not preclude a benign nature.

In summary, overall TVUS and unenhanced MR imaging display comparable diagnostic accuracy. MR imaging can allow differentiation of the nature of the mass and can therefore reliably diagnose fat-containing cystic teratoma and endometrioma, which are often difficult to diagnose by means of US. Although the use of contrast enhancement does not always improve the tissue characterization of adnexal lesions, confidence limits for diagnosing benign or malignant lesions are improved by Gd-enhanced MR imaging.

## References


Arrivé L, Hricak H, Martin MC (1989) Pelvic endometriosis: MR imaging. Radiology 171:693–696

Benacerraf BR, Finkler NJ, Wojciechowski C, Knapp RC (1990) Sonographic accuracy in the diagnosis of ovarian masses. J Reprod Med 35:491–495

Brown DL, Frates MC, Laing FC, et al. (1994) Ovarian masses: can benign and malignant lesions be differentiated with color and pulse doppler US? Radiology 190:333–336

Brown JJ, Thurnher S, Hricak H (1990) MR imaging of the uterus: low-signal-intensity abnormalities of the endometrium and endometrial cavity. Magn Reson Imaging 8:309

Buy JN, Ghossain MA, Moss AA, et al. (1989) Cystic teratoma of the ovary: CT detection. Radiology 171:697–701

Dooms GC, Hricak H, Tschoiakoff D (1986) Adnexal structures: MR imaging. Radiology 158:639–646

Finkler NJ, Benacerraf BR, Lavin PT, Wojciechowski C, Knapp RC (1988) Comparison of CA 125, clinical impression, and ultrasound in the postoperative evaluation of ovarian masses. Obstet Gynecol 72:659–664

Fleischer AC, Rogers WH, Rao BK, Kepple DM, Jones HW (1991) Transvaginal color Doppler sonography of ovarian masses with pathologic correlation. Ultrasound Obstet Gynecol 1:275–278

Gomori JM, Grossman RI (1988) Mechanisms responsible for the MR appearance and evolution of intracranial hemorrhage. Radiographics 8:427–439

Granberg S, Norstrom A, Wikland M (1990) Tumors in the lower pelvis as imaged by vaginal sonography. Gynecol Oncol 37:224–229

Granberg S, Wikland M, Karlsson B, Norström A, Friberg LG (1991) Endometrial thickness as measured by endovaginal ultrasonography for identifying endometrial abnormality. Am J Obstet Gynecol 164:47–52

Herrmann UJ, Locher GW, Goldhirsch A (1987) Sonographic patterns of ovarian tumors: prediction of malignancy. Obstet Gynecol 69:777–781

Jain KA, Freidman D, Pettinger TW, Alagappan R, Jeffrey RB, Sommer FG (1993) Adnexal masses: comparison of specificity of endovaginal US and pelvic MR imaging. Radiology 186:697–704

Keller PJ, Hunter WW, Schmaibrock P (1987) Multisection fat-water imaging with chemical shift selective presaturation. Radiology 164:539–541

Kier R, Smith RC, McCarthy SM (1992) Value of lipid- and water-suppression MR images in distinguishing between blood and lipid within ovarian masses. AJR 158:321–325

Kurjak A, Zalud I, Alfirevic Z (1991) Evaluation of adnexal masses with transvaginal color ultrasound. J Ultrasound Med 10:295–297

Lerner JP, Timor-Tritsch IE, Federman A, Abramovich G (1994) Transvaginal ultrasonographic characterization of ovarian masses with an improved, weighted scoring system. Am J Obstet Gynecol 170:81–85

Mitchell DM, Kim I, Chang TS (1991) Chemical shift phase-difference and suppression magnetic resonance imaging techniques in animals, phantoms, and humans: fatty liver. Invest Radiol 26:1041–1052

Morrow CP, Townsend DE (1987) Tumors of the ovary: general considertions, classification, the adnexal mass. In: Morrow CP, Townsend DE (eds) Synopsis of gynecologic oncology. Wiley, New York, pp 231–255

Nishimura K, Togashi K, Itoh K, et al. (1987) Endometrial cysts of the ovary: MR imaging. Radiology 162:315–318

Nyberg DA, Porter BA, Olds MO, Olson DO, Andersen R, Wesby GE (1987) MR imaging of hemorrhagic adnexal masses. J Comput Assist Tomongr 11:664–669

Osmers R, Völksen M, Shauer A (1990) Vaginosonography for early detection of endometrial carcinoma? Lancet 335:1569–1571

Outwater E, Kressel HY (1992) Evaluation of gynecologic malignancy by magnetic resonance imaging. Radiol Clin North Am 30:789–806

Prat J (1996) Female reproductive system. In: Damjanov I, Linder J (eds) Anderson's pathology, 10th edn, vol 2. Mosby, St. Louis, pp 2231–2353

Riccio TJ, Adams H, Munzing DE, et al. (1990) Magnetic resonance imaging as an adjunt to sonography in the evaluation of the female pelvis. Magn Reson Imaging 8:699–704

Rosai J (1989) Female reproductive system/ovary. In: Ackerman's surgical pathology, vol 2. Mosby, St. Louis, pp 1108–1173

Sassone AM, Timor-Tritsch IE, Artner A, et al. (1991) Transvaginal sonographic characterization of ovarian disease: evaluation of new scoring system to predict ovarian malignancy. Obstet Gynecol 78:70–76

Scully RE (1970) Tumors of the ovary and maldeveloped gland. In: Hartmann WH (ed) Atlas of tumor pathology, 2nd edn, vol 16. Armed Forces Institute of Pathology, Washington, DC, pp 252–269

Sheth S, Fishman EK, Buck JL, Hamper UM, Sanders RC (1988) The variable sonographic appearances of ovarian teratomas: correlation with CT. AJR 151:331–335

Stevens SK, Hricak H, Stern JL (1991) Ovarian lesions: detection and characterization with gadolinium-enhanced MR imaging at 1.5 T. Radiology 181:481–488

Stevens SK, Hricak H, Campos Z (1993) Teratomas versus cystic hemorrhagic adnexal lesions: differentiation with proton-selective fat-saturation MR imaging. Radiology 186:481–488

Sugimura K, Okizaka H, Imaoka I, et al. (1993) Pelvic endometriosis: detection and diagnosis with chemical shift MR imaging. Radiology 188:435–438

Talerman A (1987) Germ cell tumors of the ovary. In: Kurman RJ (ed) Blaustein's pathology of the female genital tract, 3rd edn. Springer, Berlin Heidelberg New York, pp 687–721

Taylor KJW, Schwartz PE (1994) Screening for early ovarian cancer. Radiology 192:1–10

Thurnher S, Hodler J, Baer S, Marincek B, von Schulthess GK (1990) Gadolinium-DOTA enhanced MR imaging of adnexal tumors. J Comput Assist Tomogr 14:939–949

Tien RT (1992) Fat-suppression MR imaging in neuroradiology: techniques and clinical application. AJR 158:369–379

Togashi K, Nishimura K, Itoh K, et al. (1987) Ovarian cystic teratomas: MR imaging. Radiology 162:669–673

Togashi K, Nishimura K, Kimura I, et al. (1991) Endometrial cysts: diagnosis with MR imaging. Radiology 180:73–78

Wehrli FW, Perkins TC, Shimakawa A, Roberts F (1987) Chemical shift-induced amplitude modulations in images obtained with gradient refocusing. Magn Reson Imaging 5:157–158

Weiner Z, Thaler I, Beck D, Rottem S, Deutsch M, Brandes J (1992) Differentiating malignant from benign ovarian tumors with transvaginal color flow imaging. Obstet Gynecol 79:159–162

Yamashita Y, Torashima M, Hatanaka Y, et al. (1995) Adnexal masses: accuracy of characterization with transvaginal US and precontrast and postcontrast MR imaging. Radiology 194:557–565

Yamashita Y, Hatanaka Y, Torashima M, Takahashi M, Miyazaki K, Okamura H (1994) Mature cystic teratomas of the ovary without fat in the cystic cavity: MR features in 12 cases. AJR 163:613–616

Yamashita Y, Hatanaka Y, Torashima M, et al. (1997) Characterization of sonographically indeterminate ovarian tumors with MR imaging. Acta Radiol 38:572–577

Zawin M, McCarthy S, Scoutt L (1989) Endometriosis: appearance and detection at MR imaging. Radiology 171:893–896

# 10 Transrectal Ultrasound in the Assessment of Female Pelvic Malignancies and Recurrent Disease

P. Innocenti, J. Nori, R. Santoni, G. Biti, and N. Villari

CONTENTS



## 10.1 Introduction

Transrectal ultrasound (TRUS), which is commonly used to evaluate prostatic carcinomas, also may be employed to define the local extension of cervical carcinomas (Innocenti et al. 1992; Zaritzky et al. 1979). Study of the cervix uteri and cervical disease by means of TRUS is made possible by the close relationship between the probe and the cervix. On the other hand the adnexae and the corpus uteri do not lend themselves to assessment by TRUS owing to their anterior and cephalad position; they can, however, be easily studied with a transvaginal probe (transvaginal ultrasound).

P. Innocenti, MD, Professor of Radiology; N. Villari, MD, Unit of Radiodiagnostics, Department of Clinical Physiopathology, Careggi Hospital, University of Florence, Viale Morgagni 85, I-50134 Florence, Italy
J. Nori, MD, Unit of Radiodiagnostics, Obstetric and Gynecological Clinic, Careggi Hospital, University of Florence, Viale Morgagni 85, I-50134 Florence, Italy
R. Santoni, MD; G. Biti, MD, Unit of Radiation Therapy, Department of Clinical Physiopathology, Careggi Hospital, University of Florence, Viale Morgagni, 85, I-50134 Florence, Italy

## 10.2 Materials and Methods

To evaluate the cervix uteri a high-frequency (7.5 MHz) unit equipped with an electronic linear scanner and a focusing device is used. A two-plane probe with longitudinal and transverse scanning and color Doppler may be considered optimal, though not essential, for this type of investigation.

Before the investigation the probe is covered with a disposable latex condom. It is introduced into the rectum with the patient in the lateral decubitus position. The procedure is carried out with a partially filled bladder; excessive bladder distension may affect the pelvic organs, reduce the cleavage surfaces, and cause difficulties in the interpretation of the findings.

All the pelvic structures and organs may be evaluated through longitudinal and rotatory (clockwise and anticlockwise) movements of the probe (Di Candio et al. 1984; Zaritzky et al. 1979).

## 10.3 Normal Sonographic Anatomy

When the transducer is positioned along the sagittal median plane (0° with respect to the central portion of the normal cervix), the anterior rectal wall is the nearest structure to the probe. The five-layer rectal wall is structured as follows:

1. Innermost hyperechoic layer: the mucosa–mucous interface
2. Hypoechoic second layer: mucosa
3. Hyperechoic third layer: submucosa
4. Hypoechoic fourth layer: muscular layer
5. Outermost hyperechoic layer: loose perirectal connective tissue

A hyperechoic layer separates the rectum from the cervix (uppermost portion) and the vagina (lowermost portion). This cleavage plane is formed by different structures which are not well differentiated by

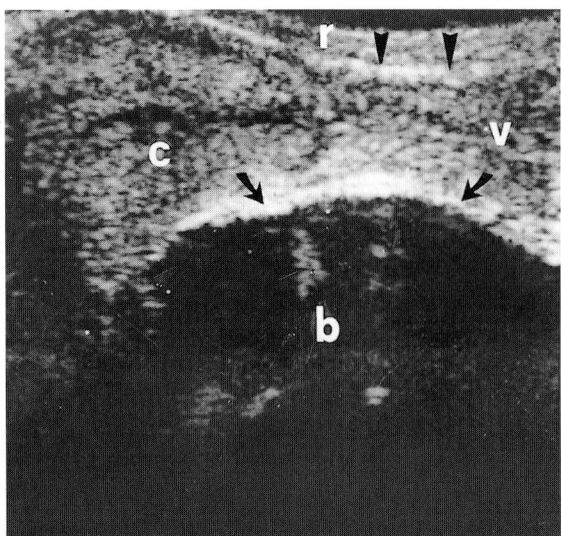


**Fig. 10.1.** Normal cervix; median sagittal scan. *b*, Bladder; *r*, anterior wall of the rectum; *c*, cervix; *v*, vagina; *arrowheads*, rectovaginal septum; *black arrows*, vesicocervical and vesicovaginal septa

ultrasound. In its uppermost portion, between the rectum and the cervix, this layer represents the peritoneal leaflets covering the posterior portion of the cervix; at the level of the vaginal fornices, it continues posteriorly toward the anterior wall of the rectum (Douglas' cul-de-sac). Distally the hyperechoic layer is formed by a connective tissue band which fades into the anterior stratum of the rectal wall (rectovaginal septum) (Fig. 10.1). The anterior and posterior vaginal walls appear as hypoechoic structures (fibrous and muscular components) separated by a hyperechoic line representing the mucosa of the anterior and posterior vaginal walls (Fig. 10.1). The vaginal walls continue into a cylindrical hypoechoic structure, representing the cervix, which is isoechoic with respect to the vaginal walls (Fig. 10.1).

The cervical canal appears as a hyperechoic central structure of varying width depending on the thickness of the mucosa, the depth of the plicae palmatae, and the amount of mucus.

The vagina and the cervix are separated from the bladder and the urethra by a hyperechoic cleavage surface. This line is formed by different structures and, in particular, distally by the extraperitoneal vesicovaginal and cervicovesical spaces and proximally by the intraperitoneal vesicouterine cavity (Fig. 10.1).

The bladder wall can be differentiated into three layers: the innermost is hyperechoic and corresponds to the mucosa and submucosa, the intermediate layer is hypoechoic and corresponds to the muscular fibers, and the outermost layer is hyperechoic and corresponds to the adipose connective tissue surrounding the bladder.

Turning the transducer clockwise or anticlockwise (15–30°), it is possible to visualize the lateral aspects of the vagina and of the fornices. Further rotation (30–80°) of the transducer allows visualization of the entire parametrium up to the pelvic wall. The parametrium is formed, mainly, by adipose connective tissue surrounding the extraperitoneal portion of the cervix and continuing upward and laterally into the broad ligaments up to the pelvic wall. The parametrium continues inferoanteriorly into the vesicovaginal and cervicovesical spaces, respectively. Posteriorly it bounds the rectovaginal space. Smooth muscular fibers and ligaments originate form the lateral part of the cervix, connecting it to the pelvic walls (cardinal ligaments) on both sides, to the anterior and posterior walls (uteropubic and uterosacral ligaments), to the anterior and lateral walls of the rectum (uterorectal muscles), and to the posterior and lateral parts of the bladder (uterovesical muscles). These ligaments and muscular structures may be visualized by sonography only in particular circumstances, i.e., when they thicken because of inflammation, endometriosis, or neoplastic involvement.

The uterine artery runs along the superior aspect of the cardinal ligament. Near the extraperitoneal portion of the cervix it branches into the uterine and cervicovaginal arteries. Venous plexuses are seen lateral to the cervix and they run upward and laterally.

The medial portion of the parametrium appears as a hyperechoic structure surrounding the cervix and the fornices, which appear relatively hypoechoic. The vessels are anechoic and, inside this structure, they appear as ribbon-like bands (Fig. 10.2). The medial and lateral segments of the parametrium have but a few vessels and appear homogeneously hyperechoic. The paravaginal tissue, into which the parametrium continues inferiorly, appear as homogeneous hyperechoic structures.

## 10.4 The Role of TRUS in the Staging and Follow-up of Cervical Tumors

The role of TRUS in the staging, treatment, and follow-up of cervical carcinomas is threefold:

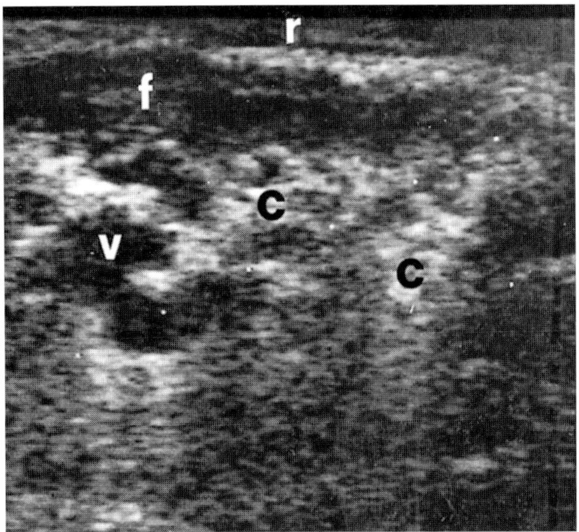


**Fig. 10.2.** Normal distal parametrium; paramedian sagittal scan. *r*, Rectal wall; *f*, lateral fornix; *v*, anechoic vascular structures; *c*, hyperechoic loose connective tissue

1. Definition of locoregional extension of cervical carcinoma before treatment
2. Evaluation of response to treatment
3. Detection of local recurrences after treatment and guidance for fine-needle biopsy of suspicious pelvic areas

**Table 10.1.** FIGO clinical stages of cervical carcinoma

| Stage | Definition |
|---|---|
| 0 | Carcinoma in situ, intraepithelial carcinoma |
| I | Carcinoma strictly confined to the cervix (extension to the corpus should be disregarded) |
| IA | Preclinical carcinoma of the cervix |
| IA1 | Minimal microscopically evident stromal invasion |
| IA2 | Lesion detected microscopically that can be measured: the upper limit of the measurement should show a depth of invasion <5 mm; a second dimension, the horizontal spread, must not exceed 7.0 mm |
| IB | Lesion of greater dimensions than stage IA2, whether established clinically or otherwise |
| II | Carcinoma extending beyond the cervix but not to the pelvic wall; the carcinoma involves the vagina but not the lower third |
| IIA | No obvious parametrial involvement |
| IIB | Obvious parametrial involvement |
| III | Carcinoma extending to the pelvic wall; on rectal examination there is no cancer-free space between the tumor and the pelvic wall, and the tumor involves the lower third of the vagina |
| IIIA | No extension to the pelvic wall but involvement of the lower third of the vagina |
| IIIB | Extension to the pelvic wall or presence of hydronephrosis or nonfunctioning kidney |
| IV | Carcinoma extending beyond the true pelvis or clinically involving the mucosa of the bladder or rectum |
| IVA | Spread to adjacent organs |
| IVB | Spread to distant organs |

## 10.4.1 Locoregional Staging of Cervical Carcinomas

The current criteria for the classification of cervical carcinomas, according to the FIGO recommendations, are reported in Table 10.1 (Pettersson 1988).

The choice of a definitive treatment modality for cervical carcinomas remains controversial, and the final decision depends primarily on the size of the tumor and its local extension. Defining the local extension of the disease only on the basis of clinical evaluation may be difficult, and staging errors range from 38.5% in patients with clinical stage I to 42.9%–89.5% in patients with stage III disease (Van Nagel et al. 1971).

As the physical examination is insufficient to properly assess extension into the paracervical tissues, a critical point is certainly the differentiation between clinical stage IB and IIB with limited parametrial involvement. In clinical stage IIB radical surgery is inadequate either alone or as the initial modality. These patients may undergo radiation therapy or neoadjuvant chemotherapy, followed by surgery, or exclusive radiation therapy. Therefore the diagnosis of limited parametrial involvement is critical in devising the therapeutic program and sequence of treatments (Averette et al. 1975; Van Nagel et al. 1971).

The criteria discussed below may be used to identify and outline tumors confined to the uterine cervix and/or tumor extension outside the cervical boundaries.

### *10.4.1.1 Stage I (Tumors Involving the Cervix Only)*

Small tumors (maximum diameter <1 cm) may be difficult to differentiate from the normal cervical structure (Innocenti et al. 1992). Tumors exceeding 1 cm in their maximum dimension produce modifications of the normal anatomy of the cervix which may be identified using TRUS (Di Candio et al. 1984; Innocenti et al. 1992; Zaritzky et al. 1979). Such modifications are represented by:

1. Increase in the transverse diameters of the cervix, up to "barrel-shaped" tumors which measure several centimeters.

2. Irregular borders of the external outline of the cervix.
3. Disappearance of the normal structure of the cervix with the presence of hypoechoic or anechoic areas with undefined borders. Focal lesions (Fig. 10.3) are significantly less frequent than diffuse tumors (Fig. 10.4). A homogeneous hyperechoic pattern of the entire cervix is exceptionally rare for cervical carcinomas whereas it is frequent in cases of cervical involvement by endometrial tumors.
4. Areas of gaseous necrosis. If present, these appear as small hyperechoic areas (Fig. 10.4). On the other hand microcalcifications inside the tumor are infrequent and they appear as small hyperechoic areas producing attenuation of the echo beam.
5. Displacement, alteration, interruption, or even effacement of the typical hyperechoic line representing the cervical canal.

### 10.4.1.2 Stages IIA and IIIA (Tumors Involving the Vagina)

The tumor may involve the vagina at different levels. When the disease is limited to its upper third, the fornices are obliterated and the cervix may not be distinguishable. Tumors involving the lower third of the vagina appear as hypoechoic irregular bands within the vaginal walls. The central hyperechoic line, corresponding to the mucous lining, may be displaced, disrupted, or not visualized at all (Di Candio et al. 1984; Innocenti et al. 1992).

### 10.4.1.3 Stages IIB and IIIB (Tumors Progressing into the Parametria)

In stages IIB and IIIB the hypo- or anechoic neoplastic tissue may be easily identified within the hyperechoic connective structures of the parametrium (Aoki et al. 1990; Tipaldi et al. 1991). In its upper portion the parametrium appears as a hypoechoic flat area including venous plexuses and the uterine artery converging toward the cervix. Its lower part is mainly composed of fibrillar connective tissue which appears homogeneously hyperechoic. When the tumor involves the proximal parametrium it may displace encase, or infiltrate the vascular structures. Further progression of the tumor toward the pelvic wall, infiltrating the lateral parametrium, produces a sonographic image characterized by a hypoechoic and inhomogeneous area which is continuous from the cervix to the pelvic wall (Figs. 10.5, 10.6).

When the tumor infiltrates the cervicovesical, rectovaginal, and vesicovaginal septa this infiltration

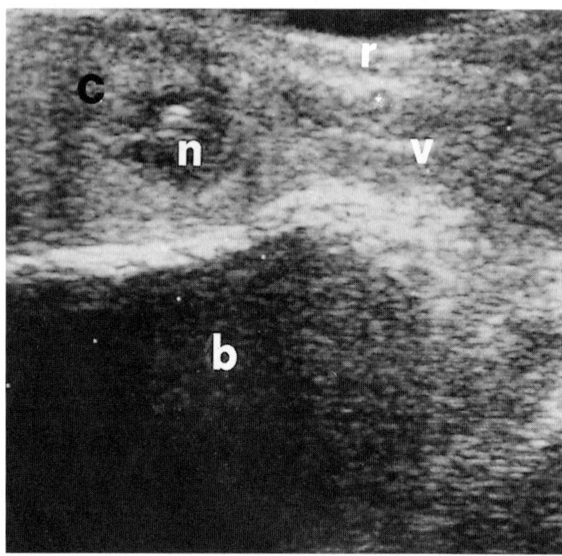


**Fig. 10.3.** Stage IB cervical carcinoma; median sagittal scan. Hypoechoic neoplastic nodule (*n*), well differentiated from the cervical stroma (*c*). *b*, Bladder; *v*, vagina; *r*, rectal wall

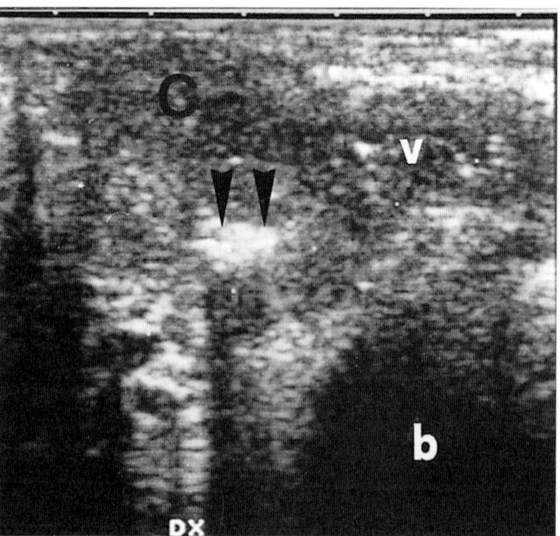


**Fig. 10.4.** Stage IB cervical carcinoma; median sagittal scan. The tumor is not distinguished from the cervical stroma (*C*). The tumor is isoechoic to the normal cervical stroma. There is evidence of gaseous necrosis within the tumor (*arrowheads*). *v*, Vagina; *b*, bladder

may be diagnosed with TRUS in spite of the relatively exiguous thickness of these structures. They are, in fact, formed by loose connective fibers and appears as hyperechoic streaks. Within the septa the tumor appears as scanty hypoechoic nodules or as a continuous band (Fig. 10.7).

The portion of the ureter running into the parametrium, behind the bladder and anterior to the cervix, is not usually visualized by ultrasound. Nonetheless, tumor infiltration of the ureter may produce obstruction and dilatation of the upper ureter, which may then be visualized by TRUS.

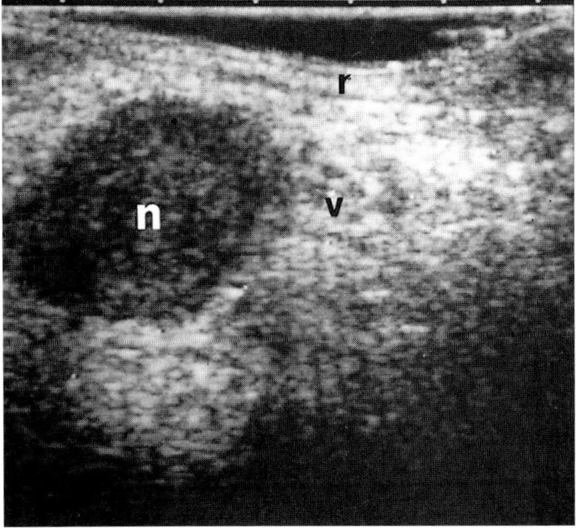


**Fig. 10.5.** Stage IIB cervical carcinoma; lateral sagittal scan. A hypoechoic neoplastic nodule (*n*) is present within the proximal right parametrium. *v*, Uterine vessels; *r*, rectal wall

#### 10.4.1.4 Stage IVA (Tumors Involving the Rectum and/or Bladder)

Conventional endoscopy (cystoscopy and proctoscopy) allows the diagnosis of neoplastic infiltration of the bladder and rectum only when the tumor penetrates the mucosa. According to the FIGO criteria, stage IVA cervical carcinoma may be diagnosed only after pathologic confirmation is obtained on biopsy of the rectum or the bladder. Nonetheless, infiltration of the rectovaginal, vesicovaginal, and cervicovesical septa without invasion of the mucosa represents relevant information before performing radical surgery. TRUS allows the diagnosis of infiltration of the external and intermediate layers of the bladder and the rectum (Innocenti et al. 1992). Under these circumstances TRUS shows the progressive disappearance of the three- or five-layer structure of the bladder and rectum respectively (Fig. 10.8). Only when the different layers of the rectal and vesical walls may be clearly identified is it possible to exclude macroscopic involvement of these structures. Bullous edema is frequently diagnosed during cystoscopy, especially in patients with bulky disease. In spite of the fact that this observation is not considered sufficient to diagnose stage IV disease, such a diagnosis may be substantiated by early invasion of the outermost layers of the bladder wall, which may be identified with TRUS.

Progressive tumor may infiltrate the mucosa, appearing as a nonhomogeneous hypoechoic mass protruding into the lumen of the bladder or rectum (Fig. 10.9).

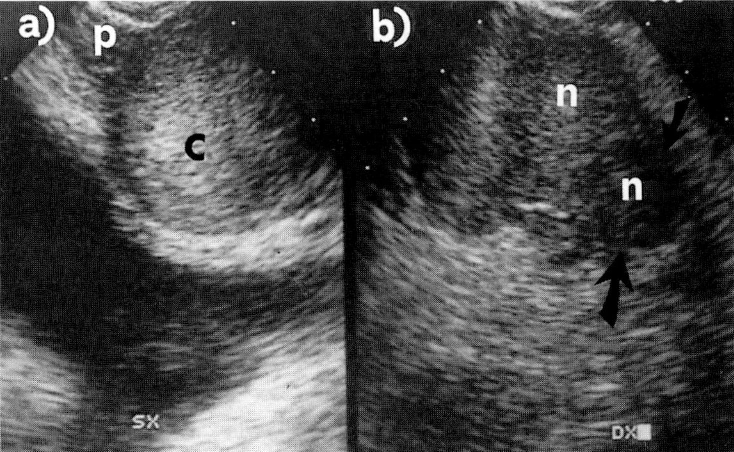


**Fig. 10.6 a,b.** Same patient as in Fig. 10.5; transverse scan. **a** Normal parametrium (*p*) on the left side. *c*, Cervix. **b** Nodules (*n*) are present within the proximal portion (*black arrows*) of the right parametrium

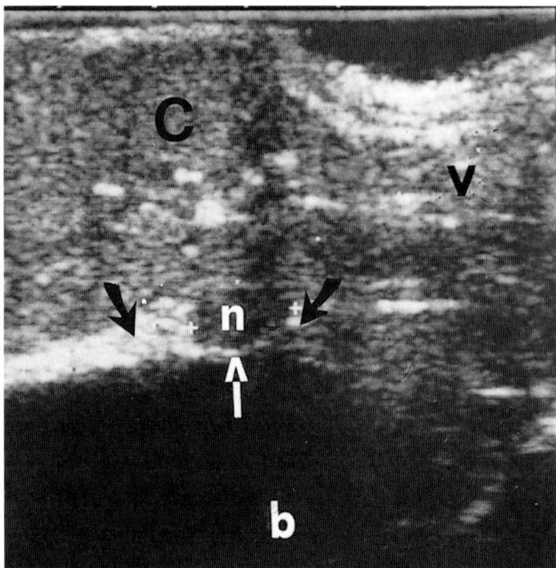


**Fig. 10.7.** Carcinoma of the cervix; median sagittal scan. There is infiltration (*n*) of the vesicocervical septum and of the wall of the bladder (*black arrows*). The bladder mucosa has a normal appearance (*white arrow*). *b*, Bladder; *c*, cervix; *v*, vagina.

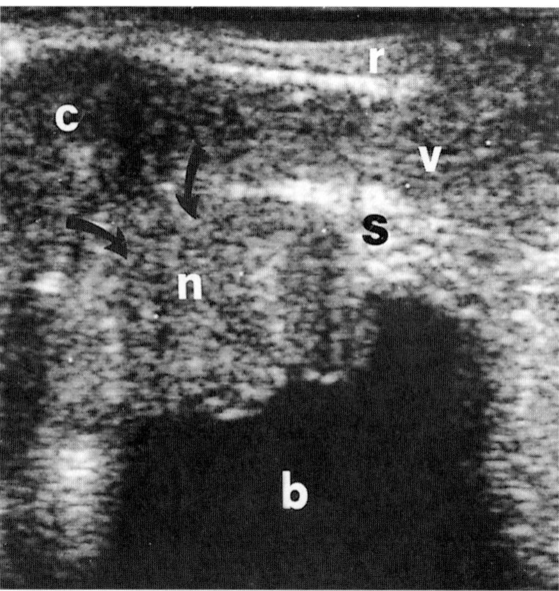


**Fig. 10.9.** Stage IVA cervical carcinoma with infiltration of the bladder; median sagittal scan. A lesion (*n*) is protruding into the bladder (*b*). The vesicocervical septum (*S*) is interrupted (*black arrows*). *c*, Cervix; *r*, rectal wall; *v*, vagina

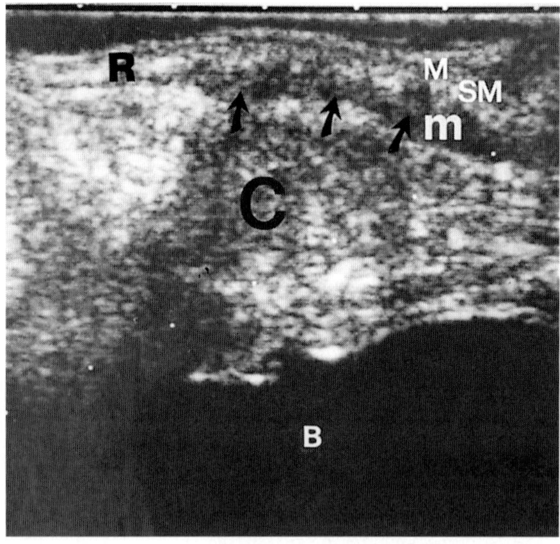


**Fig. 10.8.** Carcinoma of the cervix; median sagittal scan. There is infiltration (*black arrows*) of the wall of the rectum (*R*) with thickening of the muscular layer (*m*) and partial interruption of the submucosa (*SM*). *M*, Normal mucosa; *C*, tumor of the cervix; *B*, bladder

### *10.4.1.5 General Considerations*

In spite of the great potential of TRUS in the diagnosis of local extension of cervical carcinoma, our experience is that the method may, independently of the type of tumor growth and size, underestimate (in relation to pathology) the volume of the tumor confined to the cervix (Innocenti et al. 1992). However, other authors (Magee et al. 1991) have reached the opposite conclusion regarding determination of tumor volume by means of TRUS.

The overall accuracy of TRUS alone for determination of the locoregional extension of cervical carcinomas is 85%, which is slightly better than what may be achieved (82%) using all the diagnostic procedures suggested by the FIGO classification. The diagnostic accuracy of TRUS in clinical stage IIB cervical carcinoma (86%) is much better than the corresponding figure (57%) obtained following the recommendations of the FIGO classification in this group of patients. With regard to parametrial infiltration, TRUS shows a higher sensitivity than clinical classification (86%, vs 64%) but similar specificity (88% vs 92%), overall diagnostic accuracy (87% vs 86%), positive predictive value (67% vs 69%), and negative predictive value (96% vs 90%) (Innocenti et al. 1992).

The fact that TRUS and clinical examination of the patient under general anesthesia may be used in combination, as suggested by the FIGO staging system, indicates that the two methods need not be regarded as alternatives. TRUS should be considered for the routine workup of patients with cervical carcinoma. Errors using TRUS may be corrected by accurate clinical evaluation of the patients, and vice versa. Edema surrounding the tumor may be correctly interpreted by means of TRUS, but overestimated clinically (Averette et al. 1975; Van Nagel et al. 1971). On the other hand TRUS cannot differentiate between parametrial extension of the disease and endometriosis, which at sonography presents as isolated or confluent hypoechoic nodules involving the uterine ligaments and the connective tissues of the pelvis.

### 10.4.2 Evaluation of Response to Treatment

Transrectal ultrasound may be used to evaluate tumor response to preoperative radiation therapy or neoadjuvant chemotherapy for bulky tumors (IB, IIA, IIB) (Meanwell et al. 1985). The method allows evaluation of the volumetric modifications of the tumor–cervix "complex" following radiation and chemotherapy. Nonetheless, persistence of the tumor may not be excluded in patients showing dimensional regression as treatment produces increased echogeneity both in the tumor and in the normal tissues. While the low contrast gradient between tumor and cervical stroma is maintained there is a reduction in the echoic differences between the tumor and cervix and the loose connective pelvic tissues. As a consequence, TRUS may provide quantitative information concerning tumor–cervix complex regression, but no qualitative data regarding tumor cure.

### 10.4.3 Detection of Local Recurrences After Treatment and Guidance of Fine-Needle Biopsy

Transrectal ultrasound has an important role in the follow-up cervical carcinoma (Meanwell et al. 1987). The clinical evaluation of patients may allow the diagnosis and biopsy of recurrent or persistent tumor involving the vaginal vault after surgery, or the cervix and upper third of the vagina after exclusive radiation therapy. However, when recurrent disease is located in the center of the pelvis, clinical evaluation by itself does not allow accurate definition of the size of the recurrence and its relationship to the surrounding structures and organs.

In patients with pelvic side wall recurrences it may be difficult to obtain a clinical diagnosis of tumor relapse, depending on the site and size of the recurrence. In some cases differentiation between tumor and fibrosis is impossible, especially after exclusive radiation therapy.

After surgery, in the absence of tumor recurrence the residual vagina shows a vault-like shape with uniform thickness of all its walls and well-delineated boundaries of the vault itself. At this level two lateral and upward hypoechoic areas are frequently present at the upper lateral edges of the vault as a direct consequence of surgical resection. The surrounding loose connective tissue is homogeneously hyperechoic and devoid of vascular structures. Under these circumstances it is easy to differentiate a pelvic recurrence, with its characteristic hypoechoic features, from the surrounding structures.

As pointed out above, after radiation therapy decreased echogenicity of the pelvic structures is observed (Meanwell et al. 1987), in particular between the loose and fibrous pelvic connective tissue, the latter usually appearing hyperechoic under these paticular circumstances. In patients with clinical suspicion of pelvic recurrence, TRUS may be negative and in these cases it is advisable to perform it in association with clinical examination.

The probe can investigate the area of interest identified by digital examination of the vagina. In these patients, before may conclusions can be drawn it is necessary to obtain a tissue sample for pathology. If the recurrent tumor is not accessible from the vaginal vault a fine-needle biopsy under ultrasound guidance must be performed. Various factors may influence the choice of technique and equipment. The best way to obtain a sample for pathology is usually through the vagina using an endovaginal probe equipped with a coaxial channel for biopsy. The progression of the needle is visualized on the monitor by electronic markers and the probe is positioned abutting the area from which the sample is to be obtained. With this method it is possible to monitor the progression of the needle and to perform the biopsy of the selected site. There are certain circumstances, however, which may preclude this approach:

1. Stenosis of the vagina where the probe cannot be introduced.
2. Central pelvic recurrence located immediately above the vaginal vault: in these cases the trans-

ducer is too close to the lesion and the progression of the needle may not be monitored.
3. Low and/or lateral pelvic recurrence at an angle which is not accessible using the transvaginal approach.

In all these circumstances TRUS-guided biopsy is employed. The needle is introduced into the vagina with the rectal probe pointing toward the lesion. The vaginal needle is aligned with the probe and its progression through the vaginal vault may be monitored until it reaches the area from which a sample is to be obtained. If the recurrence is low and at an angle which is not accessible via the vaginal vault, a transperineal approach is preferred (Fig. 10.10), using the same technique as is employed to perform prostatic biopsies.

When there is no sonographic evidence of recurrent disease, but only a clinically suspicious area, the needle biopsy (transvaginal or transperineal) may be performed under digital guidance and using a Frenzen biopsy needle.

## 10.5 Conclusions

Transrectal ultrasound is a reliable, noninvasive, and relatively simple method with which to explore the pelvic structures and organs and to evaluate, in combination with the clinical examination, the local extension of cervical carcinomas. As a staging procedure its accuracy is higher than that achieved by the clinical examinations proposed by the FIGO clinical classification. In particular TRUS is more reliable in the detection of tumor extension to the proximal parametrium and allows the diagnosis of early invasion of the rectal and vesical walls. The combination of clinical examination and TRUS is able to decrease staging errors in patients with cervical carcinomas.

During treatment TRUS may be used to evaluate modifications of the tumor-cervix complex, although it is not possible to define the persistence and extension of residual tumor within the cervix.

After surgery TRUS may detect early pelvic recurrences, allowing biopsy of these areas for histopathology. Sometimes fibrosis may be differentiated from recurrent tumor by TRUS with acceptable confidence. In dubious cases, when histopathology is necessary to obtain a definitive diagnosis, TRUS may be employed to guide transvaginal or transperineal biopsy.

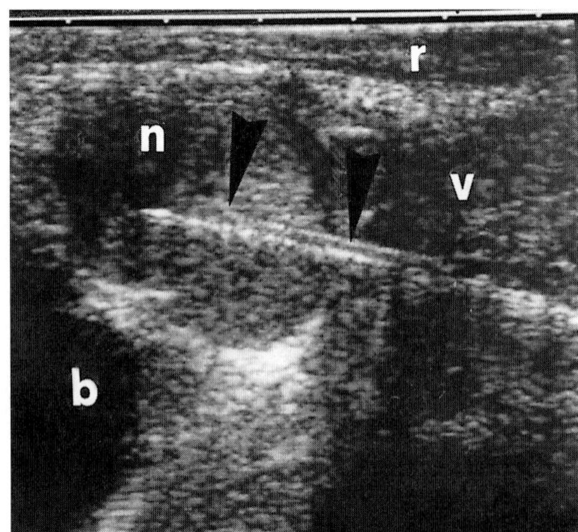


**Fig. 10.10.** Fine-needle biopsy of a side wall recurrence; lateral sagittal scan. *n*, Neoplastic nodule; *b*, bladder; *r*, rectal wall; *v*, vagina. The progression of the needle, through the perineum, is monitored with TRUS (*arrowhead*)

## References

Aoki S, Hata T, Senoh D, et al. (1990) Parametrial invasion of uterine cervical cancer assessed by transrectal ultrasonography: preliminary report. Gynecol Oncol 36:82–89

Averette HE, Ford JH, Dudan RC, et al. (1975) Staging of cervical cancer. Clin Obstet Gynecol 18:215–232

Di Candio G, Campatelli A, Mosca F, et al. (1984) Transrectal ultrasonography and cervical neoplasia: a preliminary report. Eur J Gynaecol Oncol 3:194–202

Innocenti P, Pulli F, Savino L, et al. (1992) Staging of cervical cancer: reliability of transrectal US. Radiology 185:201–205

Magee BT, Logue JP, Swindell R, et al. (1991) Tumor size as a prognostic factor in carcinoma of the cervix: assessment by transrectal ultrasound. Br J Radio 64:812–815

Meanwell CA, Rolfe EB, Blackledge G, et al. (1985) Transrectal ultrasonography in the assessment and management of recurrent cervical cancer treated with chemotherapy. Br J Cancer 51 (Suppl 4):592

Meanwell CA, Rolfe EB, Blackledge G, et al. (1987) Recurrent female pelvic cancer: assessment with transrectal ultrasonography. Radiology 162:278–281

Pettersson F (1988) Annual report on the results of treatment in gynecological cancer. Radiumhemmet Stockholm, p 30

Tipaldi L, Squillaci E, Cecconi L, et al. (1991) Il cervicocarcinoma al I e II stadio. Studio con Risonanza Magnetica ed ecografia transrettale. Radiol Med (Torino) 81:666–670

Van Nagel JR, Roddick JW, Lowing DM (1971) The staging of cervical cancer: inevitable discrepances between clinical staging and pathologic findings. Am J Obstet Gynecol 110:973–978

Zaritzky D, Blake D, Willard J, et al. (1979) Transrectal ultrasonography in the evaluation of cervical carcinoma. Obstet Gynecol 53:105–108

# 11 Radiology of the Female Bladder, Urethra, and Pelvic Floor

K.R. Mullangi, G.C. Mingin jr., and N.G. Kasabian

CONTENTS



## 11.1 Introduction

Female urology and urogynecology have become subspecialties in their respective disciplines due to the complexities of the pathology of the female bladder, urethra, and pelvic floor. This chapter complements previous chapters in *Radiology of the Lower Urinary Tract* (E.K. Lang, ed.), previously published by Springer-Verlag.

K.R. Mullangi, MD, Chief Resident, Division of Urology, Department of Surgery, UMDNJ – New Jersey Medical School, 150 Bergen Street, Newark, NJ 07103-2406, USA (*current address*: 517 North 3rd. Street, Burlington, IA 52601, USA)
G.C. Mingin, jr., MD, Resident, Division of Urology, Department of Surgery, UMDNJ – New Jersey Medical School, 150 Bergen Street, Newark, NJ 07103-2406, USA
N.G. Kasabian, MD, Director of Female Urology and Neurourology, Assistant Professor of Surgery, Division of Urology, Department of Surgery, UMDNJ – New Jersey Medical School, 150 Bergen Street, Newark, NJ 07103-2406, USA (*current address*: Urology Associates, P.C., 535 Plandome Road, Manhasset, NY 11030, USA)

## 11.2 The Bladder

### 11.2.1 Introduction

The urinary bladder is the body's reservoir for urine. It is a simple muscular bag controlled voluntarily with the necessity to void. Many bladder anomalies can be described radiologically, most of which are discussed in other parts of the book. Here, we shall focus on bladder embryology and associated congenital abnormalities; in addition, two rare disease states will be considered: endometriosis and condylomata acuminata.

### 11.2.2 Embryology

The endodermal cloaca is divided by the urorectal septum into a dorsal rectum and a ventral urogenital sinus (Fig. 11.1). The urogenital sinus is then divided into three parts: a cranial vesical part, a middle pelvic part, and a caudal phallic part. The endoderm of the vesical part is responsible for the bladder epithelium (Gyllensten 1949). The lamina propria, the muscle layers, and the serosa develop from the adjacent splanchnic mesenchyme. Initially, the bladder is continuous with the allantois, but the lumen of this vestigial structure is soon constricted. It becomes a thick fibrous cord, the urachus, attached to the apex of the bladder and the umbilicus (Matsuno et al. 1984). As the bladder enlarges, the caudal portions of the mesonephric ducts are incorporated into its dorsal wall. These ducts contribute to the formation of the mucosa of the trigone of the bladder. As the mesonephric ducts are replaced by the endodermal epithelium of the urogenital sinus with subsequent absorption, the ureters come to open separately into the urinary bladder (Gyllensten 1949). In infants and children, the bladder is in the abdomen, even when empty. It enters the pelvis at about 6 years.

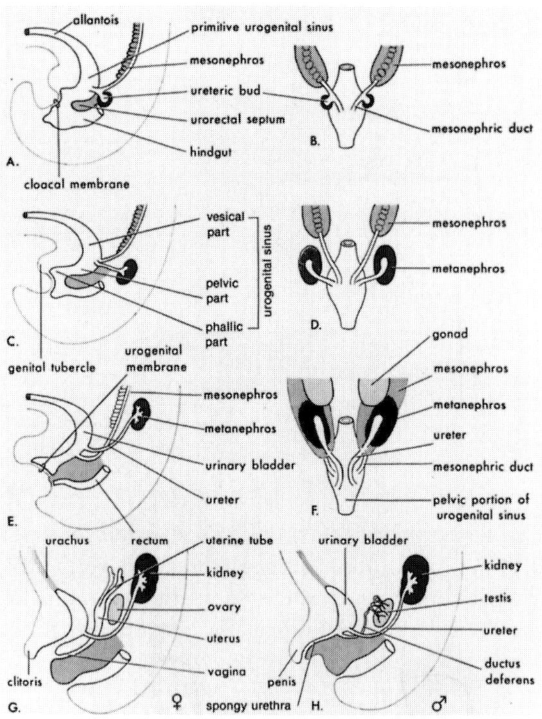


Fig. 11.1 A–H. Diagrams showing (1) division of the cloaca into the urogenital sinus and the rectum, (2) developement of the urinary bladder, urethra, and urachus, and (3) changes in the location of the ureters. A, B Lateral and dorsal views of the caudal half of a 5-week embryo showing the relationship between the mesonephros and the ureteric bud. C, D Lateral and dorsal views of the different segments of the urogenital sinus. E, F Lateral and dorsal views of the upward migration of the kidney. G Lateral view of the female genital tract. H Lateral view of the male genital tract. (From Moore 1982)

This discussion of bladder genesis will provide a foundation for understanding the mechanisms of various congenital lesions.

## 11.2.3 Congenital Anomalies

### 11.2.3.1 *Bladder Duplication*

Radiologically, bladder duplication can be divided into seven types. The most common is complete duplication of the bladder and the urethra (Kapoor and Saha 1987). Each bladder has a full-thickness muscular wall with its own ipsilateral ureter and urethra. This is more common in males than in females (Fig. 11.2). Many of these patients also have duplication of the external genitalia and lower gastrointestinal tract (Kossow and Morales 1973). In incomplete duplication, each bladder has its own muscular wall and ureter, but the two bladders communicate and drain into a common urethra (Abrahamson 1965). A rare type is the hourglass bladder, which is divided into an upper and a lower portion by a partial muscular and fibrous septum. This septum can exist as a complete sagittal septum separating the bladder vertically into two halves (Witzleben et al. 1965). One part is separated from the urethra, which develops subsequent hydronephrosis and renal dysplasia. Three other entities include incomplete sagittal septum, complete frontal septum, and multiseptate bladder (Senger and Santare 1952).

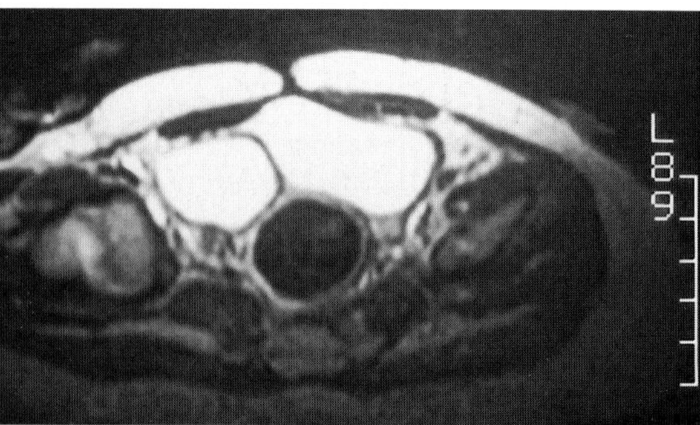


Fig. 11.2. A T2-weighted axial MRI demonstrates a duplication of the bladder. Each bladder had its own muscular wall and ureter but drained into a common urethra

### 11.2.3.2 *Urachal Abnormalities*

Incomplete obliteration of the urachus can present with various anomalies. Partially and complete patent urachi can be distinguished by examination and radiologic studies (Cherry 1950). Complete patent urachus in seen with leakage of urine at the umbilicus diagnosed with voiding cystourethrography (VCUG) with contrast extravasation at the umbilicus. VCUG will also help assess bladder dysfunction and obstruction as a cause of patent urachus. Incomplete obliteration of the urachus can lead to urachal cyst, external urachal sinus, and urachal diverticulum. Only external urachal sinus will create a wet umbilicus (Jaramillo 1990). VCUG shows no communication between the bladder and the sinus since the urachus is obliterated between the two sites. In urachal diverticulum, no open connection is present to the umbilicus. Instead, the anomaly is seen as a midline bladder outpouching extending superiorly on VCUG (BERMAN 1988). Finally, the urachal cyst is diagnosed only when infected from rupture with subsequent leakage into the umbilicus or bladder. When asymptomatic, it is detected on incidental ultrasound or computed tomographic (CT) scan (MANDEL et al. 1991).

### 11.2.3.3 Bladder Exstrophy

Bladder exstrophy is associated with absence of the lower abdominal wall and anterior bladder wall, revealing the inner surface of the posterior wall of the bladder (MARSHALL and MUCKE 1962). The pathognomic finding is present on KUB with pubic diastasis. With increased technology and radiologic experience, prenatal ultrasound can diagnose the possibility of bladder exstrophy. Key factors include absence of bladder filling with a low-set umbilicus (GEARHART and JEFFS 1988). Exstrophy is associated with epispadias, agenesis of the ureter, and rectal malformations. All variants of exstrophy have the characteristic widening of the symphysis pubis caused by the outward rotation of the innominate bones. In addition, an eversion of the pubic rami at their junction with the ischial and iliac bones occurs (CRACCHIOLO and HALL 1970).

### 11.2.3.4 Bladder Diverticula

Congenital bladder diverticula not associated with valves or neurogenic bladder are rare (BARRETT et al. 1976). They are usually solitary, occur without evidence of outlet obstruction, and are often larger than those associated with obstruction. Inherent weakness in the bladder musculature is the cause. Paraureteral diverticula incorporate the ureteral orifice and tunnel with resultant reflux (JOHNSTON 1960). Those occurring at the bladder neck can cause urethral obstruction (Fig. 11.3). Diagnosis can easily be made with VCUG. Upper tract studies will also define the anatomical and functional damage from reflux, but are not the best method for diagnosis (ALLEN and ATWELL 1980).

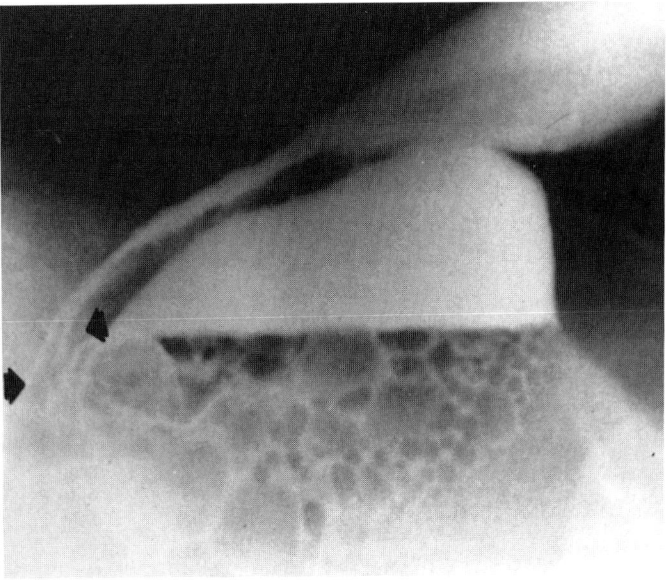

Fig. 11.3. A double-contrast cystogra, lateral projection, demonstrates a congenital diverticulum arising at the bladder neck (*arrows*) and located anterior to the bladder in the space of Retzius. (Courtesy of E.K. Lang)

## 11.2.4 Endometriosis

Endometriosis, a female disease, is defined as the presence of endometrial tissue beyond the endometrium. It is a benign disease with malignant behavior (APPEL 1988). Various mechanisms regarding the existence of ectopic endometrium in the urinary bladder include the embryonic, metaplastic, and migratory theories (KUMAR et al. 1984). The urinary tract is affected in 1.1% of cases of endometriosis, with 84% of these occurring in the bladder. A variety of constitutional symptoms can occur, with the most common being vesical discomfort (NETO et al. 1984). Sonography usually reveals a filling defect and defines the extent of the tumor. The mass is seen to extend through the wall of the bladder into the uterus. Radiologic studies localize the lesion to allow for direction of biopsy endoscopically (KUMAR et al. 1984).

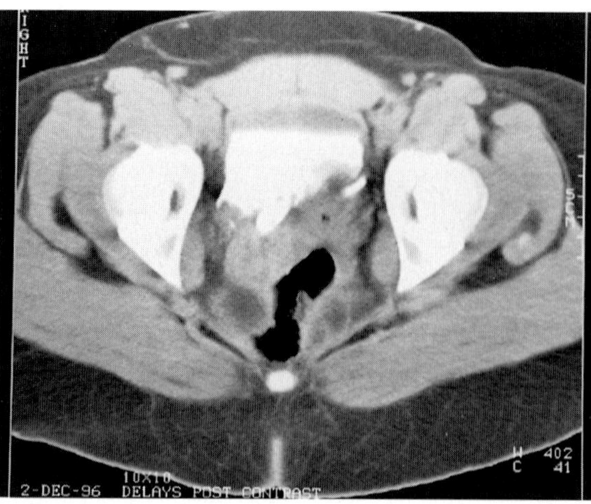


**Fig. 11.4.** Contrast-enhanced CT scan revealing pedunculated wart-like condylomatous bladder lesions

### 11.2.5 Condyloma Acuminata

Condyloma acuminata is a sexually tramsitted disease affecting the bladder rarely. The lesions can be seen cystoscopically and with CT scan as papillary, pedunculated wart-like lesions (Fig. 11.4). Bladder extension may be related to immunosuppression. Association with urothelial malignancy has been suggested. Imaging examinations can be used for monitoring the extent of involvement during treatment protocols (Murphy et al. 1990).

## 11.3 The Female Urethra

### 11.3.1 Introduction

The spectrum of disease affecting the female urethra encompasses the full range of entities seen in urologic practice. A majority of lesions go undetected or are improperly diagnosed and treated. Primary surgical treatment involves accurate diagnosis, which requires a basic understanding of the embryology, anatomy, and pathophysiology in the female urethra. Advances in diagnostic and interventional radiology demand that the physician be familiar with commonly employed excretory urography techniques as well as with advances in ultrasound (US), CT, and magnetic resonance imaging (MRI). In the current health care environment a firm grasp of the above will allow for cost-effective and intelligent decision-making.

### 11.3.2 Embryology

In the female embryo there are two pairs of genital ducts. The mesonephric or wolffian duct system and the müllerian or paramesonepheric duct system. A 6 weeks of gestation the müllerian ducts (longitudinal invaginations of the coelomic epithelium on the anterolateral surface of the urogenital ridge) are seen lateral to the mesonepheric ducts (the cranial end of the primitive mesonephros, which forms Bowman's capsule). By week 10 of gestation the müllerian ducts fuse caudally in the midline, forming the paramesonepheric or müllerian tubercle, which will later fuse with the urogenital sinus.

Further development of the above ductal systems requires their integration with the urogenital sinus. At 4 weeks of gestation the blind end of the hind gut or cloaca subdivides, forming a ventral urogenital sinus and a dorsal rectum. The mesonepheric ducts then join the urogenital sinus just lateral to the müllerian tubercle. With mesonephric regression, remnants of the duct system can be seen lateral to the fallopian tubes cranially and the vagina caudally (Gartner's duct). Portions of the degenerating ducts also extend into the urogenital sinus as sinovaginal bulbs which contribute to the vaginal plate. The pelvic portion of the urogenital sinus forms the urethra and part of the vagina (Fig. 11.5). Skene's glands are seen as ducts arising from the urethra. The müllerian tubercle from above and the urogenital sinus from below then join at the sinovaginal node to form the vagina, with the müllerian duct responsible for the formation of the upper two-thirds and the urogenital sinus for the distal portion.

### 11.3.3 Anatomy

The female urethra is a short musculomembranous tube that is well protected by the pelvic bones. The tube courses concavely downward from the trigone to the urethral meatus, the smallest portion of the tube. It is lined by squamous epithelium throughout most of its 3–5 cm length, to its junction with the transitional epithelium of the bladder (PRATT 1967). The urethral submucosa is made up of a rich vascular network which also contains connective tissue, as well as elastic and smooth muscle fibers. The musculature of the urethra is made up of an inner longitudinal and an outer circular layer of smooth muscle. The internal sphincter containing only smooth muscle is seen as an extension of the trigone. The external sphincter is made up of three elements. The first component consists of the inner longitudinal and outer circular layer of smooth muscle in the upper four-fifths of the urethra. The second part is made up of the striated urogenital sphincter, a combination of the intramural striated muscle and the distal layer of the pelvic floor muscles. The third part includes vascular elements within the urethral wall (Bo 1995).

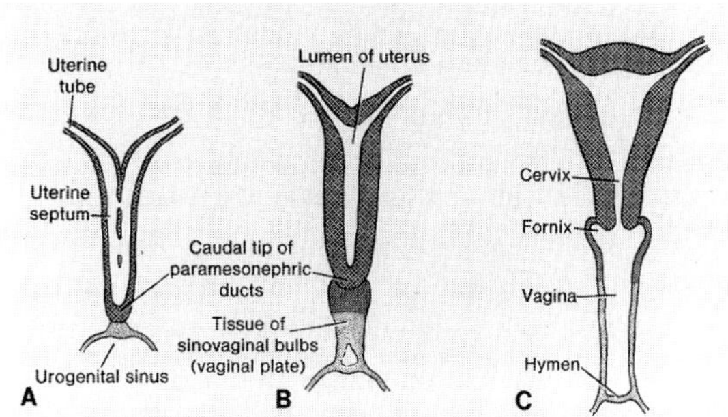


**Fig. 11.5 A–C.** Schematic drawing showing the formation of the uterus and vagina. **A** At 9 weeks. Note the disappearance of the uterine septum. **B** At the end of the 3rd month. Note the tissue of the sinovaginal bulbs. **C** Newborn. The upper portion of the vagina and the fornices are formed by vacuolization of the paramesonephric tissue and the lower portion by vacuolization of the sinovaginal bulbs. (From Sadler 1990)

## 11.3.4 Imaging: An Overview

The majority of urethral pathology is still diagnosed by means of the traditional VCUG and retrograde urethrography (RUG). Urethral ultrasonography in expert hands also gives results comparable to traditional studies (Yoder 1992). Recently transrectal ultrasounds has become an important tool in the diagnosis of urethral diverticula (Lopez Rasines 1996). CT scan is not as sensitive in delineating the urethral anatomy. Because of its multiplanar views, MRI can differentiate the urethra from the vagina and surrounding periurethral tissue.

## 11.3.5 Benign Lesions

### *11.3.5.1 Periurethral Lesions*

#### 11.3.5.1.1 Urethral Caruncle

Urethral caruncles are benign lesions which are commonly seen to affect postmenopausal women; the exact incidence is not known. The caruncle usually appears as a small soft red mass at the posterior aspect of the urethra (Fig. 11.6). The lesion is most often broad based but can appear sessile or pedunculated. The pathogenesis is suggestive of prolapse, followed by irritation, congestion, and chronic inflammation, though infection has also been speculated to have a causative role (Pratt 1967).

Caruncles may be asymptomatic; however, they usually present with pain and/or bleeding, frequency, urgency, obstruction, or rarely distention secondary to fear of voiding. The differential diagnosis includes polyp, cyst, abscess, condyloma, carcinoma, and urethral prolapse. Treatment is dependent upon symptoms. For asymptomatic women no treatment is suggested. Following this sitz baths or topical estrogens may be used. Lesions that are refractory to medical therapy require either excision by electrocautery or sharp dissection. Before surgery is performed the patient should undergo VCUG to make certain no other pathology is missed.

#### 11.3.5.1.2 Skene's Gland Abscess and Cysts

A Skene's gland cyst presents as a smooth tumor mass, which unlike the caruncle is not red or erythematous. The Skene's duct cyst is uncommon in both adults and children and is thought to be due to obstruction of the duct; however, it may occur secondary to inflammation in adults. A Skene's gland abscess appears as a tender mass lateral and inferior to the meatus (cf. appearance for Bartholin gland abscess: Fig. 11.7). The patient may present with dysuria or obstructive voiding symptoms. The differential diagnosis includes urethral diverticula and ureterocele.

On sonograms Skene's gland abscesses and cysts can be confused with diverticula. However, VCUG or RUG should prove sufficient to rule out other etiologies.

Rarely, Skene's duct cysts resolve spontaneously, necessitating treatment. In infants this consists of simple needle aspiration (Hyuk Lee 1992), while in adults excision of the gland and its duct is recommended.

11.3.5.1.3

BENIGN PERIURETHRAL MASSES

Benign periurethral masses may present as firm nontender tumors lying in the urethrovaginal septum, anterior to the urethra or intraurethrally. These tumors are rare and may be asymptomatic or produce hematuria or irritative and obstructive voiding symptoms. The two most common tumors are leiomyomas and fibromyomas. These mesothelial lesions are believed to arise from midline embryonal rests. Radiographic studies include an excretory urogram (IVP), which will show a filling defect at the bladder base. Because of their distinct anatomic, clinical, and radiographic presentation, these lesions have been likened to the male prostate. Treatment is dependent on location. Transvaginal suprapubic and transurethral excision has been utilized (SHARMA 1988).

11.3.5.1.4

FEMALE PROSTATITIS

Like the prostate gland, the periurethral glands, including the Skene's gland, can be affected by inflammatory changes caused by sexually transmitted

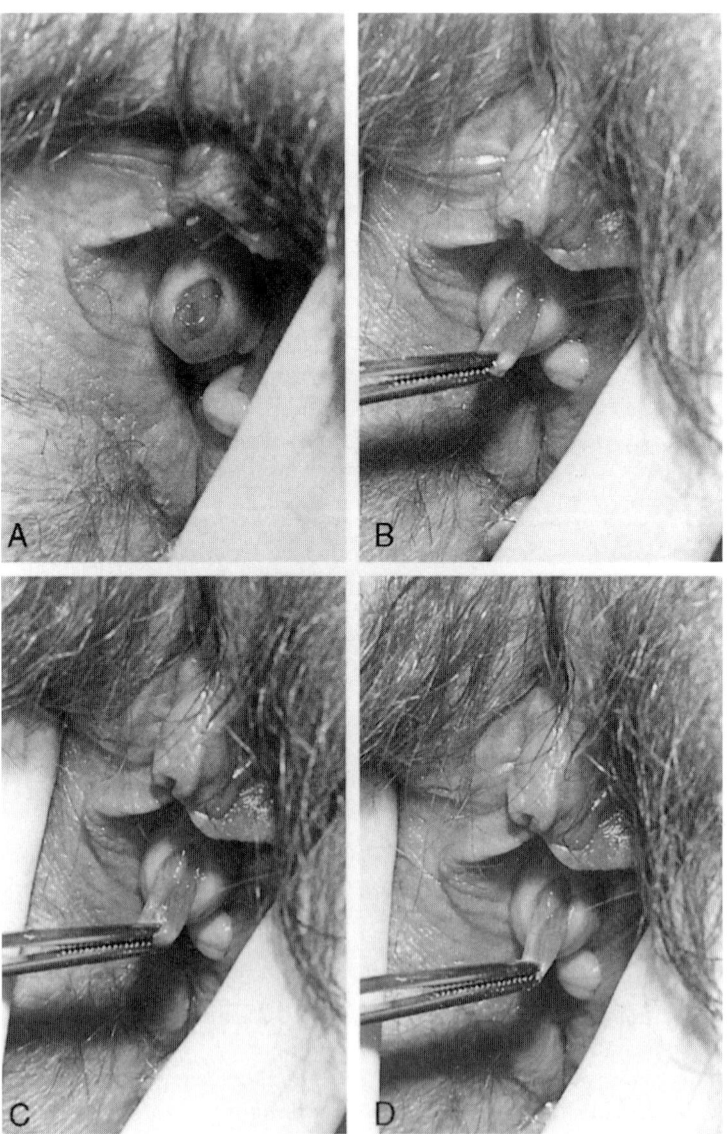


**Fig. 11.6 A–D.** Caruncle. The distal part of the urethra appears occupied by a reddish mass covering mainly the posterior lip of the meatus. (From RAZ 1996)

disease. Presenting symptoms most often include dysuria and swelling of the anterior vaginal wall.

11.3.5.1.5
MUCOSAL PROLAPSE

The appearance of prolapsed urethra may be similar to other uretheral lesions, in particular the caruncle. It may also present as a painless tumor mass. Complete circumferential prolapse of mucosa is the hallmark of this lesion (Fig. 11.8). Symptoms include bleeding, dysuria, and obstruction.

Eversion of the urethra is uncommon in middle-aged women; it is more common in young black girls and the elderly. The etiology is one of separation of the mucosal lamina from the underlying muscle, or submucosal edema. Treatment may be nonoperative including sitz baths and estrogen cream. Ligation of the mucosa with eventual sloughing, or excision and reapproximation, has yielded satisfactory outcomes.

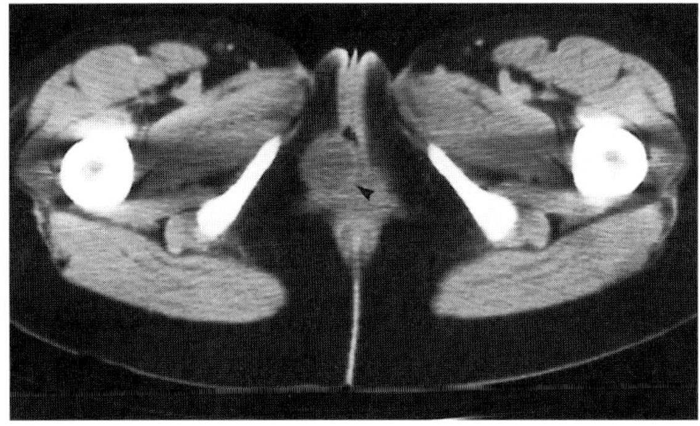

**Fig. 11.7.** A CT scan demonstrates a 2-cm cystic thick-walled mass to the right of the vaginal introitus. The appearance is typical for a Bartholin gland abscess (*arrows*). (Courtesy of E.K. Lang)

11.3.5.1.6
PROLAPSE OF A URETEROCELE

A prolapsed ureterocele presents as a smooth lesion eccentric to the meatus, it may protrude through or arise external to the meatus (Fig. 11.9). Symptoms include dysuria, bleeding, or retention. It is of note that 90% of cases are associated with a duplex system and 10% with an ipslateral single system. Radiologic investigation including ultrasound or IVP is required to demonstrate duplication. A renal scan may also prove useful to access function in a solitary system. Treatment consists of manual decompression followed by incision of the ureterocele. Definitive management of the upper tracts is dependent on the functional status of the kidney (Dmochowski 1994).

11.3.5.1.7
CONDYLOMA

The lesions of condyloma appear as irregular, firm, frond-like tumors usually in the outer third or near the meatus. A third of those with genital condyloma will have urethral lesions. The symptoms include

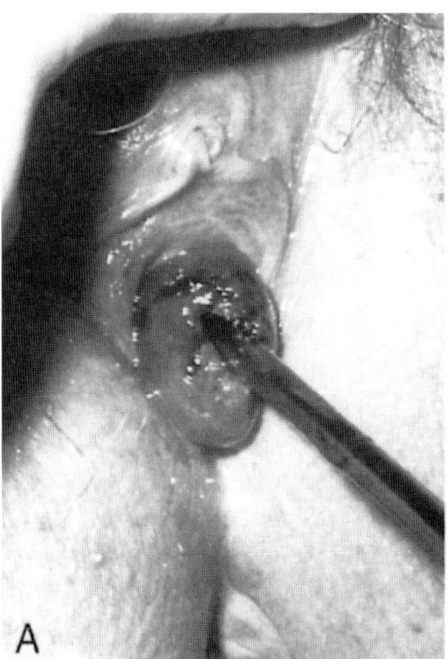



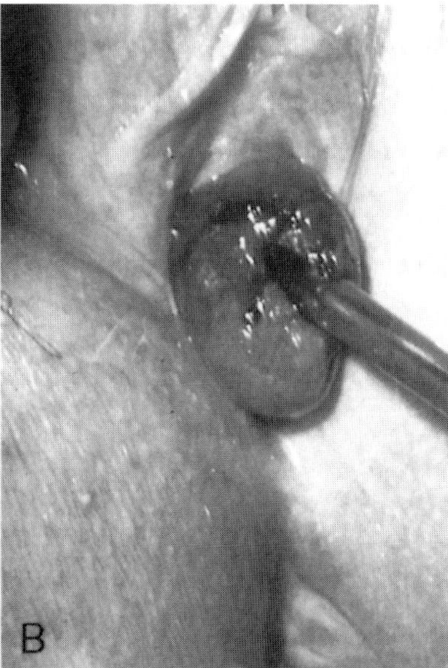



**Fig. 11.8 A, B.** Prolapse of the urethral mucosa. A mass was noticed suddenly in the vagina. The mass was pale, soft, and easily depressed by a finger. A metal sound could be passed easily into the bladder. (From Raz 1996)

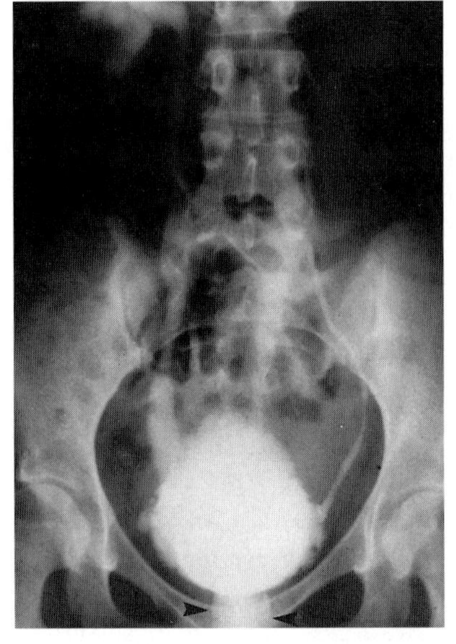

A

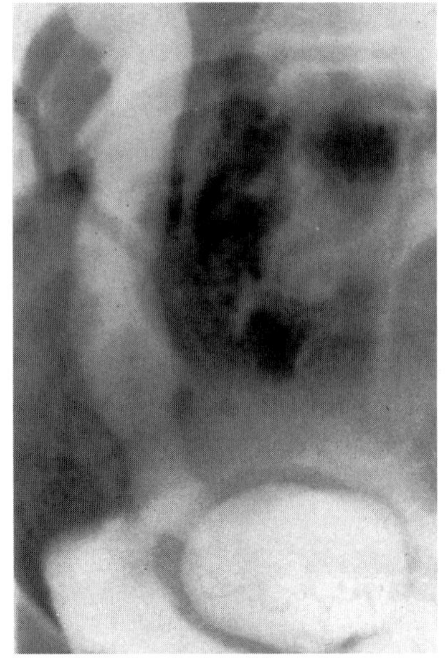

B

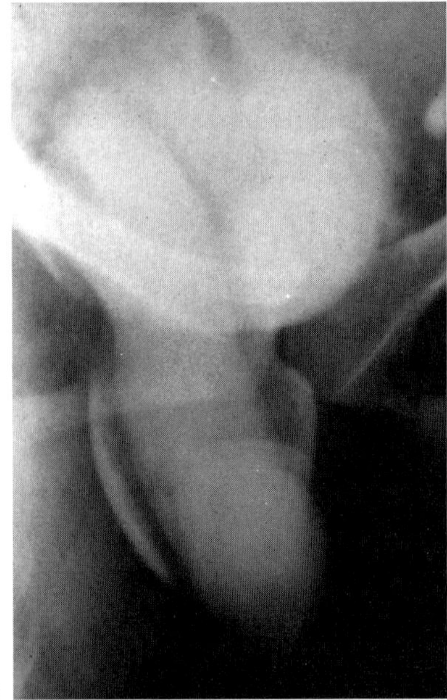

C

**Fig. 11.9.** **A** A 20-min venous urogram demonstrates mild hydronephrosis and hydroureter as well as a trabeculated bladder in this 19-year-old female. Note the presence of contrast density in the vagina (*arrowheads*). **B** A 30-min film in the same patient demonstrates the dilated distal right ureter as well as a classical ureterocele. **C** Valsalva maneuver provokes the sliding ureterocele to extend into the vagina and present at the vaginal introitus. This is the explanation for the contrast medium seen in the vagina on the IVU film and also the trabeculation of the muscularis of the bladder

dysuria, hematuria, or split stream. Urethroscopy is mandatory to delineate the proximal extent of the lesion. Therapy consists of topical and/or intravaginal 5-fluorouracil or laser ablation.

### 11.3.5.2 Urethral Lesions

#### 11.3.5.2.1 URETHRAL DIVERTICULA

A urethral diverticulum is a cystic dilatation of a portion of the periurethral ductal system. The diverticulum is most often visualized in the mid to distal urethra and measures between 0.5 and 6 cm (Fig. 11.10). Although the true incidence is not known, it appears to occur in 1%–5% of the general public (Dmochowski 1994). Rare in females under 20 years, it is most commonly seen in the third through the fifth decade. Symptoms are frequently nonspecific and a high index of suspicion is required. Presenting symptoms include from most to least common: dysuria, frequency, anterior vaginal wall mass, and stress incontinence. The etiology of urethral diverticula is incompletely understood but currently two etiologies are recognized, namely a

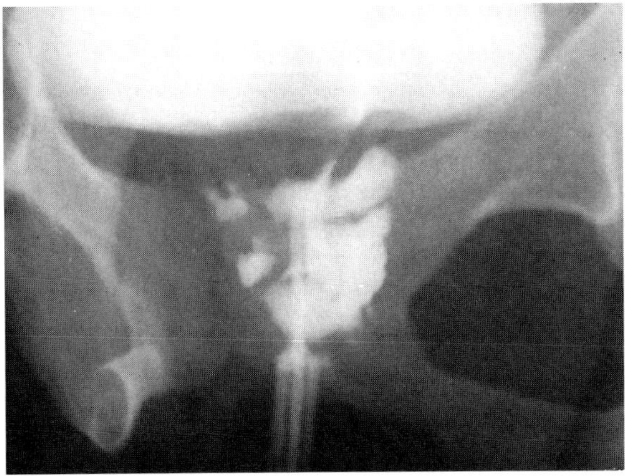

Fig. 11.10. A urethrogram performed through a double balloon Lang-Davis catheter demonstrates a multiloculated but communicating suburethral diverticulum of the female urethra. The diverticular sac is actually wrapped around the urethra. Emptying of the diverticulum of debris by massage prior to the injection ensures proper documention of the entire structure and its ramifications. (Courtesy of E.K. Lang)

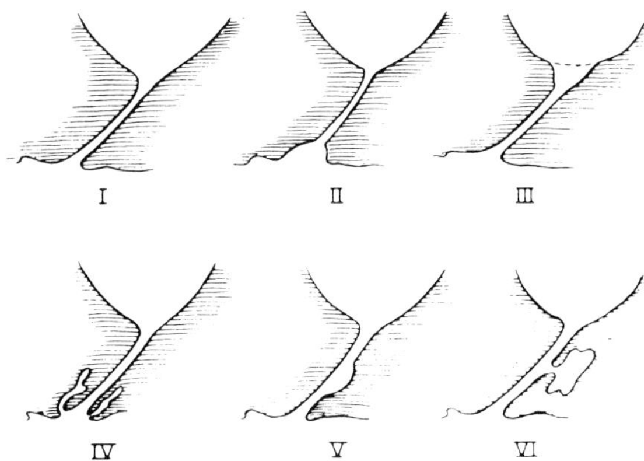


Fig. 11.11. Schematic diagram of six different appearances of the female urethra when examined by double balloon catheter. Type I = normal; type II = distal ballooning; type III = proximal ballooning; type IV = filling of periurethral glands; type V = localized outpouching; type VI = urethral diverticulum. (From GREENBERG et al. 1981)

congenital etiology as seen in newborns and an acquired etiology. In the acquired etiology the lesion arises from secondary obstruction and infection of the periurethral gland, which ruptures back into the lumen. The obstruction may be related to trauma associated with childbirth, instrumentation, or infection (DMOCHOWSKI 1994).

Currently radiologic workup includes a VCUG and positive pressure urography.

On VCUG a large percentage of urethral diverticula fill during the voiding phase and appear on the postvoid films as rounded or lobulated collections of contrast located behind the symphysis pubis (YODER 1992).

Positive pressure urography is performed using either a Davis or Trattner double balloon catheter (LANG and DAVIS 1959). The proximal balloon is filled so as to occlude the vesicle neck with the distal balloon sealing the urethral meatus. Contrast is then injected into the urethra. Six different configurations of the urethra have been reported (Fig. 11.11). Configurations I–III are considered normal, with VI being abnormal. Controversy surrounds configurations IV and V, which some authors would consider normal variants even though significant symptoms are an accompaniment. Resolution of this controversy must await further study and we suggest close correlation with the findings on history and physical examination.

Both VCUG and positive pressure urography should be used together since multiple diverticula may be obscured by the double balloon catheter. Although positive pressure urography has a 90% accuracy (KEEFE 1991), if the opening of the diverticula is occluded the aforementioned radiologic techniques may be normal. Vigorous massage of the anterior vaginal wall will empty debris and hence facilitate filling of the diverticula. Both transperineal and transrectal ultrasound have been used to improve the spatial relationship, with three-dimensional visualization of the diverticulum in relation to the urethra. Transrectal ultrasound may be superior to transperineal ultrasound because the transducer is closer to the lesion. However, ultrasound cannot differentate between diverticula and other cystic lesions (LOPEZ RASINES 1996). With MRI it is possible to delineate urethral diverticula from Gartner's duct cysts, vaginal inclusion cysts, carcinoma, and abscesses. On T2-weighted MR images, diverticula are seen as urethral enlargement with a middle zone of high signal intensity and an intact outer ring of low signal intensity. The image may be enhanced by the use of gadopentetate dimeglumine, which increases the intensity of the urethral tissue while the urine remains of low signal intensity (HRICAK 1991). MRI will not visualize the diverticular ostium nor will it differentiate between multiple diverticular sacs and a septated diverticulum. Treatment ranges from observation for asymptomatic diverticula to endoscopic or open marsupialization and diverticulectomy.

11.3.5.2.2
GARTNER'S DUCT CYSTS

Gartner's duct cysts are located from the cervix to the introitus on the anterolateral wall. The incidence in all women is 1%. Symptoms include dysuria, obstruction, incontinence, and vaginal discharge. Ureteral ectopia has also been reported, necessitating both an anatomical and a functional assessment of the upper tracts with IVP and/or renal scan. Treatment ranges from simple excision to nephroureterectomy (Dmochowski 1994).

11.3.5.2.3
URETHRAL TUBERCULOSIS

Urethral tuberculosis can present as urethritis or urethral discharge. Urethral involvement by *Mycobacterium tuberculosis* is very rare and isolation of viable mycobacteria by direct microscopy remains the gold standard for diagnosis (Induhara 1992). The etiology is most likely spread from another focus in the genitourinary tract. Upper tract radiographic evaluation is thus mandatory. Treatment is primarily medical.

### 11.3.6 Malignant Lesions

Urethral cancer is rare, accounting for only 1% of all female genitourinary malignancies. It is usually seen in postmenopausal women, with the average age of onset being 61 years. The most common symptoms are bleeding (56%), obstructive symptoms (39%), urinary frequency (25%), perineal pain, palpable mass, and vaginal discharge. Urethral cancer is locally destructive, spreading by direct invasion from as proximal as the bladder neck to as distal as the vulva, with metastasis occurring via the lymphatics. The proximal urethra drains into the pelvic nodes whereas the distal urethra drains into the inguinal nodes. On initial presentation the overall rate of inguinal node metastasis is 28%. The incidence of pelvic node metastasis is unknown. Distant metastasis occurs rarely, with lung, liver, and bone being the most common sites. Symptoms on advanced presentation include pelvic pain, weight loss, periurethral abscess, and urethrovaginal fistula. Although the etiology is not fully known, contributing factors may include trauma, intercourse, childbirth, and infection (Srinivas 1987).

Squamous cell carcinomas account for 70%–75% of urethral cancers, followed by transitional cell carcinoma, adenocarcinoma, and undifferentiated carcinoma. Melanoma is the most common primary source of metastases to the urethra. Radiologic studies initially include urethrography, but this study gives no information regarding local spread. CT scan can be used to evaluate local extension but cannot distinguish between, cervix, vagina, urethra, and intervening tissue because of its restriction to the axial plane. Any relationship of the tumor to the bladder and cervix is not appreciated. The current role for MRI in the evaluation of urethral cancer is in staging. MRI cannot differentiate between malignant and benign granulomas and inflammatory disease, thus decreasing its role as the initial diagnostic study. Once the diagnosis of carcinoma is made, MRI can be used to evaluate tumor size, location, and stage (Hricak 1991).

For staging purposes the tumor is classified according to location. Tumors in the distal third of the urethra are classified as anterior, while proximal tumors or tumors extending beyond the distal third are classified as entire. The two most common staging systems are the Grabstald, based on the pathologic criteria at the Memorial Sloan-Kettering Cancer Center, and the Prempree system (Forman 1992). Treatment is based on tumor stage and location. Early or low stage lesions of the anterior urethra or the entire urethra can be treated with local excision, transurethral resection, or interstitial radiation (iridium-192). However, for recurrent, more invasive, or entire proximal urethral lesions the treatment consists of external beam radiation with radiation implant or radical anterior exenteration. Although good local control can be achieved with radiotherapy for low stage tumors (70%–90%), control of higher stage tumors is poor (20%–30%) and the complications are significant. Presently there is no effective chemotherapy. The most important prognostic factor is location of the tumor. The overall mean 5-year survival rate is 47% for anterior lesions and 11% for posterior tumors (Srinivas 1987).

## 11.4 Continence and Voiding

### 11.4.1 Introduction

In order to fully understand the continence and voiding mechanism of the female, it is imperative to review initially the basic concepts of female pelvic anatomy, pelvic floor, and physiology. The use of both imaging and urodynamic techniques has greatly enhanced knowledge in this field. After reviewing the basic concepts, we shall examine the elements of the continence mechanism and the impact of relaxation of the pelvic floor upon emptying of the bladder. Once we have reviewed normal function, we shall concentrate on the role of urodynamics, including videourodynamics, in evaluating incontinence.

## 11.4.2 Bladder Neck Support and Continence

### 11.4.2.1 Bladder Neck

Unlike the male, the female does not possess an extensive smooth muscle sphincter at the bladder neck. It is well supplied with cholinergic fibers and relatively few noradrenergic fibers. Bladder neck support with the anterior vagina and endopelvic fascia and lateral attachments contributes to functional continence.

### 11.4.2.2 Urethra

The closure pressure and urethral length are two entities that are necessary for urinary continence. Closure pressure occurs as a result of the vasculature of the submucosal layer, fibroelastic tissues, and smooth and skeletal musculature under neurologic control. The vascular supply of the submucosa contributes to closure pressure, as does smooth muscle. The skeletal musculature that contributes constant tonus is provided by the rhabdosphincter.

### 11.4.2.3 Pubourethral Ligaments

In the midline exists a paired set of fibromuscular ligaments which anchor the anterior aspect of the urethra to the posteroinferior surface of the pubic symphysis. The pubourethral ligaments represent dense condensations of the endopelvic fascia and continue superiorly with the pubovesical ligaments. Functionally these ligaments provide support for the bladder neck and anterior aspect of the urethral wall.

### 11.4.2.4 Pelvic Floor (Levator Ani)

The levator ani is responsible for support of the urethra and bladder neck. The medial part supports the urethral wall. It provides an occlusive force on the urethral wall during increased intra-abdominal pressures. In addition, the levator ani has been shown to have a substantial quantity of type I striated muscle (Gosling et al. 1981). This provides a constant tone to the bladder neck.

### 11.4.2.5 The Perineal Body

The perineal body consists of fibromuscular elastic tissue and is found in the midline between the rectum and the vagina on a line between the ischial tuberosities. Various muscles such as the superficial and deep transverse muscles of the perineum, the bulbocavernosus muscle, the sphincter ani externus, and the levator ani insert here.

### 11.4.2.6 Urogenital Diaphragm

The urogenital diaphragm is a continuous ray of skeletal muscles oriented transversely covering the anterior surface of the urethra and distal vagina. Inferiorly the muscle wraps completely around the vagina; cranially, it is more anterior, and at the proximal third of the urethra it does not encircle the vagina but completely encircles the urethra.

### 11.4.2.7 Cardinal and Uterosacral Ligaments

The cardinal and uterosacral ligaments provide passive support of the cervix and superior vagina. They are a collection of vascular and connective tissues that originate from the anterior sacral wall and condense to form palpable paired ligaments covered by peritoneum on their superior surfaces. They insert posterolaterally on the cervix, providing posterior anchorage and elevation of the cervix and superior vagina.

## 11.4.3 Continence Mechanism

### *11.4.3.1 Bladder Neck and Urethra*

For an effective continence mechanism to work appropriately, one requires an intact urethra that is supported with appropriate anatomic support. Coaptation and compression of mucosal surfaces allows for adequate resistance to overcome incontinence. Neural stimuli also provide for resting tone. Anatomic support permits transmission of increases in intra-abdominal pressure to the bladder neck and urethra to provide adequate urinary storage. Harmoniously all these factors provide for continence during rest and stress.

The support of the lower urinary tract is a dynamic and not a static process. The bladder neck is under voluntary control. When urination begins, the bladder neck funnels and then descends. This descent of the bladder neck is attributed to contraction and relaxation of the levator ani muscles (Parks et al. 1962).

The support of the bladder neck and urethra also depends on the endopelvic fascia and anterior vagina. Three structures that are responsible for bladder neck and urethral supprt are: the arcus tendineus fasciae pelvis (white line), the levator ani, and the endopelvic fascia and anterior vaginal wall.

The pubovesical muscles are bilateral bands of detrusor muscle which connect the bladder neck to the two arcus tendinei anteriorly. These are probably responsible for assisting the bladder neck from opening (Power 1954).

### *11.4.3.2 Sphincter Mechanism*

Other factors besides pelvic support are necessary for urinary continence. The internal and external sphincter mechanisms also contribute to urinary continence. The proximal urethra, or intrinsic mechanism, must function appropriately to attain continence; appropriate bladder neck innervation is necessary for this to occur. Two bodies of smooth muscle, the detrusor loop and the trigonal ring, surround this region. The external sphincter mechanism includes the striated urogenital sphincter and circular smooth muscle. During rest, these mechanisms add to resting intraurethral pressure, and during increasing intra-abdominal pressure incontinence is prevented in cases of poor bladder neck innervation. Hypotheses concerning the function of the elements of the urinary continence mechanism have been proposed (Table 11.1).

## 11.4.4 Urodynamic Evaluation

Urodynamic studies were first described more than 100 years ago (Mosso and Pellacani 1881); since that time significant changes to technique have resulted in major contributions to the understanding

**Table 11.1.** Hypotheses concerning function of the elements of the urinary continence mechanism (from DeLancey 1991)

| Structure | Hypothetical function |
|---|---|
| Proximal urethral support | |
| Connection to levator ani | Tonic contraction maintains high position of vesical neck and contracts during cough to support vesical neck. Relaxes to change position of vesical neck to facilitate micturition. |
| Connection to arcus tendineus | Assists levators in support and limits the downward excursion of the vesical neck when the levators are relaxed, or overcome during cough. |
| Pubovesical muscles | May facilitate vesical neck opening by pulling on vesical neck when levators relax. |
| Perineal membrane | Fixes distal urethra to pubic bones. |
| Internal sphincter mechanism | |
| Trigonal ring, detrusor loop, and elastic tissue | Maintains vesical neck closure at rest and is necessary in addition to normal support for continence during cough. |
| Extrinsic sphincter mechanism | |
| Striated urogenital sphincter and circular smooth muscle | Resting tone contributes to resting urethral pressure, and contraction prevents incontinence when marginally compensated proximal mechanism leaks. |
| Longitudinal smooth muscle | Contracts during micturition to shorten the urethra. |
| Submucosal vasculature | Fills the space within the muscular tube to maintain a watertight seal. |

of the pathophysiology of the lower urinary tract. These studies, which confirm lower urinary tract dysfunction, allow one to ensure that there is a low-pressure urinary storage system and adequate bladder emptying.

#### 11.4.4.1
#### Forms of Incontinence

Incontinence, defined as the involuntary loss of urine, poses both a social and a hygienic problem. Urodynamics attempts to define the dysfunction of the lower urinary tract in order that the problem may be adequately treated. *Stress incontinence* is defined as involuntary loss of urine occurring with increases in intra-abdominal pressure. This exists when the loss of urine occurs when intravesical pressure exceeds maximum urethral pressure. *Urge incontinence* occurs in association with a strong desire to void. It is usually associated with an involuntary detrusor contraction. *Overflow incontinence* is the result of passive elevation of bladder pressure above maximum urethral pressure due to urinary retention.

#### 11.4.4.2
#### Initial Assessment

A carefully conducted history and examination will determine the investigative techniques needed to assess the problem, which will lead to appropriate diagnosis, treatment and management. A complete history is necessary which includes a detailed gynecologic and obstetric history, previous surgery, bowel and sexual function, medications, other medical or neurologic disorders, and pad usage. A voiding diary documents fluid intake, voided volumes, symptoms of urgency, and frequency and severity of urinary incontinence in a 24-hour period. Pad weight testing can also substantiate loss of urine.

Prior to a physical examination, a urinalysis is obtained to eliminate urinary tract infection as the source of the problem. Coughing or straining with a full bladder in the supine and standing position is imperative to demonstrate leakage. A Marshall test is performed to manually elevate the bladder neck without obstruction to demonstrate that incontinence stops. The Q-tip test is used to evaluate the urethral axis and for evidence of urethral hypermobility. Simultaneously, the anterior vaginal wall is examined for the presence and degree of cystocele. Coexisiting pathology is also evaluated, including vaginal atrophy, uterine prolapse, enterocele, and rectocele. Any suggestion of neurologic disorder leads to neurologic testing including deep tendon reflexes, bulbocavernosus reflex, anal sphincter tone, perineal sensation, lower extremity sensory, and motor tone.

Voiding cystourethrography (VCUG) has been used to evaluate the bladder neck position, the bladder base (cystocele), and the level of continence, and to confirm visually that stress incontinence exists. In addition, vesicoureteral reflux, evidence of bladder and urethral diverticula, or prolapsed ureteroceles can be documented. The bladder neck is evaluated for mobility, competence, and position. With VCUGs, detrusor pressures are unknown and uninhibited bladder contractions can occur, resulting in a false-positive diagnosis of stress incontinence. Pelsang and Bonney (1995) concluded that the VCUG is limited in the evaluation of stress incontinence due to detrusor instability. Kelvin and others have advocated the use of dynamic cystoproctography to evaluate disorders of the pelvic floor in women (Kelvin et al. 1994; Brubaker et al. 1993; Brubaker and Heit 1993). In short, dynamic fluoroscopy of the pelvic floor includes opacification of the small bowel, rectum, vagina, and bladder to detect sites of weakness, which are imaged at rest, during straining, and during and after evacuation. Though not specifically utilized for incontinence, this technique is useful in women who have disorders of the pelvic floor (Fig. 11.12).

#### 11.4.4.3
#### Cystoscopy

Modern technology has allowed continued refinement of urologic endoscopic equipment. Modern cystoscopes have metal sheaths in range from 8F to 26F and telescopes allowing views from 0° to 170°. The 0° or 30° lenses are best for visualizing the urethra, whereas the bladder walls are best inspected with the 70° lens. Today, fiberoptics have improved so greatly that flexible cystoscopes have emerged to sizes of 14F. In addition, with video equipment, a camera is attached to the telescope to visualize and inspect the bladder and urethra on a television screen. Typically bladder inflammation and malignancy can give rise to urge incontinence. The bladder is evaluated for trabeculation, presence of tumor or carcinoma in situ, calculi, urethral coaptation, and to confirm results of the physical

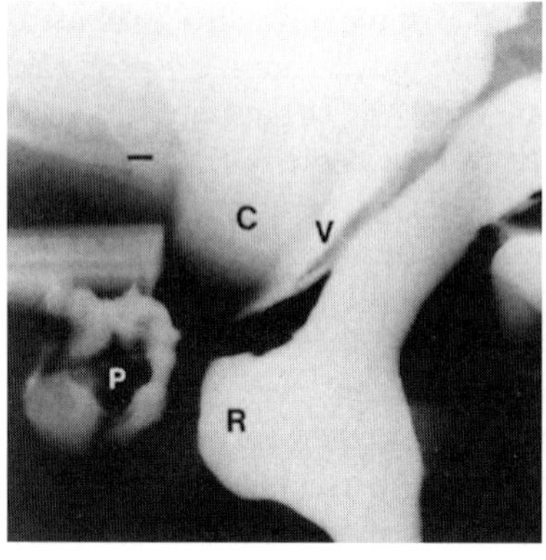

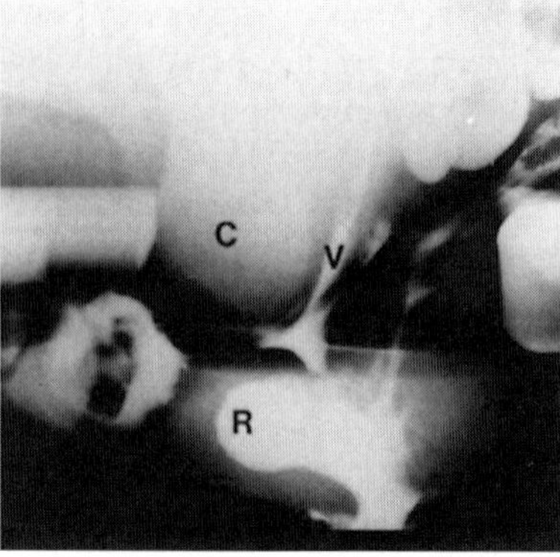

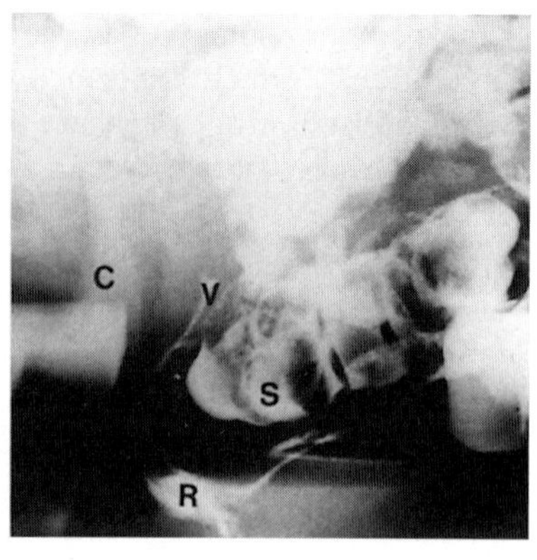


A B,C

**Fig. 11.12 A–C.** Radiographs demonstrating cystocele, rectocele, and sigmoidocele. **A** Lateral radiograph taken during rectal evacuation shows cystocele (*C*) extending well below the inferior margin of the pubic symphysis (*horizontal line*). A low rectocele (*R*) is evident. Note gauze plug (*P*) used to limit barium loss from vagina (*V*). **B** Lateral radiograph taken after rectal evacuation shows that the cystocele (*C*) has enlarged because of repeated straining, and barium is retained within rectocele (*R*). The rectovaginal space has widened but does not yet contain herniated bowel. V, Vagina. **C** After partial bladder emptying, a second postevacuation lateral radiograph shows a sigmoidocele (*S*) within a markedly widened rectovaginal space. The sigmoidocele was not detected on physical examination. *C*, Residual contrast material in cystocele; *R*, retained contrast material in rectocele; *V*, vagina. (From Kelvin FM et al. 1994)

examination. Bladder neck hypermobility and funneling are observed. With a 0° lens at the level of the mid urethra, the patient is asked to strain. During straining, the bladder neck is noted to funnel open and descend posteriorly in anatomic incontinence (hypermobility). A fixed open proximal urethra suggests intrinsic sphincter deficiency (ISD).

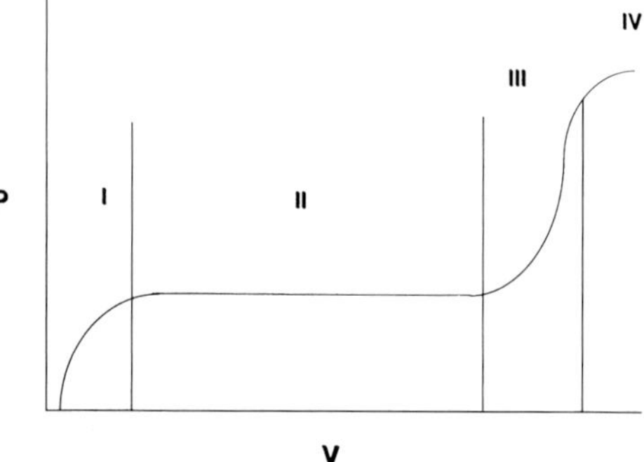


**Fig. 11.13.** Cystometrogram demonstrating the phases of filling and associated pressure (*P*)–volume (*V*) interaction. Four phases of filling are labeled. (From Dmochowski 1996)

#### *11.4.4.4 Cystometry and Videourodynamics*

Urodynamics, namely cystometry, remains the most accurate tool we possess in order to evaluate the passive filling component of bladder function. Multichannel pressure recordings allow simultaneous measurement of multiple variables. The goal of cystometry is to reproduce the patient's clinical status for improving diagnosis and therapy.

Cystometry evaluates the normal events related to bladder storage and emptying. During the initial phase (storage/filling phase: I, II, and III), one measures changes in bladder pressure with increases in volume. The second phase (voluntary contraction or voiding stage: IV) is characterized by increases in bladder pressure associated with a simultaneous decrease in outlet resistance and subsequent emptying of the bladder (Fig. 11.13). It is important to determine whether the incontinence is due to sphincter incompetence (anatomic incontinence or ISD), detrusor instability, or less commonly, overflow incontinence. Stress urinary incontinence (SUI) has been classified into three types. Types I and II are characterized by stress-induced urethral hypermobility resulting from deficient pelvic floor support. Type III SUI is defined as an open vesical neck and proximal urethra at rest with minimal or no stress-induced urethral descent; it is this latter type which is also referred to as ISD. ISD may coexist with urethral hypermobility and/or detrusor instability or poor bladder compliance.

Currently, urodynamic evaluation with abdominal or Valsalva leak point pressure (VLPP) determination is the only objective means for

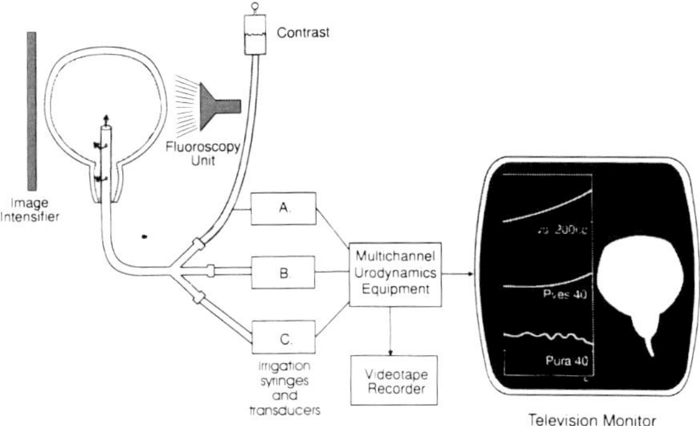


**Fig. 11.14.** Videourodynamic equipment used in a urodynamics laboratory. (From McGuire et al. 1996)

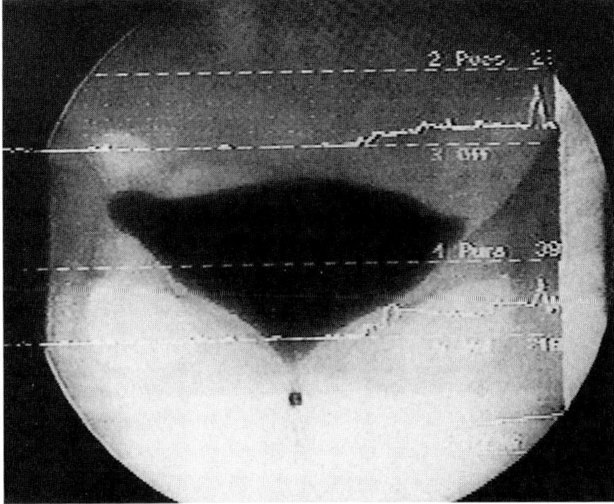

**Fig. 11.15.** An elderly lady with severe stress incontinence. Initial filling of the bladder revealed an open bladder neck. She easily leaked urine at a very low abdominal pressure of 29 cm $H_2O$, which is indicative of minimal urethral sphincter function. (From McGuire et al. 1996)

differentiating between urethral hypermobility and ISD. VLPP is defined as the lowest total intravesical pressure at which urinary leakage occurs during progressive increases in intra-abdominal pressure induced by the Valsalva maneuver, as measured urodynamically.

The most accurate means of diagnosing sphincteric incompetence or detrusor instability is by simultaneous recording of intravesical, intra-abdominal, and subtracted detrusor pressures with fluoroscopic monitoring of a contrast-filled bladder during stress maneuvers (videourodynamics) (Fig. 11.14). In many cases, an expensive videourodynamics examination can be performed by a less expensive and less invasive urodynamic study to make an appropriate diagnosis. Fluoroscopic visualization reduces artifactual errors. Since these studies are on videotape, frame by frame reexamination of the bladder can be correlated with the urodynamic findings.

Videourodynamics has allowed for better correlation with structure and function. The combination of radiographic imaging and urodynamic studies is absolutely necessary in many complex situations (Fig. 11.15).

## References

Abrahamson J (1965) Double bladder and related anomalies: Clinical and embryological aspects in a case report. Br J Urol 33:195

Allen NH, Atwell JD (1980) The paraureteric diverticulum in children. Br J Urol 52:264

Appel RA (1988) Bilateral ureteral obstruction secondary to endometriosis. Urology 32:151

Barrett DM, Malek RS, Kelalis PP (1976) Observations of vesical diverticulum in children. J Urol 116:234

Berman SM (1988) Urachal remnants in adults. Urology 31:17

Bo K (1995) Functional aspects of the striated muscles within and around the female urethra. Scand J Urol Nephrol 175:27–35

Brubaker L, Heit MH (1993) Radiology of the pelvic floor. Clin Obstet Gynecol 36:952–959

Brubaker L, Retzky S, Smith C, Saclarides T (1993) Pelvic floor evaluation with dynamic fluoroscopy. Obstet Gynecol 82:863–868

Cherry JW (1950) Patent urachus; review and report of case. J Urol 63:693

Cracchiolo A, Hall CB (1970) Bilateral iliac osteotomy. Clin Orthop 68:156

DeLancey JOL (1991) Structure and function of the continence mechanism relative to stress incontinence. In: Leach GE (ed) Problems in urology. Female urology. Lippincott Raven, Philadelphia

Dmochowski RR (1994) Benign female periurethral masses. J Urol 152:1943–1951

Dmochowski R (1996) Cystometry. In: Boone TB (ed) The Urologic Clinics of North America. Urodynamics I. Saunders, Philadelphia

Forman JD (1992) The role of radiation therapy in the management of carcinoma of the male and female urethra. Urol Clin North Am 19: no. 2

Gearhart JP, Jeffs RD (1988) Augmentation cystoplasty in the failed exstrophy reconstruction. J Urol 139:790

Gosling JA, Dixon JS, Critchley HDD, Thomson SA (1981) A comparative study of the human external sphincter and periurethral levator ani muscles. Br J Urol 53:35–41

Greenberg M, et al. (1981) Female urethral diverticula: double-balloon catheter study. AJR 136:260

Gyllensten L (1949) Contributions to embryology of the urinary bladder. Acta Anat 7:305

Hyuk Lee N (1992) Skene's duct cysts in female newborns. J Pediatr Surg 27:15–17

Indudhara R (1992) Ureteral tuberculosis. Urol Int 48:436–438

Jaramillo D, Lebowitz RL, Hendren WH (1990) Cloacal malformation: radiologic findings and imaging recommendations. Radiology 177:441

Johnston JH (1960) Vesical diverticula without urinary obstruction in childhood. J Urol 84:535

Kapoor R, Saha MM (1987) Complete duplication of the bladder, common urethra, and external genitalia in the neonate: a case report. J Urol 137:1243

Keefe B (1991) Diverticula of the female urethra: diagnosis by endovaginal and transperineal sonography. AJR 156:1195–1197

Kelvin FM, Maglinte DD, Benson JT, Brubaker LP, Smith C (1994) Dynamic cysto-proctography: a technique for assessing disorders of the pelvic floor in women. AJR 163:368–370

Kossow JH, Morales PA (1973) Duplication of bladder and urethra and associated anomalies. Urology 1:71

Kumar R, Haque AK, Cohen MS (1984) Endometriosis of the urinary bladder. J Clin Ultrasound 12:363

Lang EK, Davis JJ (1959) Positive pressure urethrography: a roentgenographic diagnostic method for urethral diverticula in the female. Radiology 72:401–405

Lopez Rasines G (1996) Female urethral diverticula: value of transrectal sonography. J Clin Ultrasound 24:90–92

Mandel J, Blyth BR, Peters CA (1991) Structural genitourinary defects detected in utero. Radiology 178:193

Marshall VF, Mucke EC (1962) Variations in exstrophy of the bladder. J Urol 88:766

Matsuno T, Tokunaka S, Koyanagi T (1984) Muscular development in the urinary tract. J Urol 132:148

McGuire EJ, et al. (1996) Videourodynamic studies. In: Boone TB (ed) The Urologic Clinics of North America. Urodynamics I. Saunders, Philadelphia

Moore KL (1982) The developing human. Saunders, Philadelphia

Mosso A, Pellacani S (1881) Sulle funzioni della vescica. Arch Ital Biol 12:3

Murphy WD, Rorner AJ, Nazinitsky KJ (1990) Condylomata acuminata of the bladder: a rare cause of intraluminal-filling defects. Urol Radiol 12:34

Neto WA, Lopes RN, Cury M, Montelatto NID, Arap S (1984) Vesical endometriosis. Urology 24:271

Parks AG, Porter NH, Melzak J (1962) Experimental study of the reflex mechanism controlling muscles of the pelvic floor. Dis Colon Rectum 5:407–414

Pelsang RE, Bonney WW (1996) Voiding cystourethrography in female stress incontinence. AJR 166:561–565

Power RMH (1954) An anatomical contribution to the problem of continence and incontinence in the female. Am J Obstet Gynecol 67:302–314

Pratt (1967) Lesions of the female urethra. Clin Obstet Gynecol 10:227–237

Raz S (1996) Female urology. Saunders, Philadelphia

Sadler TW (1990) Langman's medical embryology. Williams and Wilkins, Baltimore

Senger FL, Santare VJ (1952) Congenital multilocular bladder. J Urol 68:283

Sharma SK (1988) Benign periurethral mass lesions: The female prostate. Aus N Z J Surg 58:77–79

Srinivas V (1987) Female urethral cancer – an overview. Int Urol Nephrol 19:423–427

Witzleben DI, Chir M, Karlafitis CM (1965) Complete frontal septum of the bladder. J Urol 94:427

# 12 Hysterosalpingography in the Assessment of Congenital, Inflammatory, and Postsurgical Changes of the Uterus and Fallopian Tubes

D.B. Spring

CONTENTS



## 12.1 Introduction

About 15% of couples cannot conceive offspring. In the absence of proven inability to conceive (sterility) or the absence of demonstrated infertility of the male partner, women are considered infertile if they cannot conceive within 1 year despite unprotected coitus. Women who have never conceived are said to have primary infertility; those who have conceived in the past but appear no longer to be able to do so are considered to have secondary infertility. Women who conceive but who have repetitive spontaneous abortions are not considered infertile but rather to be habitual aborters, defined in various studies as women having two or three consecutive spontaneous abortions without a live birth.

At some point during their reproductive years approximately 1 in 4 women have an episode of infertility (Jones and Toner 1993). The National Center for Health Statistics estimated in 1988 that 8.4% of women 15–44 years of age (estimated then at 4.9 million women) had an impaired ability to have children. The problem of infertility appears to be increasing because of rising numbers of women in the 35–44 age group and an increase in couples seeking treatment of infertility.

There is great potential for medical self-deception in the investigation and treatment of infertility. Collins et al. (1983) studied pregnancies in 1145 infertile couples. They documented pregnancies in 41% (246/597) of treated couples but also in 35% (191/548) of untreated couples. Documented reasons for infertility among the "untreated" group included ovulation deficiency, endometriosis, tubal defects, seminal deficiencies, and cervical factors. Because there is a significant spontaneous pregnancy rate during the course of the workup for infertility, testing and therapy may be paced in the younger age group to take this into account. In women closer to the end of their reproductive years the speed of evaluation is increased.

The radiologist most often uses hysterosalpingography (HSG), ultrasound (US), and magnetic resonance imaging (MRI) in assessing the female genital tract for causes of infertility. Fallopian tube recanalization (FTR) may have a role in the treatment of a selected group of women with seemingly occluded fallopian tubes. In times of questioned value of health care services, infertility investigations and treatments must justify themselves.

Preliminary screening helps to identify both male and female factors which may account for infertility. Male factors account for between 28% and 46% of infertility in couples (Dor et al. 1977). Dor and colleagues, in a survey of 665 infertile couples, found that ovarian, tubal, and uterine abnormalities made up 60%, 29%, and 5% of female factors respectively. Ovulatory disorders had the highest rates of treatment success while tubal and cervical factors were the most difficult to treat successfully.

## 12.2 Routine Clinical Workup for Women

A stepwise preliminary workup reveals the cause or causes of infertility in 70%–85% of couples (Jones and Toner 1993). For the male partner this includes a semen analysis. For the female partner it includes a pelvic examination, tests for ovulation and luteiniza-

D.B. Spring, MD, Director GU Radiology, Kaiser Permanente Medical Center, 280 West McArthur Blvd., Oakland, CA 94611, USA

tion, and evaluation of tubal patency. Because HSG is a relatively simple and inexpensive procedure that provides rapid assessment of the internal structure of the uterus and fallopian tubes, infertility investigators use it early in the evaluation of infertile women. Depending upon the results of these preliminary investigations, diagnostic and/or therapeutic laparoscopy often follows next in the sequence of preliminary testing.

An abnormal pelvic examination may prompt correlation with sonography although US assessment of the pelvis is not part of the routine preliminary investigation of female infertility. Identification and assessment of pelvic masses (uterine, ovarian, adnexal) directs further investigation and therapy in these cases.

Magnetic resonance imaging provides superb morphologic information about uterine and pelvic abnormalities in many instances. MRI aids in planning uterine surgery for fibroids and in directing the diagnosis and treatment of müllerian duct anomalies.

## 12.3 Role of HSG

As mentioned above, because of its usefulness and relative simplicity, HSG remains an early investigation of infertility. It quickly provides morphologic information about the uterus and tubes as well as occasional suggestions of peritubal and cervical abnormalities. More recently hysteroscopy and falloposcopy have been added to the internal evaluation of the uterus and fallopian tubes, albeit later in the evaluation and at significantly increased cost.

Controversy persists as to an added therapeutic effect based upon the use of oil-soluble (OSCM) versus water-based (WSCM) contrast media (Rasmussen et al. 1991). Certainly both conventional water-soluble (ionic and nonionic) and oil-based agents provide useful information about the uterus, tubes, and adnexae. Opinion varies as to the diagnostic quality associated with OSCM and WSCM (Lindequist et al. 1991). Eisenberg et al. (1989) have suggested that OSCM incite a significant inflammatory reaction and question the advisability of using these agents.

The under- and overinterpretation of HSG may substantially mislead the infertility workup, making careful interpretation of HSG findings critical to the investigation. Interpretation of some of the findings associated with HSG will be discussed.

## 12.4 Uterine Factors

Intrauterine scarring or synechiae (Asherman syndrome) may follow endometritis or trauma (Fig. 12.1), almost always related to pregnancy (Toaff and Ballas 1978). The degree of scarring closely approximates the degree of hypomenorrhea. Toaff and Ballas graded intrauterine scarring on a scale of 1–4 loosely based upon the degree of cavity obliteration (<10%, <20%, <33%, >33%). Frank amenorrhea may be associated with small scars at the lower uterine segment ("cervical stenosis"). (Pregnancy, of course, must be ruled out before performing HSG when there is a recent clinical history of amenorrhea.) Other intrauterine filling defects including neoplasia, polyps, normal cornual striations, air bubbles should also be considered in the differential diagnosis.

Hypoplasia or dysplasia of the developing uterus may be associated with inutero diethylstilbestrol (DES) exposure. The now well-known "T-shaped" uterine cavity is characteristic but other HSG findings including synechiae and minor abnormalities may also be seen (Kaufman et al. 1986). There is no known increased association between inutero DES exposure and urinary tract anomalies.

Elongation or other apparent stretching of the normal uterine cavity is most often caused by submucosal fibroids. Fibroids are common but most often do not cause uterine deformities. While HSG often provides excellent indirect evidence of the presence of uterine fibroids, both US and MRI are increasingly providing more accurate assessment of leiomyomata.

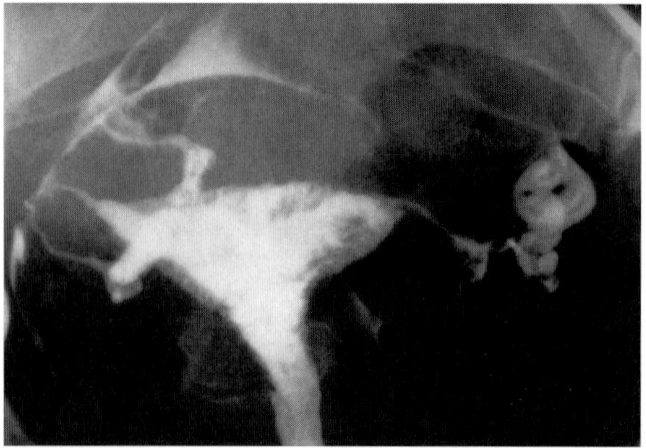

Fig. 12.1. The uterine cavity appears diffusely abnormal with no portion spared. Endometrial carcinoma, chronic endometritis, and extensive synechiae may all appear this way

Extra-endometrial filling defects may be associated with adenomyosis, postsurgical or traumatic conditions, anomalies, and intravasation. Adenomyosis is the pathologic presence of endometrium extending far into the myometrium; clinically, adenomyosis is most often associated with diffuse uterine enlargement.

Uterine anomalies are uncommon but, when present, may be associated with decreased fertility rates. HSG findings that suggest the presence of uterine anomalies include single or asymmetric uterine horns. Failure to identify both cornua should immediately suggest uterine anomalies. BUTTRAM and GIBBONS (1979) base their classification of uterine anomalies upon the degree of failure of normal development (Table 12.1).

Because of the close proximity of the developing urinary and genital tracts, anomalies often coexist in both systems. About a third of women with uterine malformations have a demonstrable urinary tract anomaly (SCHMIDT and CHAPLER 1993). Likewise, among women with major urinary tract anomalies müllerian duct anomalies are common. Up to 90% of women with unilateral renal agenesis have associated uterine anomalies.

**Table 12.1.** Buttram-Gibbons classification of müllerian anomalies (after BUTTRAM and GIBBONS 1979)

| Classification | No. of patients in series |
|---|---|
| I. Segmental müllerian agenesis/hypoplasia | 9 |
| A. Vaginal | (1) |
| B. Cervical | |
| C. Fundal | |
| D. Tubal | |
| E. Combined anomalies | (8) |
| II. Unicornuate | 19 |
| A. With rudimentary horn | |
| 1. With endometrial cavity | |
| a) Communicating | (6) |
| b) Noncommunicating | (1) |
| 2. Without endometrial cavity | (6) |
| B. Without rudimentary horn | (6) |
| III. Didelphys | 4 |
| IV. Bicornuate | 1 |
| A. Complete (division to internal os) | |
| B. Partial | (1) |
| C. Arcuate | |
| V. Septate | 67 |
| A. Complete (septum to internal os) | (14) |
| B. Incomplete | (53) |
| VI. DES-related[a] | 44 |

[a] Note: data obtained by review of records of 100 patients with diagnosed müllerian anomalies and 44 patients with a history of in utero DES exposure and abnormal HSG.

REUTER and colleagues (1989) compared HSG, US, and MRI in the differentiation of uterine anomalies. While HSG and US are often useful preliminary examinations, many believe MRI is the most accurate way to assess these anomalies.

## 12.5 Tubal Factors

The fallopian tube may appear to be diminished or increased in caliber. The site of tubal obstruction may be proximal (interstitial or isthmic portions) or distal (ampullary or fimbriated portions). One cannot assess the distal tube with HSG in those women with proximal obstruction. Tubes vary widely in apparent length and location. Care must be taken to carefully visualize freely spilling contrast media before diagnosing normal tubes, even when the rugal pattern of the distal tubes appears normal (Fig. 12.2).

SIEGLER (1974), in a review of *1000* HSGs, noted apparent tubal obstruction in 38% of studies. He observed cornual obstruction in fully 20% of studies, it being bilateral in only 5% of examinations. Siegler further observed isthmic obstruction in 5.6% and ampullary obstruction in 12.6% of HSGs.

Unilateral nonfilling of a fallopian tube in the presence of a normal contralateral tube is an acceptable, albeit unsatisfying, end point for a study. The pregnancy rate in this circumstance is similar to that found in patients with bilateral normal tubes (58%) (COLLINS et al. 1983).

There are many reasons for partial or incomplete filling of one or both fallopian tubes. While tubal disease often gives this appearance, inspissated mucoid material may cause obstruction (SULAK et al. 1987). Mucoid material in the fallopian tubes has been observed not infrequently by gynecologic surgeons at the time of pelvic surgery for unrelated reasons (e.g., hysterectomy/salpingo-oophorectomy). Cornual "spasm" has been postulated as a cause of nonvisualization of the fallopian tubes. Simple repositioning such as turning prone often results in filling of the tubes (Fig. 12.3). If the tube is not seen with prone positioning, several drugs of the prostaglandin antagonist family have been advocated to overcome cornual "spasm" (WINFIELD et al. 1982).

Salpingitis isthmica nodosa (SIN) has a characteristic appearance on HSG. Numerous small diverticula in the isthmic portion of the fallopian tube, most often bilaterally, may be seen (CREASY et al. 1985). Laparoscopy often shows a focal bulge at the medial tube (Figs. 12.4, 12.5). There is a strong asso-

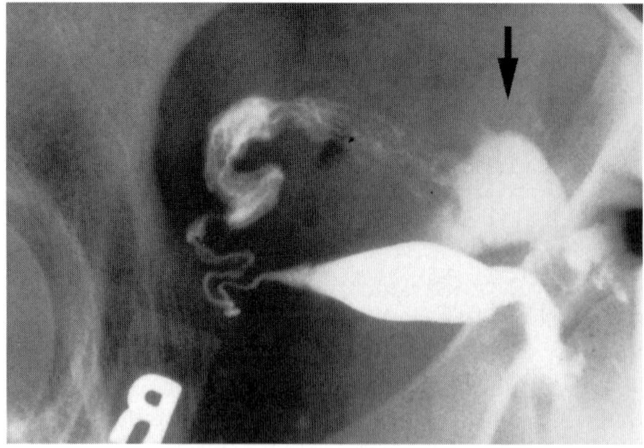

a

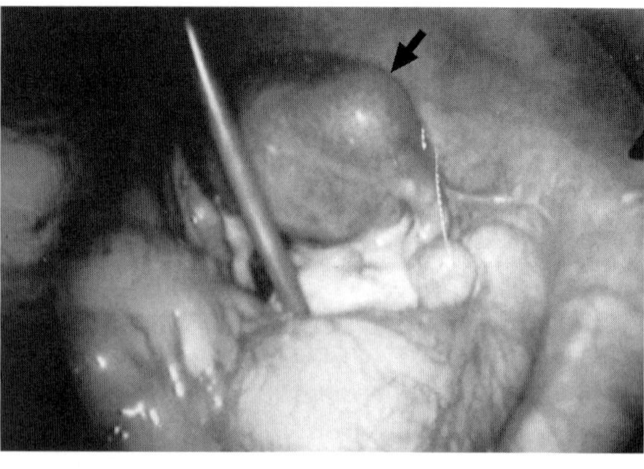

b

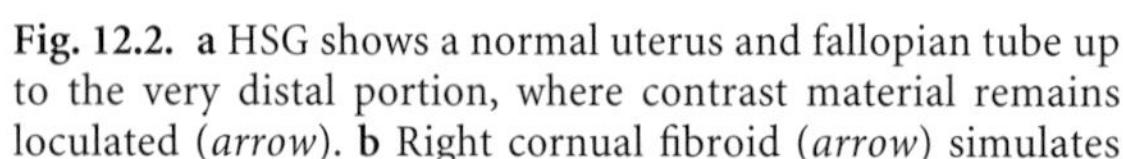

**Fig. 12.2.** **a** HSG shows a normal uterus and fallopian tube up to the very distal portion, where contrast material remains loculated (*arrow*). **b** Right cornual fibroid (*arrow*) simulates the appearance of salpingitis isthmica nodosa. The distal fallopian tubes are dilated (hydrosalpinges)

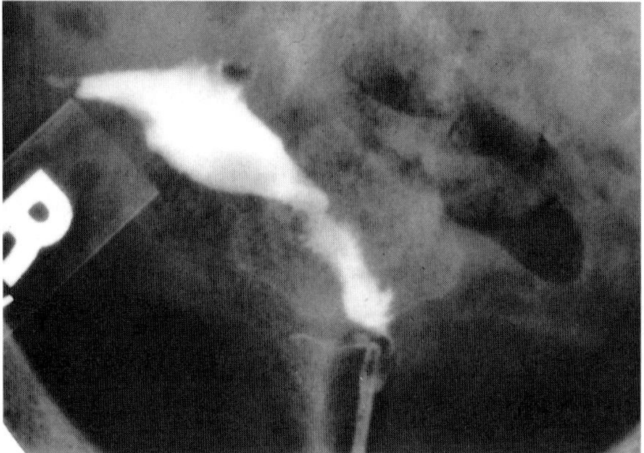

a

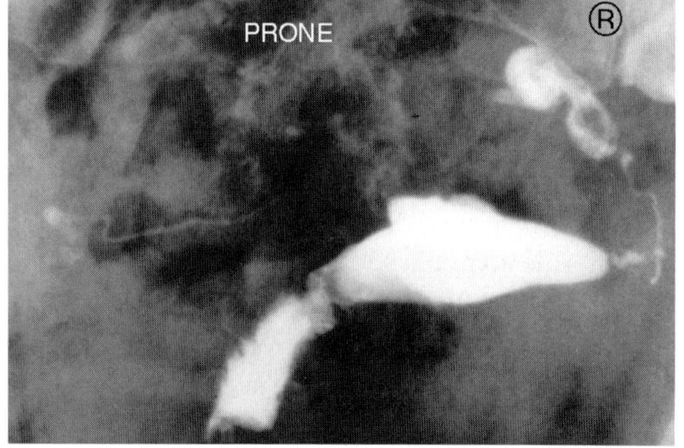


b

**Fig. 12.3.** **a** Routine frontal view of the pelvis (shown) and bilateral oblique view failed to show filling of the fallopian tubes. **b** Prone positioning shows that both tubes fill normally

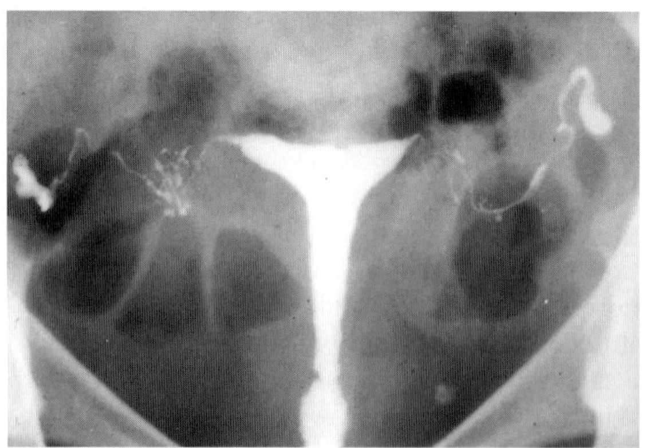

a

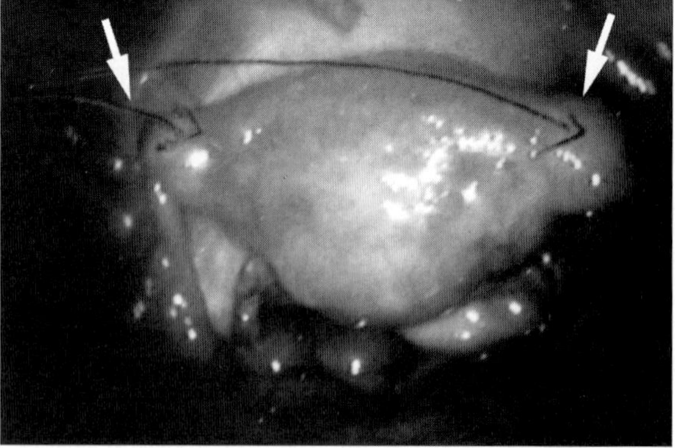

b

**Fig. 12.4.** **a** Numerous bilateral isthmic diverticula have a pathognomic appearance for salpingitis isthmica nodosa. **b** Laparoscopy shows focal isthmic bulges typical of salpingitis isthmica nodosa (*arrows*)

ciation between proximal SIN and distal tubal dilatation/obstruction. The rate of primary infertility in the presence of SIN is high (37%), as is the rate of ectopic pregnancy (9%). Tuberculosis and venous intravasation may appear similar to SIN. The diagnosis of tubal tuberculosis is often conjectural and difficult, however. In a recent review of more than 50 reported studies of SIN, its incidence among healthy,

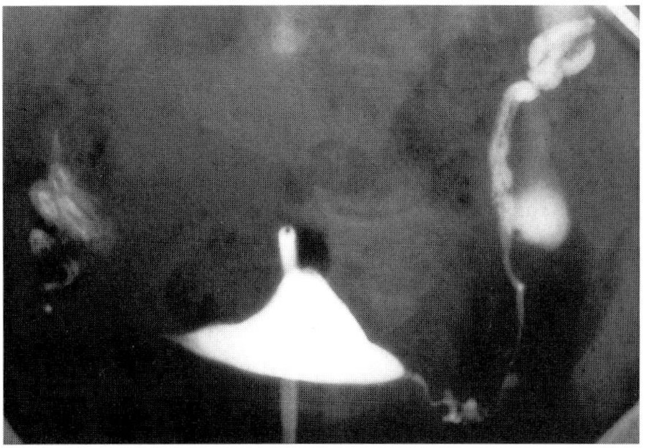

**Fig. 12.5.** The right tube is normal. The left isthmic tube has small diverticula suggestive of salpingitis isthmica nodosa. The distal fallopian tubes proved to be mildly dilated but patent

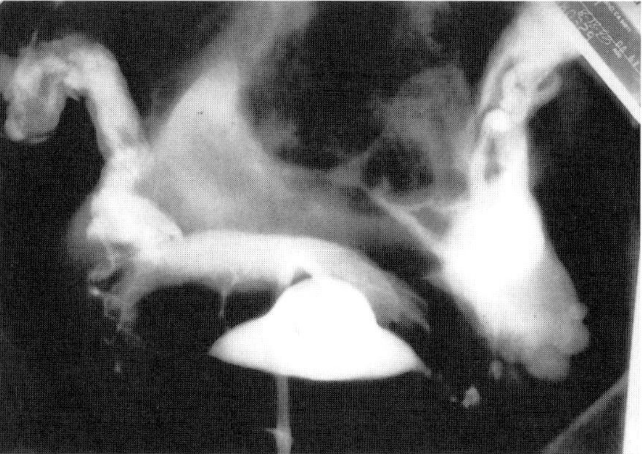

a

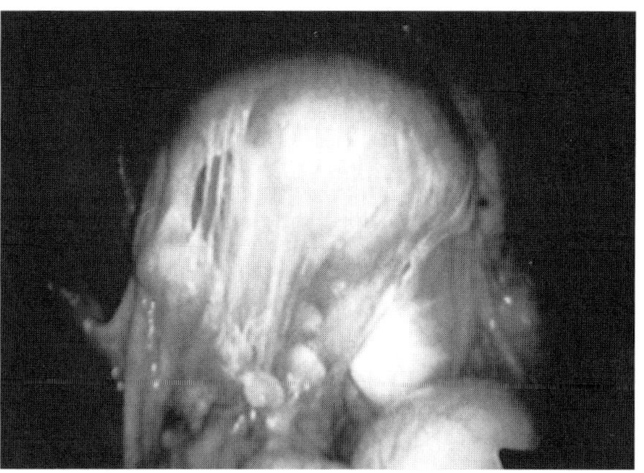

b

**Fig. 12.6.** **a** HSG shows loculated spillage of contrast media. **b** Laparoscopic view of the back of the uterus (with patient's left fallopian tube on the viewer's left-hand side). Adhesions extend from the back of the uterus and left tube over the distal fimbriated portion of the tube

fertile women was stated to be 0.6%–11% (Jenkins et al. 1993).

Microsurgical fallopian tubal reanastomosis may be performed in women with a history of prior tubal ligations. HSG is often helpful to assess the length of the residual proximal tubal segment because the length of that segment correlates well with the likelihood of successful recanalization; the pregnancy rate falls quickly when the reanastomosed tube is less than 4 cm in length (Silber and Cohen 1980).

## 12.6 Peritoneal Factors

Karasick and Goldfarb (1989) evaluated 100 patients with an HSG-based diagnosis of peritubal adhesions. They found loculated spillage of contrast material and convolution of the fallopian tubes to have the strongest association with peritubal adhesions (Fig. 12.6). They strongly believe OSCM to be far superior to WSCM for assessment of peritubal adhesions.

Endometriosis is associated with a high rate of infertility and is often associated with considerable pelvic pain during normal menses and during HSG. Because of its association with pelvic pain, endometriosis has often been misdiagnosed as pelvic inflammatory disease. Importantly, however, endometriosis may be clinically silent, except for infertility, in perhaps a third of cases.

Uncommonly HSG contrast material pools around ovarian or other pelvic masses. This diagnosis is indirect, however, and must be based on further confirmatory evidence. Cystic or solid endometriomas may be identified sonographically but must be assessed laparoscopically or at open surgery. Many significant lesions are small implants, poorly imaged by HSG, US, and MRI.

Diagnostic laparoscopy must be used to identify or confirm endometriosis as a possible cause of infertility. It may also be used to treat this disease. The American Fertility Society classification of endometriosis uses a standardized pictorial display of the pelvis with prognosis being based upon location of disease, lesion size, extent of disease, and adhesion formation.

## 12.7 The Future

What infertility services will be covered as part of traditional health insurance-mandated services and which services will be reduced in the future is being hotly debated (Jacoby 1993). Society appears ambivalent about accepting infertility as a legitimate health problem. There is no denying its importance to those who are seemingly unable to conceive and produce offspring. For many couples, the path to fertility is expensive and sometimes fruitless. Fortunately, however, the majority of infertile women may be diagnosed and treated relatively simply and inexpensively.

## References


Buttram VC, Gibbons WE (1979) Muellerian anomalies: a proposed classification (an analysis of 144 cases). Fertil Steril 32:40–46

Collins JA, Wrixon W, Janes LB, Wilson EH (1983) Treatment-independent pregnancy among infertile couples. N Engl J Med 309:1201–1206

Creasy JL, Clark RL, Cuttino JT, Groff TR (1985) Salpingitis isthmica nodosa: radiologic and clinical correlates. Radiology 154:597–600

Dor J, Homburg R, Rabau E (1977) An evaluation of etiologic factors and therapy in 665 infertile couples. Fertil Steril 28:718–722

Eisenberg AD, Winfield AC, Page DL, et al. (1989) Peritoneal reaction resulting from iodinated contrast material: comparative study. Radiology 172:149–151

Jacoby S (1993) Entitled to the embryo? (opinion) The New York Times, Nov 11

Jenkins CS, Williams SR, Schmidt GE (1993) Salpingitis isthmica nodosa: a review of the literature, discussion of clinical significance, and consideration of patient management. Fertil Steril 60:599–607.

Jones HW Jr, Toner JP (1993) The infertile couple. N Engl J Med 23:1710–1715

Kaufman RH, Adam E, Noller K, et al. (1986) Upper genital tract changes and infertility in diethylstilbestrol exposed women. Am J Obstet Gynecol 154:1312–1318

Karasick S, Goldfarb AF (1989) Peritubal adhesions in infertile women: diagnosis with hysterosalpingography. AJR 152:777–779

Lindequist S, Justesen P, Larsen C, Rasmussen F (1991) Diagnostic quality and complications of hysterosalpingography: oil-versus water-soluble contrast media: a randomized prospective study. Radiology 179:69–74

Rasmussen F, Lindequist S, Larsen C, Justesen P (1991) Therapeutic effects of hysterosalpingography: oil- versus water-soluble contrast media- a randomized prospective study. Radiology 179:75–78

Reuter KL, Daly DC, Cohen SM (1989) Septate versus bicornuate uteri: errors in imaging diagnosis. Radiology 172:749–752

Schmidt JD, Chapler FK (1993) Clinical aspects of genital and urinary tract anomalies. In: Buchasbaum HJ, Schmidt JD (eds) Gynecologic and Obstetric Urology, 3rd edn. Saunders, Philadelphia, p 116

Siegler AM (1974) Hysterosalpingography, 2nd edn. Medcom Press, New York

Silber SJ, Cohen R (1980) Microsurgical reversal of female sterilization: the role of tubal length. Fertil Steril 33:598–601

Sulak PJ, Letterie GS, Coddington CC, et al. (1987) Histology of proximal tubal occlusion. Fertil Steril 48:437–440

Toaff R, Ballas S (1978) Traumatic hypomenorrhea-amenorrhea (Asherman's syndrome). Fertil Steril 30:379–387

Winfield A, Pittaway D, Maxson W, et al. (1982) Apparent cornual occlusion in hysterosalpingography: reversal by glucagon. AJR 139:525–527

# 13 Selective Salpingography and Transcervical Recanalization of Obstructed Fallopian Tubes

E.K. LANG and H.H. DUNAWAY, JR.

CONTENTS



## 13.1 Introduction

Tubal occlusion is the cause of 25%–30% of female infertility (CONFINO et al. 1986, 1990). After excluding other factors associated with infertility or subfertility, such as diethylstilbestrol treatment, endometriosis, the male factor, immunologic factors, and anovulation, diagnostic investigations are directed to affirm or disprove tubal occlusion and to localize the site of the occlusion to the proximal or distal tube (BENADIVA et al. 1995). Based on these findings a choice is between a multitude of surgical or transcervical tuboplasty procedures, in vitro fertilization (IVF), gamete intrafallopian transfer (GIFT), intrauterine insemination, and fallopian sperm perfusion (DECHERNEY 1987). Thorough understanding of the anatomy, physiology, pharmacology, and pathophysiology of obstructed tubes is mandatory to select the optimal modality for a given patient (KARANDE et al. 1995).

E.K. LANG, MD, Professor of Radiology and Urology, Department of Radiology School of Medicine, Louisiana State University Medical Center, 1543 Tulane Avenue, New Orleans, LA 70122-2822, USA
H.H. DUNAWAY, MD, Department of Radiology School of Medicine, Louisiana State University Medical Center, 1543 Tulane Avenue, New Orleans, LA 70122-2822, USA

## 13.2 Anatomy, Physiology, and Pharmacology of the Fallopian Tubes

The oviduct can be divided into four segments: interstitial (intramural), isthmic, ampullary, and infundibular (fimbriated). The interstitial segment has a luminal diameter of only about 100 μm, as compared with approximately 400 μm for the isthmic segment and 1–2 cm for the ampullary segment. The interstitial and isthmic segments have fewer cilia on the epithelial surface than the distal region of the tubes. Fertilization likely occurs in the distal ampulla. Misalignment of mucosal folds attendant to inflammatory disease may impede transport of the egg (HERSHLAG et al. 1989).

Estrogen stimulates while progesterone inhibits muscular activity in the oviduct (ELDER et al. 1977; HODGSON and TALO 1978; KORNEGA and KADOTA 1981; LINDBLOM et al. 1980). The inhibitory response elicited by progesterone tends to relax tubal musculature and thus facilitates passage of the ovum through the fallopian tube into the uterus (SANDBERG et al. 1963). Estrogen potentiates the activation of α-adrenergic receptors while progesterone potentiates the activation of β-adrenergic receptors (HODGSON and TALO 1978; LINDBLOM et al. 1980). Because of the location of α- and β-adrenergic receptors in the inner longitudinal and outer longitudinal or spiral layers, stimulation of the α-adrenergic receptors will reduce transisthmic flow, whereas stimulation of β-adrenergic receptors will increase it (BODKHE and HARPER 1973). The known fact that terbutaline, a $\beta_2$-agonist, is more effective than $\beta_1$-agonists, indicates that the effect is mediated by $\beta_2$ receptors (STROM et al. 1983).

During estrogen dominance, α-adrenergic receptor stimulation causes isthmic contraction, while during progesterone dominance in the second part of the cycle, $\beta_2$ stimulation leads to isthmic relaxation and increased transisthmic flow (KORNEGA and KADOTA 1981; LINDBLOM et al. 1980).

Contractile response of the tube to prostaglandin varies depending on the stage of the cycle. $PGF_{2\alpha}$ stimulates while $PGE_1$ and $PGE_2$ inhibit fallopian tube contractions (SPILMAN and HARPER 1974). Moreover, $PGF_{2\alpha}$, $PGE_1$, and $PGE_2$ stimulate ciliary activity in the tubes.

Estrogen may increase the number of ciliated cells and incite ciliary activity (CROXATTO et al. 1978). Ciliary defects (tubal factor infertility) may cause infertility or ectopic pregnancy (HERSHLAG et al. 1989; VASQUEZ et al. 1984), as is attested to by pregnancies occurring in women with the Kartagener's syndrome. However, ciliary motility is not mandatory for female fertility (JEAN et al. 1979).

Human ova tend to stay in the ampulla for approximately 72 h, allowing fertilization to occur. The embryo then moves rapidly through the isthmic segment and reaches the endometrial cavity at about 80 h postovulation (CROXATTO et al. 1978). Estrogen-dependent luminal mucus facilitates migration of sperm to the ampullary segment of the tube (JANSEN and ANDERSON 1987).

## 13.3 Pathophysiology of Tubal Obstruction

The difference between tubal obstruction and tubal occlusion was recognized as early as 1954, based on observations of uterotubal insufflation (RUBIN 1954). SULAK et al. (1987) first described amorphous material, probably the result of menstrual backwash, as a cause for nonfilling of the tubes during hysterosalpingography. On histopathologic examination of a small series of 18 patients, obstruction by amorphous material occurred in 50% of the patients, causing nonfilling of the tubes on hysterosalpingograms.

Spasm of the uterotubal junction during the estrogen phase is another common cause for nonfilling of the tubes (KORNEGA and KADOTA 1981). Since $PGE_1$ and $PGE_2$ inhibit while $PGF_{2\alpha}$ stimulates fallopian tube contractions, the use of prostaglandin antagonists will reduce the degree of spasm at the uterotubal junction (LANG 1991a; SANDBERG et al. 1963). Aspirin, a very mild prostaglandin antagonist, or terbutaline given intramuscularly has been advocated for this purpose (LANG et al. 1990; LANG 1991a; LANG and DUNAWAY 1996; THURMOND et al. 1988b). In our experience, approximately one-third of patients with nonfilling of the tubes on the initial hysterosalpingogram will show normal filling following the use of aspirin or terbutaline to mitigate the existing spasm (LANG 1990, 1991a,b; LANG and DUNAWAY 1996; LANG et al. 1990, 1992). Glucagon given intravenously has likewise been reported to successfully abate spasm at the uterotubal junction (WINFIELD et al. 1982).

Occlusion of the tubes may be caused by inflammatory disease, salpingitis isthmica nodosa, tuberculosis, or endometriosis. Intentional tuboligation and strictures attendant to failed reconstructive surgical interventions are today a major cause of tubal occlusion.

## 13.4 Indications for Selective Salpingography and Transcervical Recanalization of the Fallopian Tubes

Selective salpingography increases the diagnostic value of hysterosalpingography and in many instances obviates the need for diagnostic laparoscopy and chromopertubation (CAPITANIO et al. 1991; MOVSEPIAN et al. 1994; LANG 1991a; LANG and DUNAWAY 1996; LANG et al. 1990; THURMOND 1994; THURMOND et al. 1988a). Laparoscopy is then reserved for assessment of the periovarian space, and salpingoscopy for microscopic evaluation of the ciliated epithelium of the fimbriated segment of the tubes (KERIN et al. 1990; SHAPIRO et al. 1988; SNODEN et al. 1984).

In our experience selective salpingography demonstrated patency in 131 of 318 patients in whom hysterosalpingography had failed to show patent tubes after use of prostaglandin antagonists (LANG and DUNAWAY 1996) (Fig. 13.1).

Transcervical recanalization of the fallopian tube can alleviate obstruction of the proximal tubes in a substantial number of patients. Obstruction due to inflammatory disease such as salpingitis isthmica nodosa or tubal fibrosis, as well as strictures occurring at the site of reimplantation (tubocornual anastomosis), is amenable to this treatment. Moreover, ability to then perform a selective salpingogram renders valuable information on the status of the distal tubes. Disease of the distal tubes such as hydro- or pyosalpinx or adhesions near the ovaries almost always necessitates surgical intervention in the form of fimbrioplasty or fimbriolysis (ROCK et al. 1978).

The risk due to radiation exposure is not considered a deterrent since the average absorbed ovarian

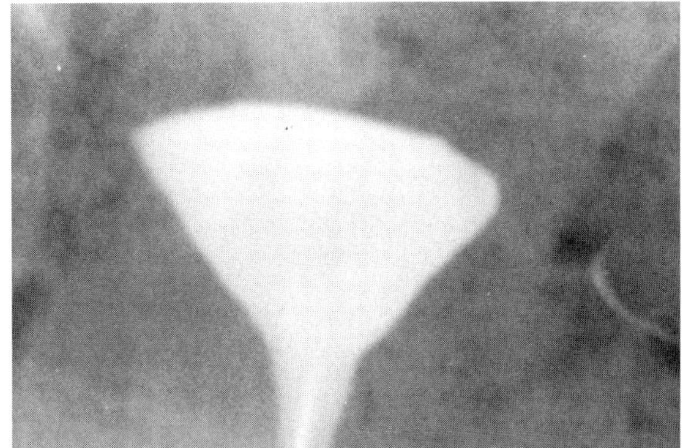
a

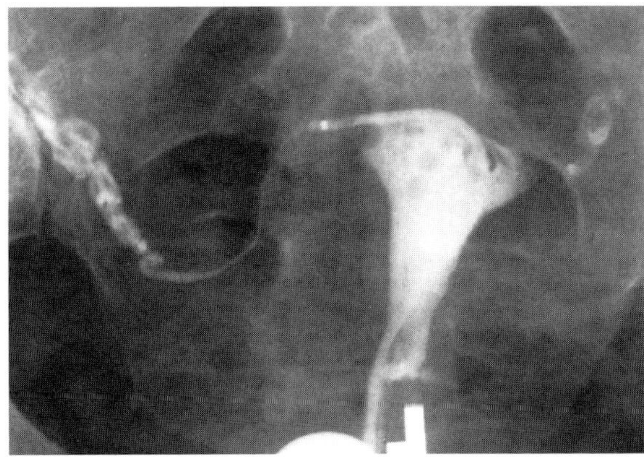
b

**Fig. 13.1. a** A hysterosalpingogram after administration of prostaglandin antagonists fails to opacify the right tube. **b** A selective salpingogram demonstrates an entirely normal right tube; initial nonfilling was probably due to spasms, debris, or a combination thereof

radiation dose is about 8.5–15.6 nGy (HEDGPETH et al. 1991; NAKAMURA et al. 1996). The risk of reaction to contrast media is likewise minimal. Based on experience derived from rabbit studies, the inflammatory reaction of the fallopian tube lining provoked by both oily and aqueous ionic and nonionic contrast media appears to be of limited duration and usually subsides by the 4th day (THURMOND et al. 1991).

Transcervical catheterization of the fallopian tubes can also be expanded to serve the purpose of sterilization (MAUBON et al. 1994; SCHMITZ-RODE et al. 1994). Custom-designed platinum microcoils, hydrogel combined with sclerosing agents, and microspindles have been advocated for this purpose (MAUBON et al. 1994; SCHMITZ-RODE et al. 1994). These sterilization techniques offer the advantage of relative ease, noninvasiveness, and low cost. However, their safety has not been confirmed in either humans or animals. Reversal of some of the chemical sterilization procedures by transcervical tube catheterization and application of quinacrine has been reported (THURMOND et al. 1995). However, reversibility for most of these techniques has not been established. Since the method is nonsurgical and, therefore, less expensive and perhaps potentially safer, delivery of a device or chemical to the fallopian tube via transcervical catheterization for the purpose of temporary or permanent sterilization has been advocated as an alternative method (THURMOND et al. 1995).

## 13.5 Selective Salpingography

As has been suggested by Sulak and others, nonfilling of the fallopian tubes on hysterosalpingography may be caused by spasm with debris lingering in the fallopian tubes (SULAK et al. 1987). Use of prostaglandin antagonists such as aspirin, glucagon, or terbutiline will eliminate a substantial number of false-positive hysterosalpingograms due to spasm. In our experience approximately 20% of patients reexamined after premedication with a prostaglandin antagonist will show normal filling of previously obstructed tubes (LANG 1991a,b; LANG and DUNAWAY 1996).

Selective salpingography in which aqueous contrast medium is injected under some pressure into the tubal orifice will unveil a further substantial number of false-positives. In our experience false-positives accounted for approximately 33% of all patients presenting with uni- or bilateral nonfilling of the tubes on hysterosalpingography (LANG 1991a; LANG and DUNAWAY 1996). Many of these obstructions may be due to inspissated debris back-washed from prior menstruation (CONFINO et al. 1988, 1990; LANG et al. 1990; SULAK et al. 1987). However, some patients with spasm may be refractory to amelioration by prostaglandin antagonists. CONFINO et al., in their original report in 1988, utilized selective salpingography performed by placing a balloon into the cornu and pressure injection of the tubal ostium, and by this means restored patency in 57% of their patients with obstructed tubes. This is very similar to our experience, patency of initially obstructed tubes being demonstrated in 53% of patients (213/400) after use of either prostaglandin antagonists or selective salpingography (LANG and DUNAWAY 1996). Some obstructions are due to a pathologic process in the uterus, leiomyomas, synechiae, or webs in the cornua (Figs. 13.2, 13.3).

The true incidence of obstruction secondary to spasm or inspissated material is difficult to establish

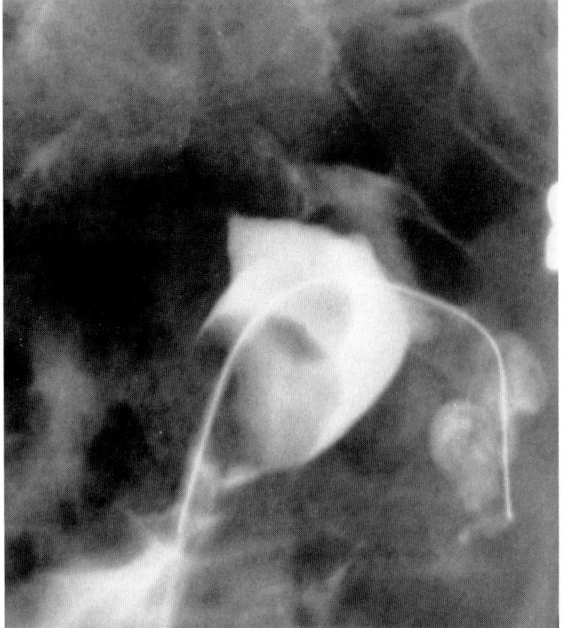

**Fig. 13.2.** The initial salpingogram failed to show filling of either tube. Selective catheterization made possible placement of a guidewire and catheter bypassing multiple submucosal fibroids in the endometrial cavity. The injection shows a normal left tube to the fimbriated end and unabated spillage

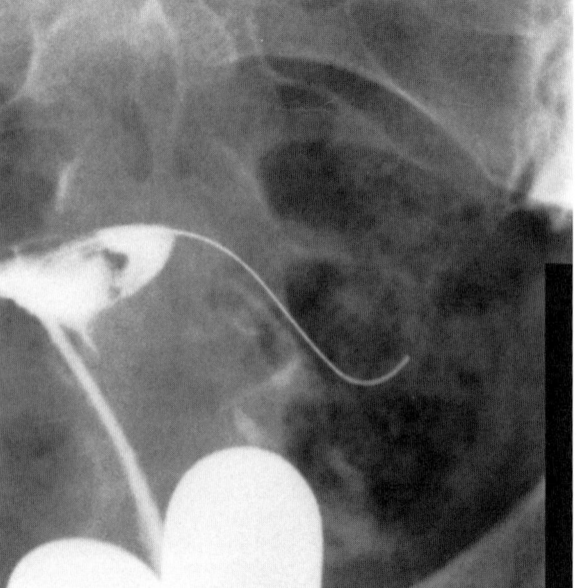

a

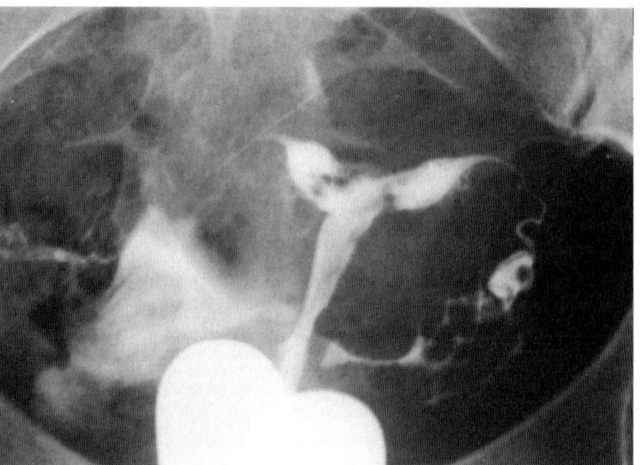

b

**Fig. 13.3.** **a** Selective placement of a guidewire into the ampullary segment of the left tube was possible despite extensive synechiae in the uterine fundus. **b** Subsequent selective injections demonstrate normal right and left tubes

from reports in the literature (SWART et al. 1995; WADIN et al. 1994). THURMOND et al. in 1990 reported successful recanalization in 86%. However, there was no breakdown of patients with successful opacification of the tubes on selective salpingograms alone or only after catheterization with a mandrill guidewire and 3-French Teflon dilator. KUMPE et al. (1990) likewise reported a technical success rate for recanalization of 98% but did not give a breakdown of whether this was achieved by salpingography or only after recanalization with a guidewire and catheter.

In our series, tubes that remained obstructed after administration of prostaglandin antagonists and use of selective salpingography were recanalized by transcervical selective catheterization using a 0.015-in. platinum tip guidewire and a 1.2- to 3.0-French tracker catheter in 145 patients (LANG and DUNAWAY 1996). In 88 patients we were able to recanalize one tube, in 57 both. Forty-two of our 400 patients proved refractory to combined pharmacologic manipulation, selective salpingography, and transcervical recanalization.

In our experience a combination of residual debris, spasm, and mild inflammatory disease may be the cause of nonfilling in some patients (16 of 400 in our series). Only on selective salpingography and sometimes laparoscopy could one appreciate the presence of mild inflammatory disease (Fig. 13.4). In the 187 patients in whom we diagnosed an organic occlusion of the tubes, one tube was afflicted in nine patients and both in 178. The reasons for organic tube obstruction were failed microsurgical procedures in 43 patients, salpingitis isthmica nodosa in 62, endosalpingitis in 71, and endometriosis in only eight patients. In three patients the precise etiology was never established (LANG and DUNAWAY 1996) (Figs. 13.5, 13.6).

Transcervical recanalization was technically successful in 145 of 187 patients or 202 tubes. Forty-two patients were refractory to attempts at transcervical recanalization (HAYASHI et al. 1994). Fibrous

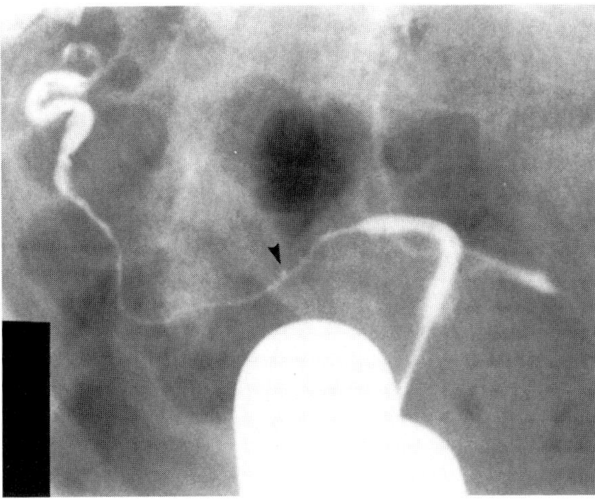

**Fig. 13.4.** A selective salpingogram shows a near-normal lumen of the isthmic segment. Only a small extraluminal collection of contrast medium (*arrowhead*) indicates the presence of salpingitis isthmica nodosa

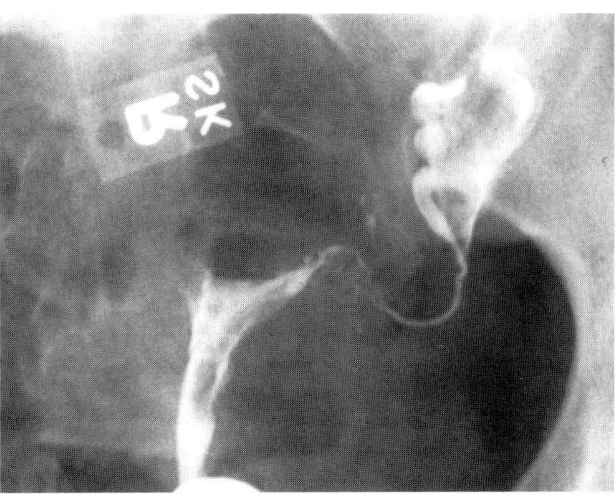

**Fig. 13.6.** Recanalization of the isthmic segment of the left tube by guidewire and bougie dilator was successful. However, there remain considerable irregularities in the lumen of the isthmic segment of the tube, raising the question of high risk for tubal pregnancy

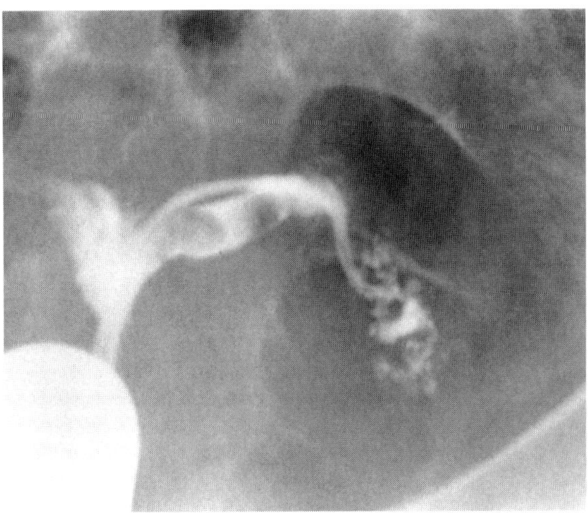

**Fig. 13.5.** Note extensive pudding of contrast medium along the isthmic segments of the right and left tube, characteristic of salpingitis isthmica nodosa

stenosis with lymphoplasmocytic infiltrates have been identified by LETTERIE and SAKAS (1991) as a common cause for failure of tubal recanalization. Intrauterine pregnancies were attained in 24 patients (LANG and DUNAWAY 1996).

## 13.6 Technique of Fallopian Tube Catheterization and Recanalization

Transcervical fluoroscopic recanalization was introduced by PLATIA and KRUDY in 1985. A variety of techniques have been advocated, all principally designed to pass a guidewire via a transcervical approach into at least the isthmic segment of the fallopian tube. Generally, fluoroscopic guidance has been favored (CAPITANIO et al. 1991; CONFINO et al. 1986, 1988, 1990; KUMPE et al. 1990; LABERGE et al. 1990; LANG 1990, 1991a,b, 1995; LANG and DUNAWAY 1994, 1996; LANG et al. 1990, 1992; THURMOND et al. 1988a; THURMOND and ROSCH 1990). However, ultrasound guidance for fallopian tube catheterization has also been advocated by some (LISSE and SYDOW 1991; THURMOND 1992). A plethora of different devices have been proposed for access through the cervical canal. These have included vacuum cup devices, double-balloon catheters, and self-retaining cannulas (LABERGE et al. 1990; MEYEROVITZ 1991; THURMOND et al. 1990). All of the devices have in common the concept that the shaft is placed through the endocervical canal to allow coaxial passage of a catheter with a curved tip to facilitate engagement of the cornua and subsequent selective catheterization of the tubes. Stabilization of the shaft in the endocervical canal is achieved either by a vacuum cup or by multiple balloons seated in the endocervical canal, the rostral end of the endocervical canal, and the endometrial cavity.

Governed by the availability of devices from manufacturers, such as Bard, (Billerica, Mass.), Cook, (Bloomington, Ind.), Target Therapeutics, (Santa Monica, Calif.), and Conceptus, (Santa Monica, Calif.), we have principally used a coaxial system consisting of a straight endocervical cannula, a catheter with a curved tip to engage the cornua, a highly flexible, platinum-tipped 0.014- to 0.016-in. guidewire, and a second coaxial catheter, 1.2–3.0 French, used as bougie dilator and to perform the selective study.

All our patients were referred to our gynecoradiology service after hysterosalpingograms performed at an outside institution or at our clinics had failed to fill the fallopian tubes. The patients were scheduled for a repeat hysterosalpingogram and follow-up selective salpingography if needed, after preparation with a prostaglandin antagonist (aspirin 325 mg daily for 2 days) and antibiotics (doxycycline hyclate) (Chilcott Lab, Morris Plains, N.J.) 100 mg twice daily for 2 days. Transcervical tuboplasty was generally performed as an outpatient procedure. The patients were premedicated with 25 mg of Demerol (Winthrop Pharmaceuticals, New York, N.Y.) and Fentanyl 25 µg (Elkins-Sinn, Cherry Hill, N.J.) intravenously. A standard hystersalpingogram using a balloon catheter placed in the endocervical canal was then performed. If this study again failed to opacify the tubes, selective salpingography was carried out. The cervix was stabilized with a single-tooth tenaculum. A 7-French Teflon sheath was then introduced through the endocervical canal into the endometrial cavity. Through the Teflon sheath a 3.5- to 5.5-French, torque-controlled catheter equipped with either a 120° or a 90° angled tip was advanced into the right and left cornua. Engagement of the cornua was facilitated by exercising traction on the tenaculum as well as by slightly rotating the uterus by tortion traction exerted on the tenaculum. Engagement of the ostium could be further facilitated by tracking the tip of the catheter under fluoroscopic control over a 0.035-in. guidewire engaged in the ostium of the tube.

If engagement of the cornua was not possible with a 90° or a 120° angle tip, custom reshaping of the tip of the catheter was recommended. Various angulations deemed optimal for engagement of the cornua according to information derived from the preceding hystersalpingogram could be obtained by steaming the tip of the catheter and modifying its curve.

Once the catheter was seated in the ostium, a selective injection of the tube was carried out. Water-soluble contrast medium, usually Conray-60 (Mallinckrodt, St. Louis, Mo.), was utilized for this purpose in amounts of 1.5–2.5 ml. If this injection again failed to visualize the tubes, selective catheterization of the tubes via the catheter engaged in the tubal ostium and utilizing a 0.015-in. guidewire with a 7-cm highly flexible platinum tip (Target Therapeutics, Santa Monica, Calif.) was attempted. If the guidewire could be advanced only for a short segment and encountered obstruction, sheathing of the guidewire with a 1.2- to 3.5-French Target Therapeutic catheter (Target Therapeutics, Santa Monica, Calif.) to stiffen it could be used to bougie dilate a partial obstruction and facilitate further retrograde advancement of the guidewire tip. Advancement of the catheter to the very end of the wire and then repeated probing with the guidewire usually allowed gradual advancement through a partially obstructed segment (Fig. 13.7). Forceful injection of 0.5 ml of aqueous contrast medium through the Target Therapeutic catheter was sometimes used to hydrodilate the narrowed segment.

For refractory lesions a 0.018-in. guidewire with a central channel was introduced. Contrast medium was injected through the central channel while attempting advancement. The relatively high pressure injection hydrodilated the stricture and facilitated further advancement of the guidewire. Once the 0.018-in. guidewire had been successfully passed, the same segment was negotiated with a central channel 0.025-in. guidewire.

Bougie dilatation is advocated to negotiate all stenotic or partially obstructed segments of the interstitial, isthmic, and ampullary segments of the fallopian tube. A controlled "to and fro" probing motion of the guidewire will gradually advance the tip. Often a "crunching" sensation is experienced when passing a partial or near-complete obstruction

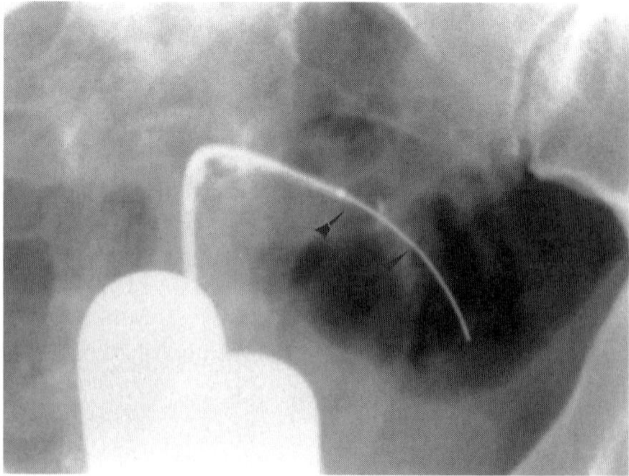

**Fig. 13.7.** The metallic ring indicating the end of the 5.5-French curved catheter is firmly seated in the tubal ostium. The guidewire has been gradually advanced into the distal isthmic segment, utilizing a "to and fro" probing motion. Note the 2.2-French coaxial catheter that had been threaded over the guidewire to stiffen it and facilitate passage through the partially obstructed segment (*arrowheads*)

due to inflammatory disease (salpingitis isthmica nodosa) (Fig. 13.8). In the presence of synechiae at the cornual ostium impeding access to the tube, disruption by balloon dilatation is recommended (Confino et al. 1986, 1990; Daniell and Miller 1987; Thurmond et al. 1988a) (Fig. 13.9). For this purpose a 0.035-in. guidewire is advanced until it has engaged the ostium of the tube. A 2-mm coronary balloon catheter is then tracked over the guidewire, the balloon inflated and the synechiae ruptured. Backward migration of the balloon into the uterine fundus may be prevented by advancing the curved 3.5-French coaxial catheter against the balloon and retaining it in position (Thurmond 1994).

After the desired position for the tertiary catheter, usually in the isthmic segment of the tube, has been reached, 0.5–1.5 ml of aqueous contrast medium is injected to document the distal tube, its patency, and spillage from the fimbriated end of the distal tube (Fig. 13.10). To properly evaluate the more proximal segments of the tubes that may have been subjected to recanalization, the tertiary catheter is gradually withdrawn to the interstitial segment and multiple injections with aqueous contrast medium are carried out to document the interstitial and isthmic segments of the tube. Finally, the tertiary catheter is removed and another global evaluation of the tube is carried out by injecting 3 ml of aqueous contrast medium through the catheter seated in the cornu (Fig. 13.10) (Swart et al. 1995).

This injection is designed to study the distal tubes. Disease of the distal tubes – hydrosalpinx, pyosalpinx, fimbrial adhesions, loss of normal fold pat-

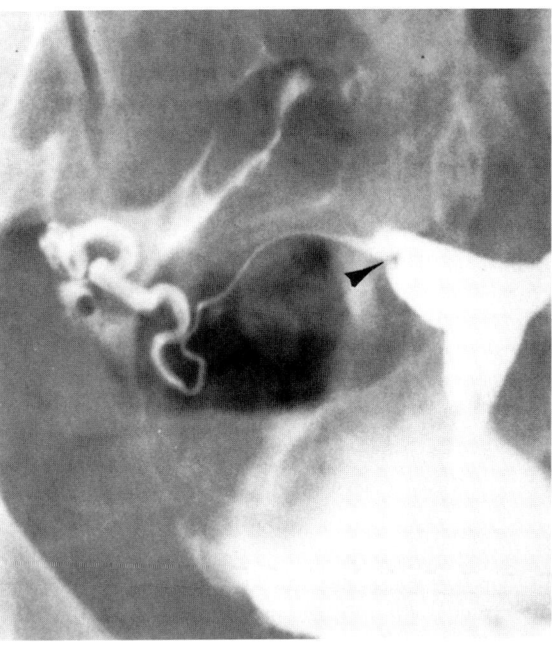

**Fig. 13.9.** A hysterosalpingogram demonstrates a small remnant of an obstructive membrane in the right cornu (*arrowhead*). This membrane was disrupted by placing and distending a 2-mm coronary balloon catheter advanced over a relatively stiff 0.018-in. guidewire anchored into the isthmic segment

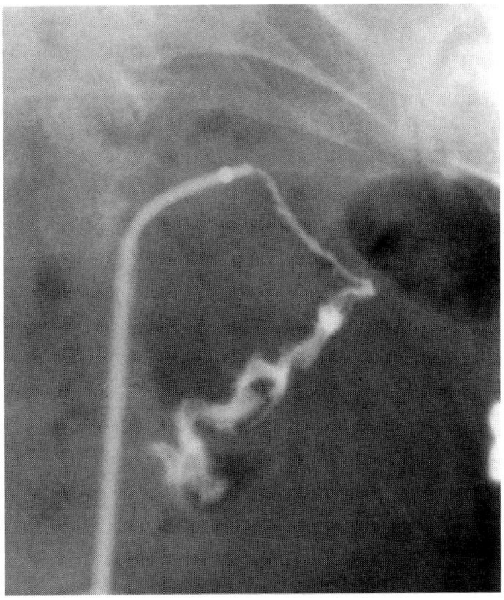

**Fig. 13.8.** Following successful recanalization by bougie technique an injection is carried out through the catheter wedged in the tubal orifice for global evaluation of the results. Note residual irregularities in the interstitial and isthmic segments of the tube, which are the result of strictures attendant to endosalpingosis. Such changes predispose to tubal pregnancy

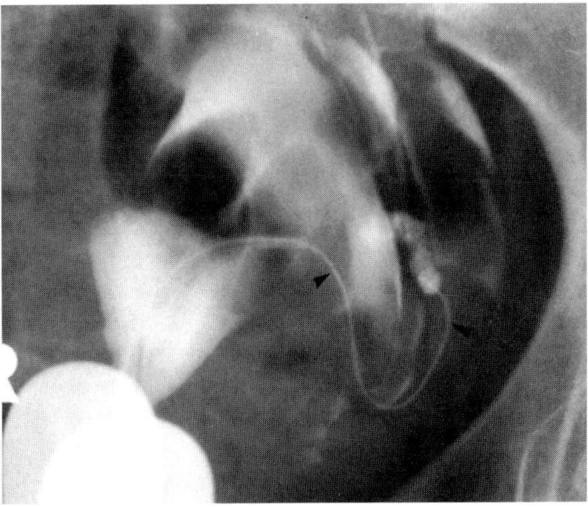

**Fig. 13.10.** After bougie dilatation the tertiary coaxial catheter has been advanced passed the isthmic segment into the ampullary segment. An injection of 1.5 ml of aqueous contrast medium demonstrates a normal distal tube and unabated spillage

tern, or hydropic degeneration – indicated by a "cobblestone pattern" and indicative of loss of ciliated epithelium, can be assessed (Fig. 13.11). Disease of distal tubes was found in 18 of 62 patients with underlying salpingitis isthmica nodosa, in 16 of 72 patients with salpingitis and perisalpingitis, in 1 of 8 with endometriosis, in 8 of 25 after failed microsurgical correction of inflammatory etiology, and in 4 of 18 after failed reversal surgery (Lang and Dunaway 1996). Endosalpingosis is a diagnosis that must usually be established by laparoscopy or salpingoscopy (Keltz et al. 1995; Shapiro et al. 1988). Measurement of the greatest diameter of hydro- or pyosalpinx is obtained as a prognostic indicator of irreversible damage of the ciliated epithelium (Carey and Brown 1987; Jacobs et al. 1988) (Figs. 13.12, 13.13).

Antibiotic coverage with doxycycline hyclate 100 mg twice daily for 2 days prior to and for a further 3 days after selective salpingography or a recanalization procedure is recommended. However, if the selective salpingogram demonstrates a marked hydro- or pyosalpinx, a potent polyvalent intravenous antibiotic effective particularly against gram-negative bacteria may be administered during or immediately after the procedure. Any symptoms of a gram-negative septicemia induced by the procedure mandate hospitalization and energetic treatment by intravenous antibiotics and administration of intravenous fluids.

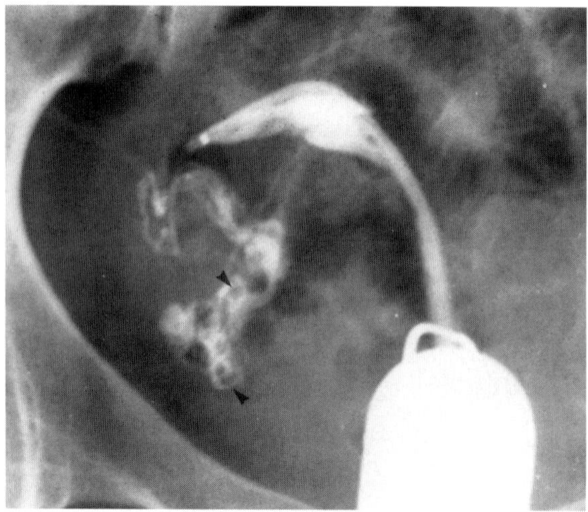

**Fig. 13.11.** After successful recanalization of the isthmic segment, selective salpingography shows filling to the fimbriated end of the right tube. However, a "cobblestone" appearance suggests irreversible changes afflicting the ciliated cells of the distal tube and, hence, a low probability for normal ovum transport. IVF may be indicated as the next procedure

Selective injections of the fallopian tubes should be recorded in AP as well as multiple oblique projections to show all segments satisfactorily. After spillage of contrast medium from the fimbriated end has occurred, a pumping action effected by the exertion of intermittent traction on the tenaculum tends to distribute contrast material over the outside of the uterus and thereby facilitate anatomic delineation particularly of the interstitial segment of the tube (Thurmond 1994). Spillage of contrast medium also

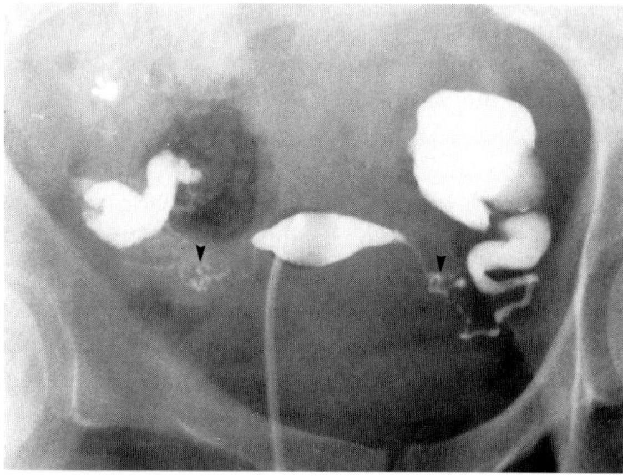

**Fig. 13.12.** Following successful recanalization a hysterosalpingogram demonstrates patency of the isthmic segments despite evidence of extensive salpingitis isthmica nodosa (*arrowhead*) but also bilateral pyosalpinx. Minimal spillage from the fimbriated end of the left tube is contained by periovarian adhesions. Moreover, the distal tube is dilated to more than 2 cm, suggesting damage to the ciliated epithelium

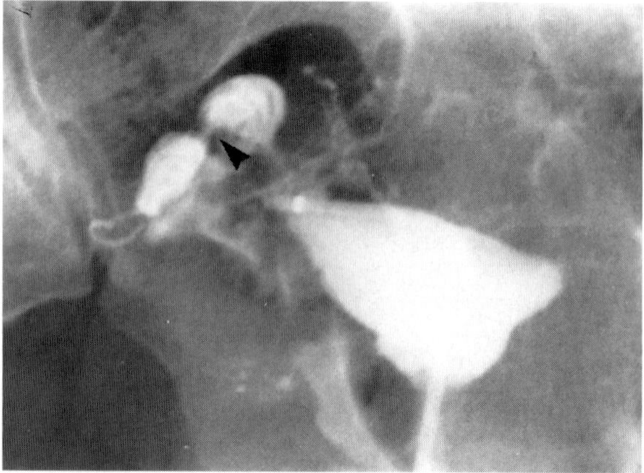

**Fig. 13.13.** After successful recanalization of the isthmic segment a selective salpingogram shows a stricture at the ampullary fimbriae junction of the tube (*arrowhead*). Since longitudinal folds in the segment are normal, laparoscopic surgery can easily correct this lesion

delineates periovarian adhesions and locculated collections around the fimbriae (Fig. 13.14).

In our group of 145 patients who underwent bougie transcervical recanalization, 13 complications occurred: perforation without sequelae in nine patients, gram-negative septicemia in one, and temperature elevation greater than 38°C in three (LANG and DUNAWAY 1996). Gram-negative septicemia occurred in a patient in whom we demonstrated bilateral pyosalpinx after successful recanalization of the proximal tubes. Septic shock developed within 2h and had to be treated vigorously with IV fluids, corticosteroids, and antibiotics (Fig. 13.15). Based on this experience we advocate restraint when injecting contrast medium into dilated distal tubes suspected of pyosalpinx. Increased pressure could force bacteria into the circulation and cause a gram-negative septicemia. If possible, advancement of the tracker catheter into the dilated distal tube should be attempted to aspirate a sample for bacteriologic identification and antibiotic sensitivity studies. In our experience the cultures in the majority of the patients tend to be sterile. However, *Chlamydia trachomatis*, enterococcus, *Enterobacter, Klebsiella, Proteus, E. coli* and *Streptococcus viridans* may be cultured (LANG and DUNAWAY 1996). Perforations are another complication of transcervical recanalization but are almost always without late sequelae (CAPITANIO et al. 1991; CONFINO et al. 1986, 1988; MOVSEPIAN et al. 1994; KUMPE et al. 1990; LABERGE et al. 1990; LANG 1990; PETERSEN and ROSCH 1994; PLATIA and KRUDY 1985; RISQUESZ and CONFINO 1993; THURMOND and ROSCH 1990; THURMOND et al. 1988a, 1990; THURMOND 1992, 1994). The incidence of tubal pregnancy after transcervical recanalization varies widely and may in fact be relate to the underlying pathology (CONFINO et al. 1988, 1990; KUMPE et al. 1990; LANG 1990; LANG et al. 1992; LANG and DUNAWAY 1996; PETERSEN and ROSCH 1994; PLATIA and KRUDY 1985; THURMOND 1992, 1994; THURMOND and ROSCH 1990). The average indicence rate of ectopic pregnancy is 3%–5% (CONFINO et al. 1986, 1988, 1990; KUMPE et al. 1990; LANG 1990, 1991a,b, 1995; LANG and DUNAWAY 1994, 1996; LANG et al. 1990, 1992; THURMOND 1994;

a

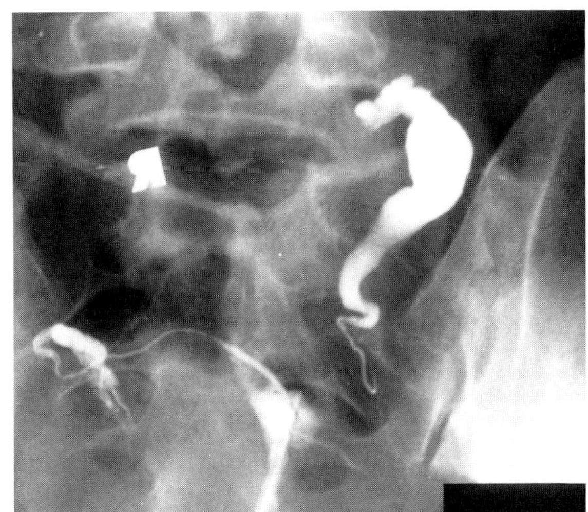

b

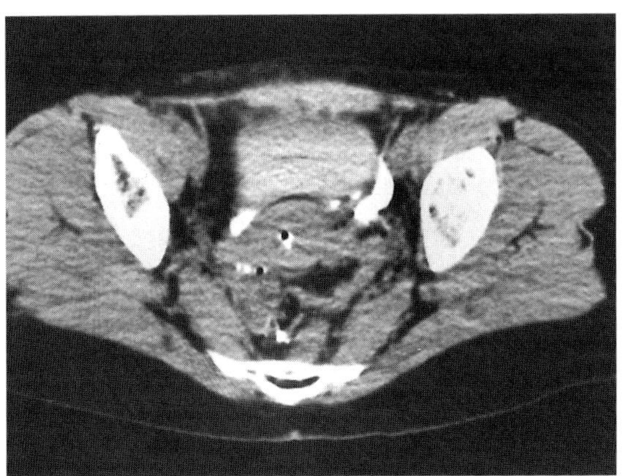

**Fig. 13.14. a** Selective right and left salpingograms demonstrate a left pyosalpinx with contrast medium spilling from the fimbriated end into a space limited by periovarian adhesions. Likewise, on the right side there is no free spillage. **b** A follow-up computed tomogram demonstrates puddles of contrast medium in the periovarian space contained by adhesions

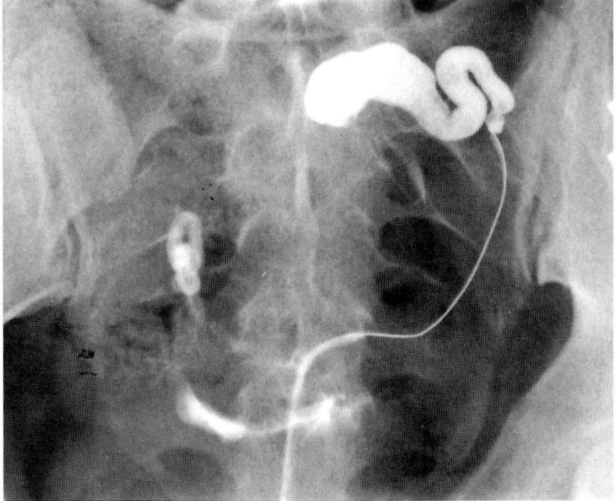

**Fig. 13.15.** A 0.025-in. guidewire with a central channel has been advanced through a selective catheter into the ampullary segment across an area of stricture due to salpingitis isthmica nodosa. The injection demonstrates a huge pyosalpinx. The patient experienced a febrile reaction associated with gram-negative septicemia provoked by the injection. (Courtesy of LANG 1991a)

THURMOND and ROSCH 1990; THURMOND et al. 1988a).

Among 120 patients who had failed to become pregnant and were reexamined 6 months after the initial transcervical recanalization, patency of one or both tubes was demonstrated in 69 (48 one tube, 21 both tubes). This is similar to the reocclusion rates reported by GLACER (44%), CONFINO (32%), KUMPE (37%), and THURMOND (48%) (CONFINO et al. 1986, 1988; HAYASHI et al. 1994; KUMPE et al. 1990; THURMOND 1994; THURMOND and ROSCH 1990).

Although repeat transcervical recanalization successfully reconstituted the lumen in 11 of our 19 patients, none of these patients became pregnant during a follow-up of 12 months (Fig. 13.16). This contrasts with the relatively high rate of pregnancy, two of eight patients, reported after successful repeat recanalization by THURMOND and ROSCH (1990).

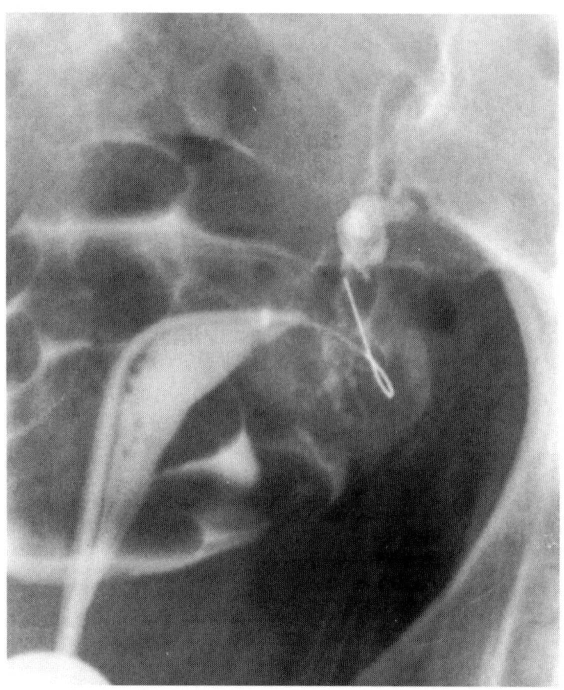

a

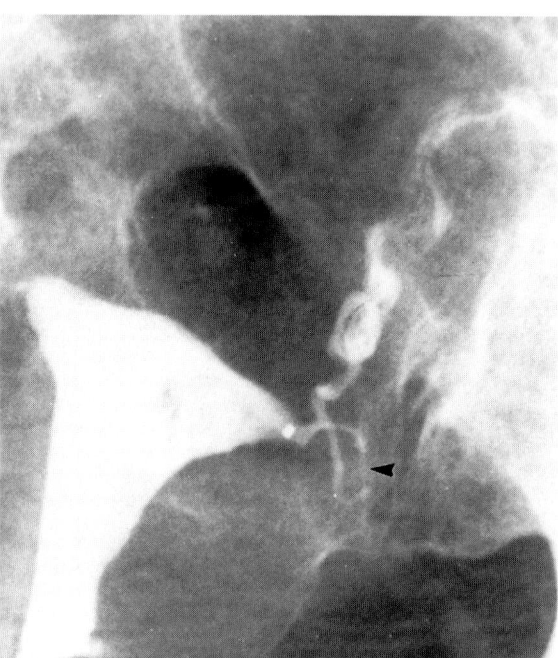

c

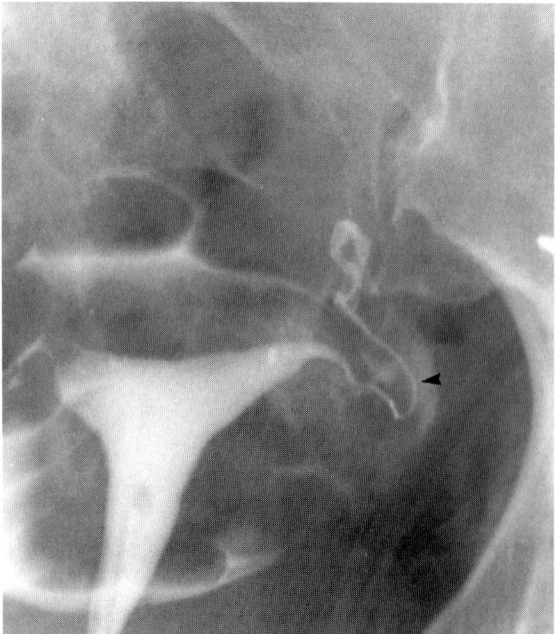

b

**Fig. 13.16.** **a** A strictured segment of the isthmic portion of the left tube is successfully dilated with a guidewire and bougie dilator. **b** A subsequent selective salpingogram shows a near-normal lumen. **c** A repeat selective salpingogram 3 years later shows stenosis of the previously successfully dilated segment of the left tube

The explanation for this disparity may lie in differences in underlying pathology. In their series of 100 consecutive patients, THURMOND and ROSCH identified only nine with obstruction due to salpingitis isthmica nodosa. Therefore, a disproportionately high percentage of the patients may have had nonfilling of the tubes due to spasm or inspissated debris, conditions which inherently permit a higher rate of pregnancy as compared with organic disease of the tubes.

## 13.7 Transcervical Recanalization of Strictures in the Postoperative Fallopian Tube

Surgical procedures advocated for restitution of patency of the proximal segment of the fallopian tube are accompanied by a relatively high incidence of secondary stricture formation or occlusion. Tubouterine anastomoses in particular have been associated with frequent secondary stenoses at the anastomotic site (ROCK 1983). However, the interstitial isthmic and interstitial ampullary anastomoses favored today for the correction of inflammatory occlusion of the isthmic segment may also result in secondary stenoses and/or occlusion. Isthmic-isthmic and isthmic-ampullary anastomoses, employed to reverse sterilization procedures in particular, have a high rate of stricture and dehiscence and sometimes cause fistula formation (ROCK 1983).

Obviously, reocclusion of the proximal tubes can be treated by repeat tuboplasty (CANIS et al. 1991; LAURITSEN et al. 1982; URMAN et al. 1992). The second intervention, however, is fraught by technical difficulties. If the tube has been shortened to 3–4 cm from prior surgical intervention, no further length can be sacrificed as this would disturb the relationship of the fimbriated end to the ovary.

Transcervical recanalization of postoperative fallopian tubes has been successful in a substantial number of patients with a prior history of underlying inflammatory disease but also in a smaller number with surgical procedures reversing a sterilization procedure.

## 13.8 Technique

Patients are prepared for the procedure akin to our protocol for transcervical recanalization. For sedation, we prefer intravenous administration of midazolam hydrochloride (Versed, Hoffmann-Laroche, Nutley, N.J.) and/or fentanyl citrate (Sublimaze, Janssen Pharmaceuticals, Piscataway, N.J.). This endocervical canal is cannulated with a 7-French Teflon sheath and a 3.5-French catheter with an appropriately curved tip is advanced through the sheath and positioned under fluoroscopic control in the respective cornu. Selective catherization is first attempted with a highly flexible 0.014-in. platinum tip guidewire (Target Therapeutics, Santa Jose, Calif.). If an obstruction is met that cannot be negotiated, a 0.018-in. guidewire with a central channel is introduced and advanced to the obstruction, and an injection of contrast medium is carried out through the central channel. This injection may show complete blockage or extravasation along the fistular tract or sometimes may successfully hydrodilate the stricture and allow further retrograde passage of the guidewire (LANG 1995; LANG and DUNAWAY 1994). In patients with a uterotubal ampullary or isthmic anastomosis, the posterior wall of the uterus is investigated by moving the curved catheter across its surface (Fig. 13.17a). If an opening can be engaged, selective advancement of the guidewire is again attempted, akin to the procedure described above (Fig. 13.17b). After the guidewire has been threaded across the stenosis, bougie dilatation with a 1.4- to 3.5-French catheter is attempted, executing a gentle "to and fro" motion of the catheter across the stricture (Fig. 13.17c,d). Finally, an injection of contrast medium is carried out with the tip of the catheter positioned in the isthmic segment to investigate the condition of the distal tube (Fig. 13.17c).

Having demonstrated patency of the distal tube, a routine balloon hysterosalpingogram is performed to a affirm that the stricture has indeed been adequately dilated.

Demonstration of a fistular tract originating from the site of the microanastomosis is an ominous finding generally predicting failure of any further transcervical recanalization attempts (Fig. 13.18). Surgery appears to be the only modality capable of correcting this complication.

In our experience transcervical recanalization succeeded in 14 of 16 patients with postsurgical stenoses (Fig. 13.19). Three of these patients became pregnant within 16 months after recanalization and two more after IVF and embryo transfer (ET). Reexamination of the 11 patients who failed to become pregnant 6–42 months after recanalization showed that reocclusion had occurred in three.

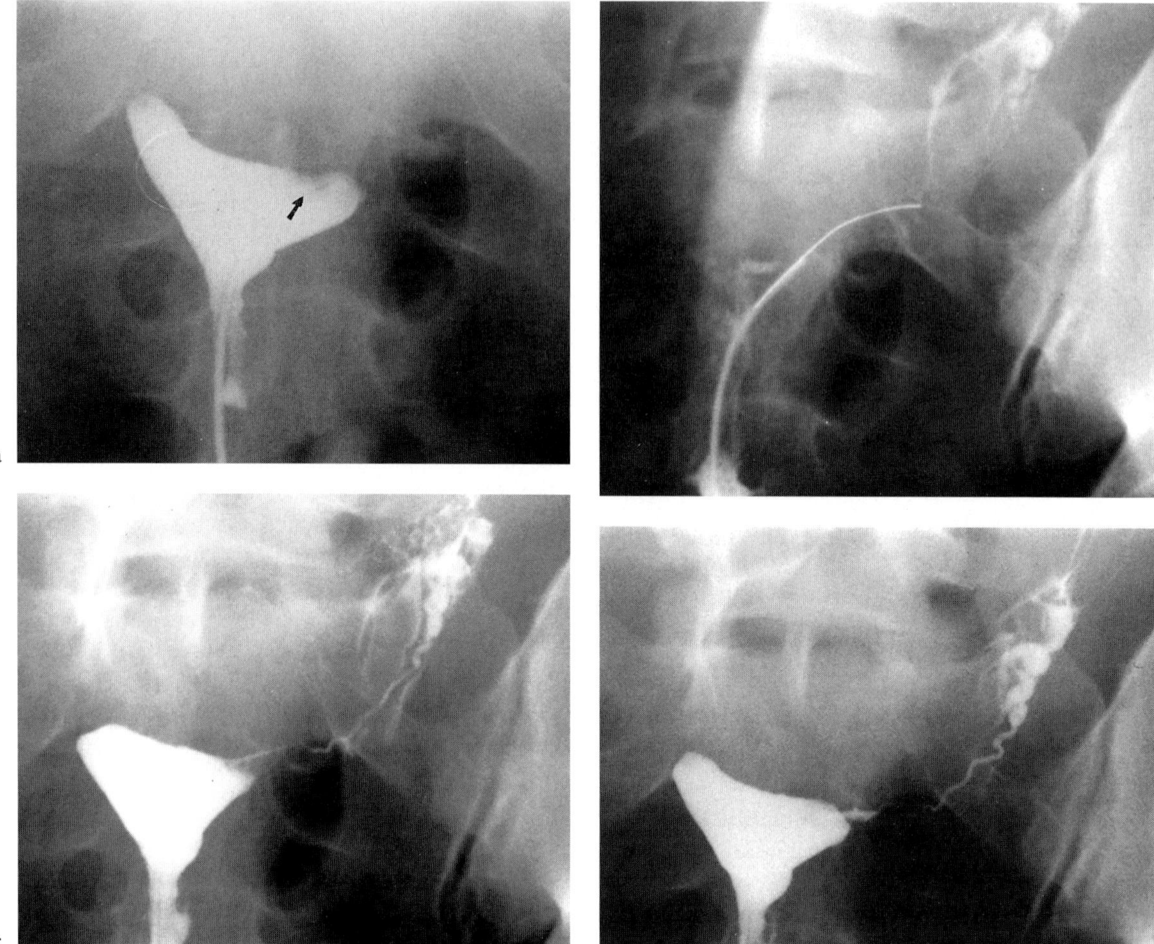

**Fig. 13.17. a** A hysterosalpingogram fails to show filling of either tube. Note an area of reduced density (*arrow*) indicating the probable site of a prior uterotubal anastomosis. **b** The anastomosis was engaged with a curved catheter and a guidewire with a central channel was advanced through the stenotic segment. The injection through the central channel demonstrates a normal distal tube. **c,d** The stenotic segment of the anastomosis is progressively dilated with a 1.8- and a 3.0-French bougie dilator. The injection demonstrates a normal distal tube. The patient became pregnant during the second cycle and delivered a well baby. (Courtesy of Lang and Dunaway 1994)

## 13.9 Reconstructive Surgery of the Fallopian Tube

Tubal surgery for infertility has a longstanding, time-honored history. As long ago as 1884 a unilateral ampullary cuff procedure was utilized to maintain apposition to the ovary (Schroder 1884). Principally, surgical interventions can be grouped into two types: those directed at conditions affecting the proximal tubes and those directed at conditions affecting the distal tubes.

Tubouterine implantations utilizing the isthmic or the ampullary segment or a combination thereof used to be widely practiced for correction of proximal tube obstruction (Jones and Rock 1983; Rock 1983). Tubal anastomosis of the interstitial, isthmic, and ampullary segments was the other type of intervention used to correct stenosis or occlusion of proximal tubes.

Salpingoplasty, fimbrioplasty, salpingoneostomy, and salpingolysis are surgical procedures for correction of lesions in the distal tubes (Bateman et al. 1987; Carey and Brown 1987; DeCherney and Kase 1981; Russeu et al. 1986). Lesions afflicting the distal tubes lie exclusively within the domain of surgical and laparoscopic intervention (Schlaff et al. 1990). Conversely, transcervical recanalization competes with surgical procedures in the management of obstructive lesions of the proximal tubes.

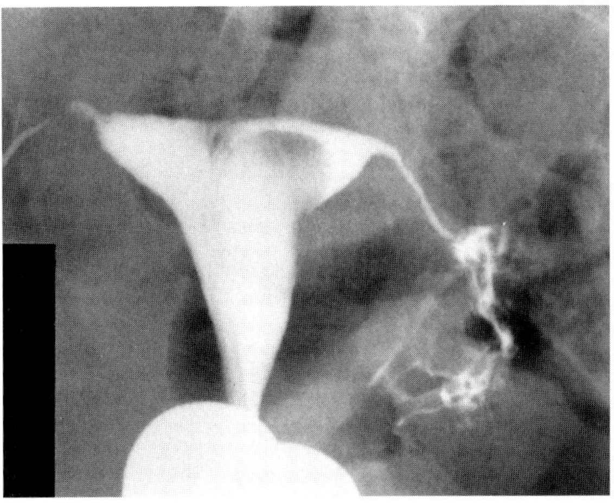

**Fig. 13.18.** A hysterosalpingogram shows extravasation of contrast medium at the site of an end-to-end microanastomosis of the isthmic and ampullary segments, correcting a prior tuboligation

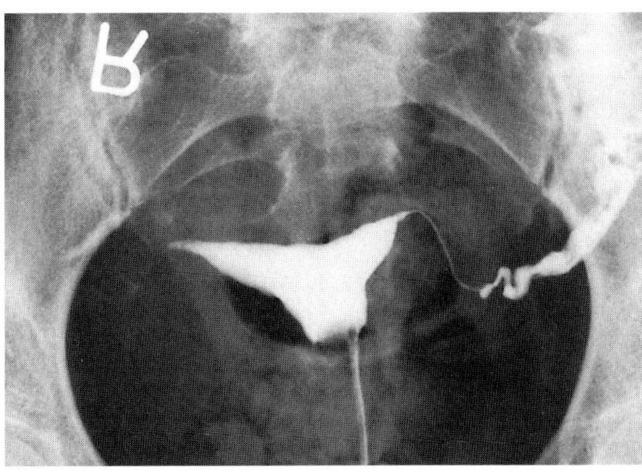

**Fig. 13.19.** After premedication with antibiotics a stricture at the anastomosis was successfully negotiated with a guidewire and a 1.8-French tracker catheter was advanced into the ampullary segment of the left tube. An injection through that catheter shows a normal distal tube. Following bougie dilatation of the stricture at the anastomotic site, the tube remained patent at 6 months' follow-up

Fimbrioplasty is defined as lysis of fimbrial adhesions or dilatation of fimbrial phimosis (DeCherney and Kase 1981) (Fig. 13.12). Most of these procedures are now carried out with laparoscopic surgical techniques. Creation of a new ostium (salpingoneostomy) is a procedure maintaining the fimbriae and reestablishing their relationship to the ovary. Success of this procedure hinges upon an intact ciliated epithelium. Hence, the procedure has a success rate, i.e., attained pregnancy, of about 86% in patients with mild hydrosalpinx but of only 8% in patients with severe hydrosalpinx (Rock 1983; Rock et al. 1984). Severe hydrosalpinx is associated with a loss of ciliated cells which appear to have a major role in the capture of oocytes (Bateman et al. 1987). Microsurgical techniques achieve a more consistent and slightly higher term pregnancy rate than do conventional surgical techniques (Bateman et al. 1987; DeCherney and Kase 1981; Fayez and Suliman 1982). Laser surgery may offer a further advantage in attaining term pregnancy (Tulandi and Vilos 1985). However, the spontaneous abortion rate and ectopic pregnancy rate tend to be high after salpingoneostomy procedures (32% live birth, 12% spontaneous abortions, 11% ectopic pregnancies) (Jacobs et al. 1988). The fimbrioplasty group shows somewhat better results (72% conception rate, 57% live birth, 11% spontaneous abortion, 7% ectopic pregnancy) (Jacobs et al. 1988). If combined surgical interventions for proximal and distal disease are carried out, the conception rate has been reported to be as low as 25%, with a live birth rate of 11% (Movsepian et al. 1994; Patton et al. 1987). This emphasizes the need for accurate assessment of the distal tubes in patients with proximal disease, which is often difficult by laparoscopy alone (Patton et al. 1987) (Fig. 13.12).

Patients treated by lysis of adhesions only, tend to have a higher rate of intrauterine pregnancy (41%) than those treated with salpingostomy (18%) (Carey and Brown 1987). Reocclusion appears to be a common problem, since Carey and Brown found that after 16 months almost all pregnancies in this group were ectopic gestations. The single most important prognostic factor appears to be the presence of a normal rugal pattern (Fig. 13.13). Neosalpingostomy is credited with a pregnancy rate of 60.7% in patients with normal rugae versus 7.3% in those in whom rugae were absent (Schlaff et al. 1990). The fact that some authors have reported an increase in intrauterine pregnancy rate over a prolonged follow-up time after neosalpingostomy suggests that there may be ciliogenesis (Russell et al. 1986; Vasquez et al. 1984). In his series, Russell reported an intrauterine pregnancy rate of 27.7% between 1 and 2 years after surgery, but of 41.6% in the subsequent 5- to 6-year follow-up study. Laparoscopic distal tuboplasty does not appear to offer a significant advantage in attaining intrauterine pregnancies, the results reflecting closely the severity of damage to the ciliated epithileum (Canis et al. 1991). Operative difficulty as related to the mobility of the fimbriae mandates a high degree of skill and experience. Theoretically postoperative adhesion formation should be reduced since laparoscopy avoids drying of the peritoneum and hence decreases the potential for infections (Canis et al. 1991).

Proximal oviductal disease accounts for only 20% of operations done for tubal occlusions (Patton et al. 1987). In a series of some 295 patients with postinflammatory oviductal disease reported from the Mayo Clinic, 27 showed primarily proximal oviductal disease which was corrected surgically. The probability of conception resulting in a live birth was 53.2% within 3.5 years after operation (Patton et al. 1987). Three patients had ectopic pregnancies.

Microsurgical cornual anastomosis was found to result in a pregnancy rate of 44% (Donnez and Casanas-Roux 1986). The pregnancy rate was highest in patients with an undamaged intramural portion (55%) and lowest in those who had multiple diverticular lesions (16%) (Donnez and Casanas-Roux 1986). Histologic examination reveals persistent lymphoplasmocytic inflammation, such as occurs with chronic salpingitis, fibrous stenosis, and endosalpingosis; all of these conditions cause occlusions throughout the smooth muscle, which are different from the changes seen with tubal endometriosis. In the experience of Donnez and Casanas-Roux (1986), multiple diverticula, i.e., loculated puddles of contrast medium, always equated with tubal endometriosis. This mandated excision of large segments of the tube. Maximal tubal length, preservation of the intramural segment, absence of chronic inflammation, absence of tubal inclusion in the tubal wall, and absence of tubal endometriosis emerged as favorable prognostic factors (Donnez and Casanas-Roux 1986).

Tubocornual anastomoses have been found to produce a pregnancy rate of 53%–63%. The results are slightly better in the group operated on for infection (62.5%) than in the group operated on for prior sterilization (42.9%) (Lavy et al. 1986). Tubocornual anastomosis offers the advantage of better preservation of the length of the reconstructed tube and lack of disruption of tubal blood flow via the tubouterine implantation (Lavy et al. 1986; Rock et al. 1984). The group of patients with resulting short tubes have a significantly lower viable pregnancy rate (33%). A tubal pregnancy rate of 12% has been reported in patients with tubocornual anastomosis; it is possible that fistulas formed in these occluded segments prior to surgery may contribute to the development of tubal pregnancies.

Isthmic-isthmic and intramural-isthmic tubal anastomoses appear to have the highest rate of intrauterine pregnancies, at 70%–75% (Jones and Rock 1983; Rock 1983; Winston 1977). However, intramural-ampullary, isthmic-ampullary, and ampullary-ampullary anastomoses result in a statistically similar pregnancy rate (Jones and Rock 1983; Rock 1983).

Pregnancy success (live birth rate) after reversal of sterilization is in the range of 55%–60%, with an ectopic pregnancy rate approaching 3%–4%. The Pomeroy procedure and monopolar cautery used for sterilization appear to adversely influence subsequent reversal surgery (Rock 1983; Rock et al. 1978).

Uterotubal implantation, a technique no longer widely practiced, was found by Rock (1983) to result in a lower pregnancy rate of approximately 37%. Peritubular and periovarian adhesions adversely influence the success rate of this surgical procedure and in the presence of dense pelvic adhesions the pregnancy rate dropped to 8% (Rock 1983). This reemphasizes the point that a tubocornual anastomosis with deep resection of the intramural segment of the tube is better suited to cope with extensive inflammatory disease than a uterotubal anastomosis (Gillett and Herbison 1989; Lavy et al. 1986).

In the even of failure of a macrosurgical tuboplasty, repeat microsurgical tuboplasty may be considered in the management of postinflammatory tubal disease (Thie et al. 1986). Pregnancy rates of up to 18% have been achieved in the repeat tuboplasty group (Thie et al. 1986). However, a further improvement in pregnancy rate after microsurgery cannot be expected since the problem in these patients does not tend to be patency but rather loss of function of tubal mucosa (Thie et al. 1986). ET or IVF ET, therefore, represents a viable alternative in this group of patients.

## 13.10 In Vitro Fertilization

Microsurgery, if successful, offers multiple cycles in which to attempt conception and, therefore, the possibility of achieving more than one pregnancy (Benadiva et al. 1995). Based on published data, minimal to moderate tubal disease might best be handled by reconstructive surgery first, particularly in young patients. However, in patients with severe pelvic adhesions, IVF might be considered as the primary approach (Fig. 13.20). Obviously IVF is the only therapeutic action for patients with inoperable tubes (absent tubes, tubercular salpingitis, etc.)

(BENADIVA et al. 1995). In older patients the status of the tubes should be evaluated expeditiously and treatment chosen in the light of contemporary expectations of producing conception by means of the available modalities. The patient should be informed of the "take home baby" rate per cycle of IVF as well as the cumulative rate for multiple cycles.

In vitro fertilization should also be considered in patients with male subfertility. Pregnancy rates per cycle as high as 35% have been reported for this technique as well as for intracytoplasmatic sperm injection (ICSI) (SHUSHAN et al. 1995). With the advances in assisted reproductive technology improving results for IVF and GIFT may be expected (DECHERNEY 1995; NEUMANN et al. 1994). Continued cycles of menotropins may result in a "take home baby" rate of 36%, similar to the 38% rate of three IVF cycles (SHUSHAN et al. 1995). In cases of endometriosis without tubal involvement, GIFT may be useful.

The cost of IVF is today less than or the same as that of tubal surgery (DECHERNEY 1995; HOLTZ et al. 1991). Holtz calculated the cost for life birth as $17000 after tubal surgery, compared with $12000 after IVF (MOVSEPIAN et al. 1994).

Immunologic infertility may be difficult to alleviate by IVF. Even washing of oocytes in a suspension of bovine serum albumin did not substantially reduce the effect of female antisperm antibodies and failed to reverse impairment of fertility in immunologically infertile patients (VASQUEZ et al. 1984).

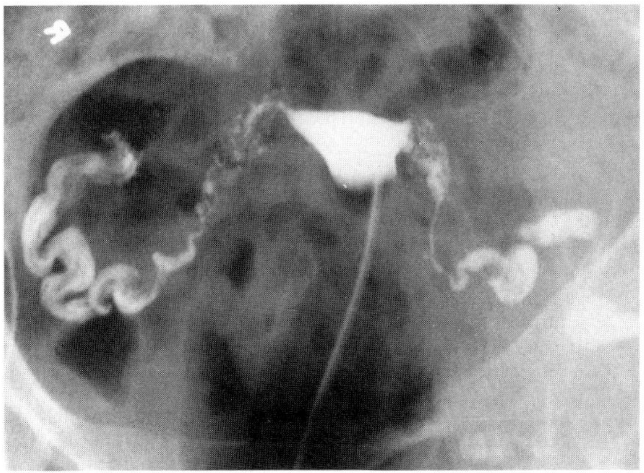

Fig. 13.20. A hysterosalpingogram demonstrates severe salpingitis isthmica nodosa involving both the right and the left tube. Moreover, adhesions cause loculation of contrast medium in the peri- ovarian space. The severity of the disease militates against reconstructive surgery and attempts at reconstruction by transcervical recanalization. IVF might be considered as the primary approach

The ultimate decision regarding treatment must take into consideration factors such as the high rate of ectopic pregnancy and the high cost of hospitalization in patients treated by neosalpingostomy, which has a success rate of 25% with regard to pregnancy. The success rate for a first GIFT attempt has been reported to be 31%, rising to 43% after second and third attempts (COLLINS et al. 1995; MOLLOY et al. 1995). However, GIFT is a procedure by which eggs and sperm are placed in patent fallopian tubes and GIFT generally requires laparoscopy.

The cumulative pregnancy rate following tubal surgery in patients with tubal factors has been reported as 28.9% (BENADIVA et al. 1995). However, a significant falloff is noted with advancing age: less than 30 years, 48.4%; greater than 42 years, 4.3%. The cumulative pregnancy rates for IVF cycles 1–4 are 32%, 59%, 70%, and 77% respectively in patients with only a tubal factor, while in patients with a tubal factor and associated infertility factors they are 28%, 55%, 62%, and 75% (BENADIVA et al. 1995). Thus BENADIVA et al. conclude that 70% of women with a tubal factor infertility will have a live birth within four cycles of treatment with IVF. This compares favorably with tubal reconstructive surgery. Because of the rapid decline in fertility with advancing age, in older women treatment methods that provide the highest likelihood of success, such as IVF, should be used (BENADIVA et al. 1995; DECHERNEY 1987, 1995).

After removal of adhesions or partial blockage of the tube or rejoining by microsurgery, GIFT may have a better chance of success than a single cycle IVF. GIFT birth rates are 20%–25% per cycle (DECHERNEY 1987; NOVY 1994; Society Assisted Reproductive Technology 1996). IVF rates are 5%–10% higher. Transfer of an IVF embryo to a recipient uterus is more difficult. Surrogate mothers can be utilized for either technique.

The cost per IVF cycle was $6233 in the United States in 1993 (COLLINS et al. 1995; NEUMANN et al. 1994). The addition of insurance coverage to the typical employer health plan insurance would be at a cost of $3.14 per year (BURNER et al. 1992; COLLINS et al. 1995).

Within the framework of reproduction medicine, selective salpingography and transcervical recanalization occupy an important position in the critical diagnostic workup of a patient and offer a cost-effective first attempt at recanalization of obstructed proximal segments of the fallopian tubes.

## References


Bateman BG, Nunley WC Jr, Kitchin JV III (1987) Surgical management of distal tubal obstruction – are we making progress? Fertil Steril 48:523–542

Benadiva CA, Kligman I, Davis O, Rosenwaks Z (1995) Invitro fertilization versus tubal surgery: is pelvic reconstructive surgery obsolete? Fertil Steril 64:1051–1061

Bodkhe RR, Harper MJK (1973) Mechanism of egg transport: changes in the amount of adrenergic transmitter in the genital tract of normal and hormone treated rabbits. In: Segal N, Crozier SJ (eds) Regulation of mammalian reproduction. Thomas, Springfield, Illinois, 364

Breckenridge JW, Schinfeld JS (1991) Technique for ultrasound guided fallopian tube catherization. Radiology 180:569–570

Burner ST, Waldo BR, McKusick DR (1992) National health expenditure projections through 2030. Health Care Financing Review 14:1–29

Canis N, Mage G, Pouly JL, Manhes H, Wattiez A, Bruhat MA (1991) Laparoscopic distal tuboplasty: report of 87 cases and a 4 year experience. Fertil Steril 56:616–621

Capitanio GL, Ferraiolo A, Croce S, Gazzo R, Anserini P, DeCecco L (1991) Transcervical selective salpingography; a diagnostic and therapeutic approach to cases of proximal tubal injection failure. Fertil Steril 56:1145–1150

Carey M, Brown S (1987) Infertility surgery for pelvic inflammatory disease; success rates after salpingolysis and salpingostomy. Am J Obstet Gynecol 156:296–300

Collins JA, Bustillo N, Visscher RV, Lawrence LB (1995) An estimate of the cost of invitro fertilization services in the United States in 1995. Fertil Steril 64:538–545

Confino E, Friberg J, Gleicher N (1986) Transcervical balloon tuboplasty. Fertil Steril 46:963–966

Confino E, Friberg J, Gleicher N (1988) Preliminary experience with transcervical balloon tuboplasty. Am J Obstet Gynecol 159:370–375

Confino E, Tur-Aspa I, DeCherney A, et al. (1990) Transcervical balloon tuboplasty; a multi-center study. JAMA 264:2079–2082

Croxatto HB, Oritz ME, Diaz S, et al. (1978) Studies on the duration of egg transport by the human oviduct; ovum location of various intervals following luteinization hormone peak. Am J Obstet Gynecol 132:629–641

Daniell JF, Miller W (1987) Hysteroscopic correction of cornual occlusion with resultant term pregnancy. Fertil Steril 48:490–493

DeCherney AH (1987) Anything you can do, I can do better – or differently. Fertil Steril 48:374–376

DeCherney AH (1995) Infertility; we're not taking new patients. Fertil Steril 64:470–474

DeCherney AH, Kase N (1981) A comparison of treatment for bi-lateral fimbrial occlusion. Fertil Steril 35:162–167

Donnez J, Casanas-Roux F (1986) Prognostic factors influencing the pregnancy rate after micro-surgical cornual anastomosis. Fertil Steril 46:1089–1092

Elder MG, Myatt L, Chandhun G (1977) The role of prostaglandin in the spontaneous motility of the fallopian tube. Fertil Steril 28:86–92

Fayez JA, Suliman SO (1982) Infertility surgery of the oviduct; comparison between macro-surgery with micro-surgery. Fertil Steril 37:73–78

Gillett WR, Herbison GP (1989) Tubo-cornual anastomosis; surgical considerations and co-existent infertility factors in determining the prognosis. Fertil Steril 51:241–246

Hayashi N, Kimoto T, Sakai T, et al. (1994) Fallopian tube disease; limited value of treatment with fallopian tube catheterization. Radiology 190:141–144

Hedgpeth PL, Thurmond AS, Fry R, Schmidgall JR, Rosch J (1991) Radiographic fallopian tube recanalization; absorbed ovarian radiation dose. Radiology 180:121–122

Hershlag A, Diamond MP, DeCherney AH (1989) Tubal physiology; an appraisal. J. Gynecol Surg 5:3–25

Hodgson BJ, Talo A (1978) Spike burst in rabbit oviduct; effects of estrogen and progesterone. Am J Physiol 334:E439

Holtz N, Maltau JN, Forstahl F, Hansen LJ (1991) Handling of tubal infertility after introduction of in vitro fertilization; changes and consequences. Fertil Steril 55:140–143

Jacobs LA, Lapthie J, Patton PE, Williams TJ (1988) Primary micro-surgery for post-inflammatory tubal infertility. Fertil Steril 50:855–859

Jansen RPS, Anderson JC (1987) Catheterization of the fallopian tubes from the vagina. Lancet II:309–310

Jean Y, Langlais J, Roberts KB, Chapdelaine A, Bleu T (1979) Fertility of women with non-functional ciliated cells in the fallopian tubes. Fertil Steril 31:349–354

Jones HW Jr, Rock JA (1983) Reparative and constructive surgery of the female generative tract. Williams & Wilkins, Baltimore, MD.

Karande VC, Rao R, Pratt VE, et al. (1995) A randomized perspective comparison between intrauterine insemination and fallopian sperm perfusion for treatment of infertility. Fertil Steril 64:638–640

Keltz MD, Kliman HJ, Arici AM, Olive VL (1995) Endosalpingosis found at laparocolostomy for chronic pelvic pain. Fertil Steril 64:482–486

Kerin J, Dayhovsky L, Grundfest W, Surrey E (1990) Falloscopy a micro-endoscopic transvaginal technique for diagnosing and treating endo-tubal disease incorporating guidewire canulation and direct balloon tuboplasty. J Reprod Med 35:606–612

Kornega M, Kadota T (1981) Changes in mechanical properties of the circular muscles of the isthmus of the human fallopian tube in relation to hormonal domination and postovulatory time. Fertil Steril 36:343–351

Kumpe DA, Zwerdlinger SC, Rothbarth LJ, Durham JD, Albrecht BH (1990) Proximal fallopian tube occlusion; diagnosis and treatment with transcervical fallopian tube catheterization. Radiology 177:183–187

LaBerge JM, Pomec VJ, Gordon RL (1990) Fallopian tube catheterization; modified flouroscopic technique. Radiology 176:283–284

Lang EK (1990) Selective salpingography and transvaginal bougie dilation of strictures of the fallopian tubes. Digitale Bildgebung. Schneider, Berlin, pp 347–352

Lang EK (1991a) Organic versus functional obstruction of the fallopian tubes; differentiation with prostaglandin antagonist and beta agonist mediated hysterosalpingography and selective ostialsalpingography. AJR 157:77–80

Lang EK (1991b) Ostialsalpingography and transvaginal fallopian tube recanalization. Contemp Diagn Radiol 14:1–5

Lang EK (1995) Transvaginal recanalization of occluded fallopian tubes. Minimally Invasive Therapy 4:129–135

Lang EK, Dunaway HH (1994) Transcervical recanalization of strictures of the post-operative fallopian tube. Radiology 191:507–512

Lang EK, Dunaway HH (1996) Recanalization of obstructed fallopian tube by selective salpingrography and transvaginal bougie dilation; outcome and cost analysis. Fertil Steril 66:210–215

Lang EK, Dunaway HE, Roniger WE (1990) Selective ostialsalpingography and transvaginal catheter dilatation in the diagnosis and treatment of fallopian tube obstruction. AJR 154:735–740

Lang EK, Doody MC, Dunaway HH (1992) Ostialsalpingography and transcervical percutaneous recanalization of the proximal tubes. Lippincott's Review Radiology 1:547–561

Laŭritsen JP, Pagel JD, Vangsted P, Starŭp J (1982) Results of repeated tuboplastics. Fertil Steril 37:68–72

Lavy G, Diamond MP, DeCherney AH (1986) Pregnancy following tubocornual anastomosis. Fertil Steril 46:21–25

Letterie GS, Sakas EL (1991) Histology of proximal tubal obstruction in cases of unsuccessful tubal canalization. Fertil Steril 56:831–835

Lindblom B, Hamberger L, Ljumg B (1980) Contractile patterns of isolated oviductal smooth muscle under different hormonal conditions. Fertil Steril 33:283–294

Lisse K, Sydow P (1991) Fallopian tube catheterization and recanalization under ultrasound observation; a simplified technique to evaluate tubal pregnancy and open proximally obstructed tubes. Fertil Steril 56:198–201

Molloy D, Doody ML, Breen T (1995) Second time around: a study of patients seeking second assisted reproduction pregnancies. Fertil Steril 64:546–551

Maubon A, Thurmond A, Laurent A, Honiger J, Scanlan R, Rouanet JP (1994) Selective tubal sterilization in rabbits; experience with hydrogel combined with sclerosing agent. Radiology 193:721–723

Meyerovitz MF (1991) Hysterosalpingography and fallopian tube cannulation; use of double balloon introducing catheters. Radiology 181:901–902

Movsepian DM, Eschelman DJ, Shapiro MY, Sullivan Kl, Cardiver GA Jr (1994) Fallopian tube recanalization in an unrestricted patient population. Radiology 190:137–141

Musich J, Behrman S (1983) Surgical management of tubal obstruction at the utero-tubal junction. Fertil Steril 40:423–440

Muzii L, Marana R, Mancŭso S (1996) Distal fallopian tube occlusion: false diagnosis with hysterosalpingography in cases of tubal diverticula. Radiology 199:469–472

Nakamura K, Ishŭgŭchit T, Maekoshi H, et al. (1996) Selective fallopian tube catheterization in female infertility and absorbed radiation dose. Eur Radiol 6:465–469

Neumann PJ, Weinstein MC, Gharib ST (1994) The cost of a successful delivery with invitro fertilization. N Engl J Med 331:329–343

Novy MJ (1994) Concurrent tuboplasty and assisted reproduction. Fertil Steril 62:242–245

Patton PE, Williams TJ, Coulam CB (1987) Micro-surgical reconstruction of the proximal oviduct. Fertil Steril 47:35–39

Petersen BD, Rosch T (1994) Complications of fallopian tube recanalization. Cardiovasc Intervent Radiol 11:237–239

Platia MP, Krudy AG (1985) Transvaginal fluoroscopic recanalization of proximally occluded oviduct. Fertil Steril 44:704–706

Risquesz F, Confino E (1993) Transcervical tubal recanalization of past, present and future. Fertil Steril 60:211–226

Rock JA (1983) Reconstruction of the fallopian tube. In: Jones HW Jr, Rock JA (eds) Reparative and constructive surgery of the female genital tract. Williams and Wilkins, Baltimore, MD, pp 381–410

Rock JA, Katyama P, Martin EJ, Wodruff JD, Jones AW Jr (1978) Factors influencing the success of salpingostomy techniques for distal fimbrial obstruction. Obstet Gynecol 52:591–596

Rock JA, Bergquist CA, Kimball AW Jr, et al. (1984) Comparison of the operating microscope and loupe for microsurgical tubal anastomosis; a randomized clinical trial. Fertil Steril 41:229–235

Rubin IC (1954) Utero-tubal insufflation; value in treatment of tubal obstruction to ovular migration. Fertil Steril 4:311–323

Russell JB, DeCherney AH, Laufer N, Poland ML, Naftolin F (1986) Neosalpingostomy; comparison of twenty-four and seventy-two months follow-up time shows increased pregnancy rate. Fertil Steril 45:296–298

Sandberg FA, Ingelman-Sandberg A, Ryden G (1963) The effects of prostaglandin E on the human uterus and on the fallopian tubes invitro. Acta Obstet Gynecol Scand 42:269–278

Schlaff WD, Hassiagkos DK, Damewood MD, Rock JA (1990) Neosalpingostomy for distal tubal obstruction; prognostic factors and impact of surgical technique. Fertil Steril 54:984–990

Schmitz-Rode T, Ross P, Timmermans H, Thurmond AS, Gunther R, Rosch J (1994) Experimental non-surgical female sterilization; transcervical implantation of microspindels in fallopian tubes. J Vasc Intervent Radiol 5:905–90a

Schroder C (1884) Die Excision von Ovarientumoren mit Erhaltung des Ovarium. Zentralbl Gynakol 8:716–721

Shapiro BS, Diamond MP, DeCherney AH (1988) Salpingoscopy, an adjunct technique for evaluation of the fallopian tube. Fertil Steril 49:1176–1181

Shushan A, Eisenberg VH, Schenker JG (1995) Sub-fertility in the area of assisted reproduction; changes and consequences. Fertil Steril 64:459–469

Snoden EU, Jarrett JC, Dawood MY (1984) Comparison of diagnostic accuracy of laparoscopy, hysteroscopy and hysterosalpingography in evaluation of female infertility. Fertil Steril 41:709–713

Spilman GH, Harper MJK (1974) Comparison of the effects of adrenergic drugs and prostaglandins on rabbit oviductal motility. Biol Reprod 10:549–556

Society Assisted Reproductive Technology (1996) Assisted reproductive technology in the United States and Canada: 1994 results generated from the American Society for Reproductive Medicine – Reproductive Technology Registry. Fertil Steril 66:697–705

Strom CH, Dahlstron A, Lindblom B, Ahlman H (1983) Effects of intra-luminal administration of adrenoreceptor agonists on transisthmic flow in the rabbit oviduct. Biol Reprod 29:295–316

Sulak PJ, Letterie GS, Coddington CC, Hayslip CC, Woodward JE, Klein TA (1987) Histology of proximal tubal occlusion. Fertil Steril 48:437–440

Swart P, Mol BWJ, Van der Veen F, Van Beurden M, Radekap WK, Bossuyt PMM (1995) The accuracy of hysterosalpingography in the diagnosis of tubal pathology: a meta-analysis. Fertil Steril 64:486–491

Thurmond AS (1992) Transcervical fallopian tube recanalization. Semin Intervent Radiol 9:80–86

Thurmond AS (1994) Pregnancy after selective salpingography and tubal recanalization. Radiology 190:11–15

Thurmond AS, Rosch J (1990) Non-surgical fallopian tube recanalization for treatment of infertility. Radiology 174:371–374

Thurmond AS, Rosch J, Patton PE, Burry KA, Novy MJ (1988a) Fluroscopic transcervical fallopian tube catheterization for diagnosis and treatment of female infertility caused by tubal obstruction. Radiographics 8:621–640

Thurmond AS, Novy MJ, Rosch J (1988b) Terbutaline in diagnosis of interstitial fallopian tube obstruction. Invest Radiol 23:209–210

Thurmond AS, Uchida BT, Rosch J (1990) Device for hysterosalpingography in fallopian tube catherization. Radiology 174:571–572

Thurmond AS, Hedgpeth PL, Scanlan RM (1991) Selective injection of contrast medium; inflammatory effects on rabbit's fallopian tube. Radiology 180:97–99

Thurmond AS, Torres MK, Mullik B, Kessel E (1995) Reversal of sterilization due to application of quinacrine by means of transcervical tubal catheterization. J Vasc Intervent Radiol 6:147–150

Thie JL, Williams TJ, Coulam CD (1986) Repeat tubo-plasty compared with primary micro-surgery for post inflammatory tubal disease. Fertil Steril 45:784–788

Tulandi T, Vilos GA (1985) A comparison between laser surgery and electro surgery for bi-lateral hydrosalpinx; a two-year follow-up. Fertil Sertil 44:846–851

Urman B, Gomel B, McComb P, Lee N (1992) Mid-tubal occlusion; etiology management and outcome. Fertil Steril 57:747–750

Vasquez G, Vemer HM, Boeckx WD, Brasens IA (1984) Ciliogenesis following salpingostomy of rabbit hydrosalpinx. Eur J Obstet Gynecol Reprod Biol 18:103–107

Wadin K, Lonuemark M, Rasmussen C, et al. (1994) Frequency of proximal tubal obstruction in patients undergoing infertility evaluation. Acta Radiol 35:357–362

Winfield AC, Pittaway D, Maxson W, Daniell J, Went AC (1982) Apparent cornual occlusion in hysterosalpingography; reversal by glucagon. AJR 139:525–527

Winston RML (1977) Micro-surgical tubo cornual anastomosis for reversal of sterilization. Lancet 1:284–288

# 14 Interventional Radiologic Procedures in the Management of Inflammatory and Neoplastic Conditions in the Female Pelvis

E.K. Lang, P. Baharamipour, and Y.T. Patel

CONTENTS



E.K. Lang, MD, Professor of Radiology and Urology, Department of Radiology School of Medicine, Louisiana State University Medical Center, 1543 Tulane Avenue, New Orleans, LA 70122-2822, USA
P. Bahramipour, MD, Assistant Professor of Radiology, Department of Radiology, UMDNJ – New Jersey Medical School, 150 Bergen Street, Newark, NJ 07103, USA
Y.T. Patel, MD, Associate Professor of Clinical Radiology, Director, Division of Vascular and Interventional Radiology, UMDNJ – New Jersey Medical School, 150 Bergen Street, Newark, NJ 07103-2406, USA

## 14.1 Percutaneous Drainage of Pelvic Abscesses

Surgical drainage in conjunction with antibiotic therapy has been the accepted treatment for deep pelvic abscesses for the past 5 decades. With the advent of imaging modalities such as ultrasound and computed tomography (CT), permitting precise localization and characterization of abscess cavities, percutaneous drainage by guided interventional radiologic techniques has become popular. Percutaneous drainage techniques have been shown to be safe, efficacious, and inexpensive and to entail little morbidity. In most instances, percutaneous drainage is instituted with the intent of definitive eradication of the abscess. Palliative drainage may be indicated in some complex abscesses with the intent of improving the patient's general condition to make possible definitive eradication of the process by a later surgical intervention (Mueller et al. 1987).

### 14.1.1 Selection of Patients

Tubo-ovarian abscesses deep pelvic abscesses caused by a variety of conditions such as pelvic inflammatory disease, diverticulitis, appendicitis, Crohn's disease, pancreatitis, visceral perforations, prior surgical interventions, necrotic pelvic tumors, pyometria, infected hematomas, or necrotic and infected tumors – are generally amenable to percutaneous drainage (Johnson 1994; Mueller et al. 1989; Nunez et al. 1986).

### 14.1.2 General Concepts of Percutaneous Drainage

Following established surgical dictums, the drainage tube should enter the abscess cavity at its most dependent point. Violation or perforation of other organs should be avoided. If at all possible the drainage route should be extraperitoneal (McDowell and Mueller 1995). In female patients, the following drainage routes to deep pelvic abscesses are feasible: (a) transabdominal, (b) transvaginal, (c) transrectal, (d) transgluteal, and (e) transperineal. Transvaginal drainage is often the preferred route for abscesses located in the cul-de-sac, tubo-ovarian abscesses, abscesses originating from the parametria, or other inflammatory processes of the female genital organs (Alexander et al. 1994; Feld et al. 1994; McGahan et al. 1996; Nosher et al. 1987; Tyrrel et al. 1990; VanDerKolk 1991; van Sonnenberg 1991a). Most of the abscesses, however, are also drainable via a transabdominal, transrectal, transperineal, or transgluteal approach (Bennett et al. 1992; Butch et al. 1968; Carmody et al. 1993; Casola et al. 1992; Gazelle et al. 1991; Longo et al. 1993; Mauro et al. 1985; Nosher et al. 1986; Pereira et al. 1996; Tyrrel et al. 1990). Abscesses representing complications of diverticulitis, appendicitis, or Crohn's disease are frequently best drained via a transabdominal approach (Johnson 1994; Mueller et al. 1987; Nunez et al. 1986) (Fig. 14.1).

### 14.1.3 Indications

Fever, elevated white cell count, presence of fluid collection in the pelvis and sometimes lower abdominal pain, dysuria, frequency of micturition, and change in bowel habits are indications for guided percutaneous aspiration and usually drainage. Needle aspiration of fluid under ultrasound, CT, or magnetic resonance imaging (MRI) guidance, is the first step, with examination of the aspirate for presence of bacteria (Gram stain) and culture and sensitivity studies (Feld et al. 1994). Recently aspiration of the abscess followed by lavage with reduced amounts of saline (less than 50% of the fluid aspirated) has been advocated as a sole intervention to treat deep-seated pelvic abscesses (Kuligowska et al. 1995). In general, however, aspiration alone is advocated only if the aspirate is not overly turbid and the Gram stain negative. Particularly in the presence of thick pus, placement of a drainage catheter followed by drainage for a prolonged period is advocated (Johnson 1994).

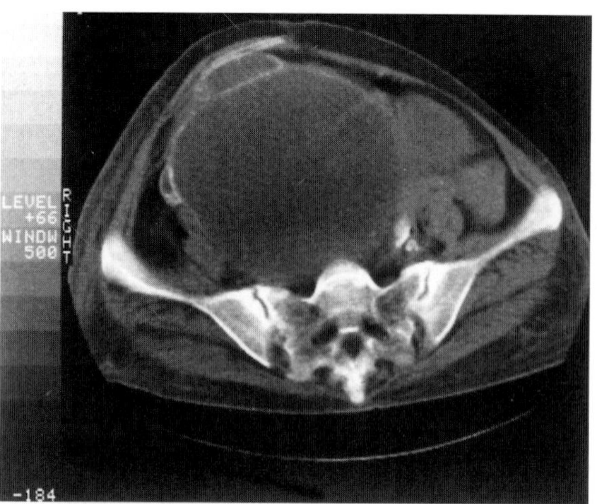


a

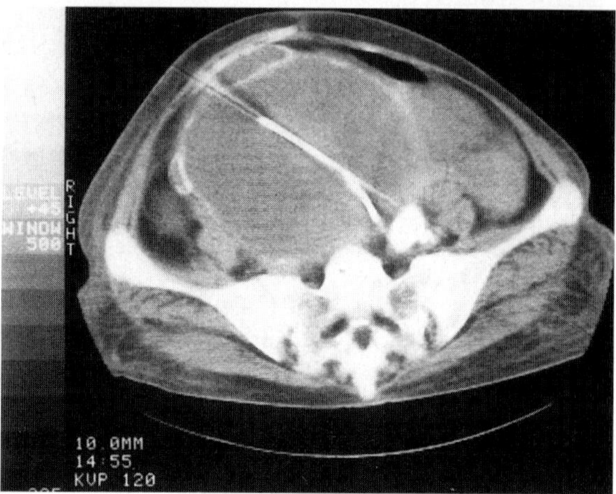


b

**Fig. 14.1.** **a** A huge abscess is demonstrated in the true pelvis adhering to the anterior abdominal wall. **b** A percutaneous drainage catheter has been introduced via an anterior transabdominal approach. A firm adhesion of the abscess membrane to the anterior abdominal wall makes this an "extraperitoneal" approach

### 14.1.4 Technical Considerations

Computed tomography, particularly after enhancement with intravenous contrast medium, offers criteria for assessment of the age, maturity, and thickness of the abscess membrane. Whether an abscess should be drained by a single catheter or by placement of multiple catheters depends on the accessibility of loculated components and the degree of compartmentalization of the abscess. Layering of debris alerts the physician to the need for a large-bore catheter to evacuate such accumulations effectively. The presence of gas bubbles in an abscess may indicate the presence of a gas-forming abscess or communication to the bowel, bladder, vagina, uterus, or, rarely, fallopian tubes (Papanicolaou et al. 1987; Schuster et al. 1992). In general the abscess is accessed under imaging guidance with an 18- or 20-gauge needle and some of its contents aspirated. The aspirate is assessed for turbidity and viscosity and a Gram stain is performed. Unless sterile fluid collection is indicated by the above-mentioned indicators, one should proceed to place a permanent drainage device. Technically this can be accomplished utilizing a Seldinger technique, i.e., introducing a guidewire through the needle, establishing a tract by successive dilation with Teflon dilators and finally placing a drainage catheter of appropriate size. Another option is to place a catheter utilizing a trocar device and to enter the abscess cavity "in tandem," i.e., parallel to the needle that has established the presence of the abscess (Eschelmann and Sullivan 1993).

Initially as much of the abscess content as possible is aspirated. The amount of the aspirate is recorded and can be correlated to the volume calculated on the prior diagnostic computed tomogram or sonogram. Both the initial needle and the catheter are placed such as to avoid injury and/or transection of other organs and bowel loops and damage to vessels or nerves. Whenever possible an extraperitoneal path is preferred (Johnson 1994).

After 1–2 days of successful drainage, lavage of the abscess cavity with saline may be instituted. The amount of lavage fluids utilized should never exceed 50% of the amount aspirated in the prior 24-h period. In the presence of extremely viscous aspirate or aspirate containing blood clots, 100 000–200 000 units urokinase and/or high osmolar compounds may be administered to liquefy the content. After 2–4 days of drainage, reassessment of the residual abscess cavity is indicated. If CT is utilized a small amount of a water-soluble contrast medium (1 ml of contrast medium in 5–10 ml of saline) should be introduced into the cavity 1 h prior to obtaining the scan and retained by clamping of the catheter. This serves to identify whether loculation has occurred or whether the abscess cavity has been effectively drained from the present catheter position. If loculated components are identified, placement of a second catheter or adjustment of the catheter position after penetrating the septa is necessary.

Defervescence will occur in most patients within 24–48 h. Drainage, however, should be pursued until there is cessation of drainage. The presence of fistulas to the bowel, bladder, or uterus may mandate prolonged drainage of up to 3 months (Papanicolaou et al. 1987; Schuster et al. 1992).

Triple antibiotic therapy should be initiated just prior to attempted abscess drainage and maintained until results of cultures from the aspirate or of blood and urine cultures mandate the use of different antibiotics. Antibiotic therapy should be continued for at least 10 days even though there may be defervescence and cessation of drainage after 1 or 2 days.

### 14.1.5 Drainage Routes

Transabdominal drainage can be performed under ultrasound, CT, MRI, or sometimes even fluoroscopic guidance. An extraperitoneal path avoiding the bowel and vascular and genitourinary structures should be selected (McDowell and Mueller 1995). All sideholes of the drainage catheter should be within the abscess cavity to avoid inadvertent contamination of other spaces. The drainage catheter should be advanced to the cephalad-most extent of the abscess and gradually retracted, commensurate with progressive shrinkage and diminution of the abscess cavity under drainage.

### 14.1.6 Transvaginal Drainage

The transvaginal route is ideal for drainage of abscesses in the cul-de-sac, tubo-ovarian abscesses, and other deep pelvic abscesses (Alexander et al. 1994; Bret et al. 1992; Eschelmann and Sullivan 1993; Feld et al. 1994; McGahan et al. 1996; Nosher et al. 1987; Sanchez et al. 1992; VanDerKolk 1991; vanSonnenberg et al. 1991a,b). It can be performed under CT guidance, visual colposcopic guidance, or ultrasound guidance, or using an ultrasound probe with an interventional channel. Endovaginal ultrasound provides excellent images of the internal detail of such abscesses. The location of the vaginal surface to the abscess can be accurately established (Nosher et al. 1987; VanDerKolk 1991; vanSonnenberg et al. 1991a). Generally the wall of the abscess is no further than 2 cm from the transducer (Fig. 14.2). Most interventional probes are equipped with an instrument channel through which the needle can be advanced (VanDerKolk 1991). If not, the probe should have a channel that provides a deep longitudinal groove through which the needle can be introduced (Alexander et al. 1994). The tip

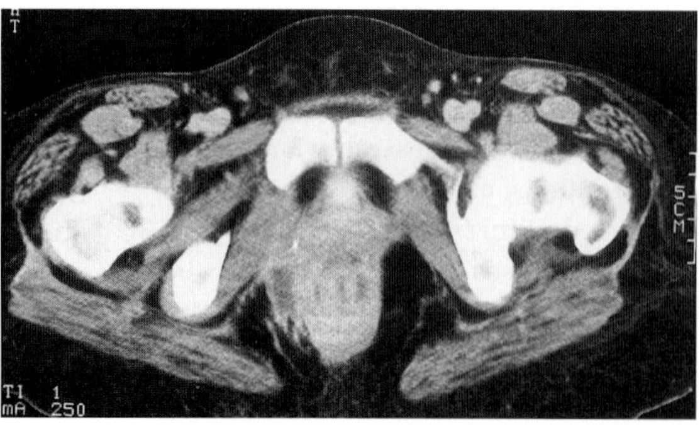

Fig. 14.2. An abscess with a relatively thick wall is identified to the right of the vaginal wall. Separation is by approximately 1.2 cm

of the needle should be etched to facilitate visualization with the endovaginal probe and confirmation of the position of the tip (VANSONNENBERG et al. 1991a). Generally the patient is placed in a lithotomy position. The fornix is sterilized with a povidone-iodine solution and the transducer advanced into the posterior fornix. A local anesthetic is injected and then the needle is advanced under ultrasound guidance into the cavity. If an 18-gauge thin needle is used, a stiff Amplatz or glide guidewire can be advanced into the abscess cavity and coiled. After removal of the endovaginal probe, the tract is dilated with a 6- and 7-French Teflon dilator. A small stab incision along the guidewire tends to facilitate this task. Thereafter a catheter of appropriate caliber is seated and attached to straight drainage. The catheter can be secured with tape against the leg of the patient. Drainage under CT, transabdominal ultrasound, or visual guidance through the colposcope is performed in a similar fashion, identifying the posterior fornix visually and advancing the tip of the perforating needle to its location in the abscess under transabdominal ultrasound or CT guidance (Fig. 14.3).

### 14.1.7 Transrectal Drainage

The problem of interposed bowel, genitourinary, or vascular structures can be addressed by transrectal drainage under radiologic guidance (BENNETT et al. 1992). An endorectal ultrasound probe or transabdominal ultrasound or CT can be used for localization (BENNETT et al. 1992; CARMODY et al. 1993; GAZELLE et al. 1991; KASTAN et al. 1996; LOMAS et al. 1992; MAURO et al. 1985; NOSHER et al. 1986; PEREIRA et al. 1996; SAVADER et al. 1990).

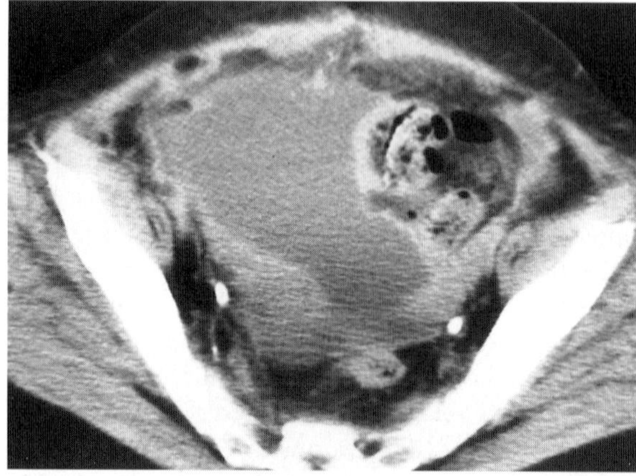

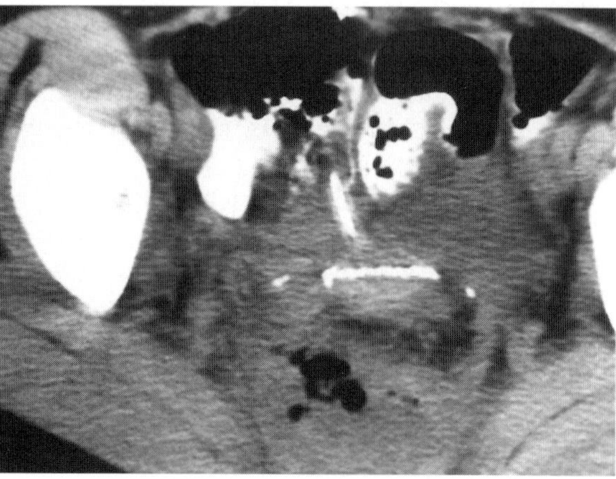

Fig. 14.3. **a** A large abscess extends from the cul-de-sac posteriorly and anteriorly, displacing the sigmoid colon to the left. **b** Under CT control a drainage catheter has been advanced through the anterior vaginal fornix into the abscess, which has been decompressed by aspiration of 120 ml of pus. Contrast medium has been injected to assess for loculated components

Transrectal abscess drainage is a time-honored surgical technique with an excellent performance and safety record. Although transrectal ultrasound guidance provides the easiest access, transabdominal ultrasound and CT have been used successfully for guidance (GAZELLE et al. 1991; NOSHER et al. 1986) (Fig. 14.4).

Transrectal drainage under transabdominal ultrasound or CT control can be performed by introducing a standard barium port tube into the rectum and occluding the barium port with an appropriately sized rubber stopper (BENNETT et al. 1992). The patient is then placed in a left lateral decubitus position and the rectum distended with air. Fluoroscopic, CT, or ultrasound guidance establishes the appropriate trajectory to the abscess, which usually can be seen bulging into the anterior or sometimes the posterior rectal wall. The enema tip is advanced and placed

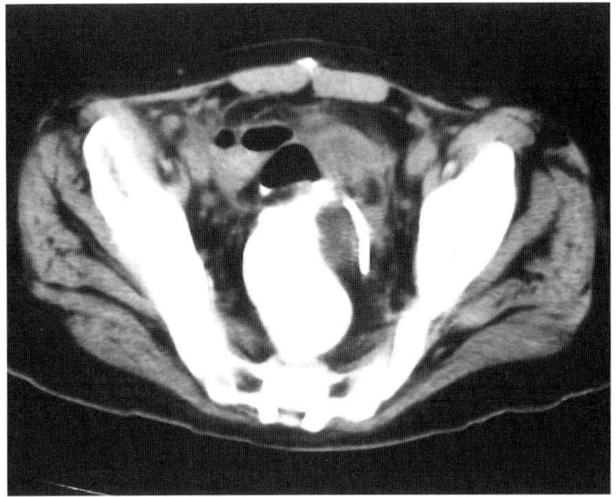

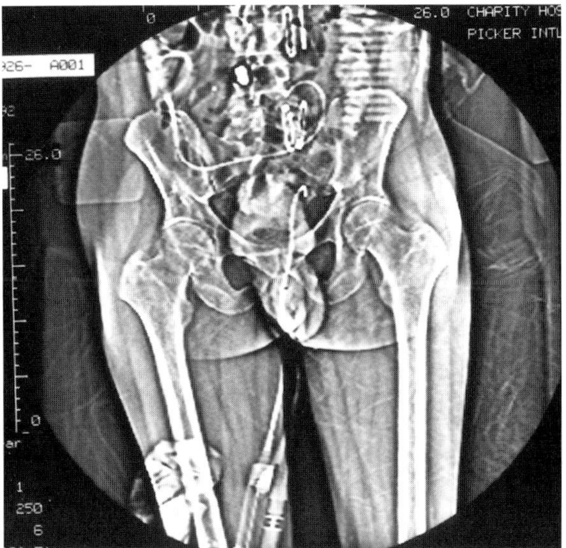

**Fig. 14.4.** **a** A drainage catheter has been introduced into an abscess via a transrectal route under rectal ultrasound guidance. The position is now confirmed on appropriate CT slices. **b** A topogram demonstrates the position of the catheter, which is taped to the thigh of the patient

against the bulging component of the rectal wall and an 18-gauge, thin-wall, 20-cm-long needle is then introduced through the barium port and advanced into the abscess cavity (BENNETT et al. 1992). A distinctive give and pop is felt as the abscess wall is transgressed. Once again a stiff 0.038-in. Amplatz guidewire is then advanced, the tract dilated with 6-, 7-, and 8-French Teflon dilators, and ultimately a self-retaining catheter placed over the guidewire within the abscess. Transrectal ultrasound-guided drainage is most easily accomplished by utilizing an end-firing transrectal ultrasound probe. Once the abscesses have been identified by the transrectal probe and the probe has been appropriately angled, a 20-cm-long 18-gauge needle is advanced along the biopsy guide and the abscess punctured. After removal of the probe a sample is aspirated for culture and sensitivity studies and Gram stain. A 0.038-in. Amplatz guidewire is introduced and coiled in the abscess cavity. After removal of the transrectal ultrasound probe the tract is dilated with Teflon dilators and finally a self-retaining catheter placed within the cavity. Number 10- to 12-French catheters are usually deployed but up to 14-French Malecot catheters can be safely introduced by this procedure. Intermittent suction, drainage, and flushing every 6h with normal saline has been advocated. CT is most useful in identifying the precise location of the abscess in relation to the anterior, lateral, or posterior rectal wall and thus facilitates appropriate puncture and entry into the abscess cavity (BENNETT et al. 1992).

The transrectal approach often offers the shortest and most direct access route to deep-seated pelvic abscesses. However, surgical drainage may not be feasible if the abscess is not palpable by rectal examination. The use of CT or ultrasound eliminates the prerequisite that the abscess be palpable by rectal examination and allows localization of the abscess on the basis of the imaging studies as well as guidance of the needle into the abscess (LONGO et al. 1993).

Premature expulsion of the drainage catheter has been one of the drawbacks of this technique (BENNETT et al. 1992). However, if necessary drainage catheters can be reintroduced to complete the drainage protocol.

### 14.1.8 Transgluteal Drainage

The transgluteal route has been advocated if safe access via the anterior abdominal wall cannot be mapped out. An approach through the greater sciatic foramen is utilized (BUTCH et al. 1968; KELLER 1992; LONGO et al. 1993; VANSONNENBERG, 1992). Once pus is returned a tract is created to accommodate a self-retaining pigtailed catheter using a Seldinger technique (Fig. 14.5). Unfortunately the technique has met with difficulties: hemorrhagic complications as well as excessive pain and even paresis, due to proximity to the nerve, have been reported (KELLER 1992; KOPECHY 1992; MALDEN and PICUS 1992; VANSONNENBERG 1992). Frequent irritation of the sciatic nerve when utilizing a transgluteal approach has often necessitated premature removal of the

a
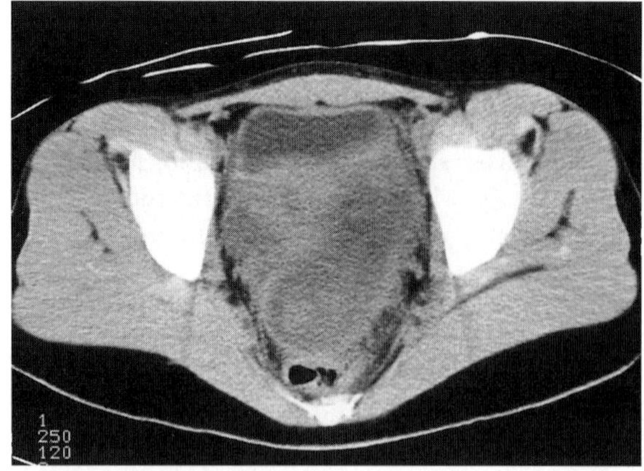


b
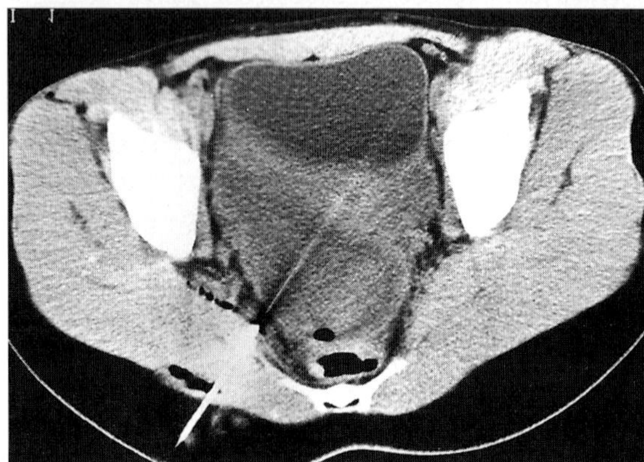

c
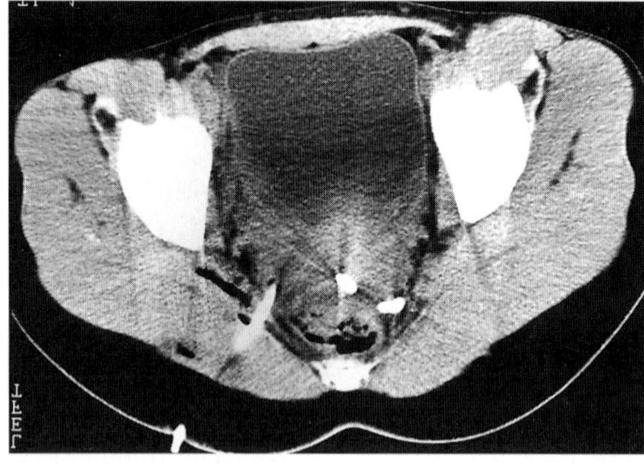

**Fig. 14.5.** **a** CT shows a large abscess in the cul-de-sac. Access via a transabdominal approach seems difficult. **b** An 18-gauge needle has been advanced via a transgluteal route into the abscess. **c** After dilating the tract, a self-retaining pigtail catheter is seated in the abscess. Note the relatively anterior position of the catheter in relation to Alcock's canal and the sciatic nerve

drainage catheter (Casola et al. 1992). Even a posterior approach attempting to avoid the sciatic nerve, which is located posterior to the acetabulum, has not eliminated the problem of nerve irritation, which sometimes may be accentuated by drainage along the catheter and secondary phlegmon in the region of the sciatic notch (Butch et al. 1968; Keller 1992; Bennett et al. 1992; Longo et al. 1993; vanSonnenberg 1992). Hemorrhage following the removal of the drainage catheter is an ominous sign indicating injury to the arterial wall. In at least one patient, transcatheter embolization of the right internal pudendal artery was necessary to control bleeding (Keller 1992). The possibility of traversing vessels when using this concealed approach and the frequency of pain incurred by the position of the catheter next to the sciatic nerve have curtailed the use of this approach. A paracoccygeal route is said to avoid these problems (Longo et al. 1993).

### 14.1.9 Transperineal Drainage

A transperineal route offers ready access to the cul-de-sac in female patients and can be used as an alternative to transvaginal or transrectal drainage (Lomas et al. 1992). This route offers the advantages of better retention of the drainage catheter and lack of expulsion of catheters, which is common with transvaginal and transrectal drainage routes.

### 14.1.10 Tubo-ovarian Abscess Drainage

Tubo-ovarian abscesses may be uni- or bilateral. Most commonly they are drained under CT or transabdominal ultrasound guidance (Tyrrel et al. 1990). Vaginal ultrasound guidance is another excellent modality for drainage of tubo-ovarian abscesses.

Indications for their drainage are persistence of fever, leukocytosis, and pain despite intravenously administered triple antibiotic therapy. If possible antibiotics should be administered intravenously for at least 48 h prior to the procedure. Triple antibiotic therapy is recommended until the offensive organisms are identified from the aspirated sample. Two mg of versed (Midazolan HC) or fentanyl 25 µg is used for conscious sedation. Local anesthesia is accomplished by instillation of 2% lidocaine. A seldinger technique or trocar catheter insertion parallel to a guide needle is commonly favored. Although percutaneous drainage of the tubo-ovarian abscess tends to be highly successful (94% or better), follow-up surgery to remove a pyosalpinx or a phlegmonous uterus may often be necessary

(CASOLA et al. 1992). The mean duration of catheter drainage in such patients is 1 week. The drainage catheter may be removed after defervescence, cessation of drainage and documentation of no residual walled-off abscess cavity on follow-up CT (Fig. 14.6).

Organisms cultured tend to be *Escherichia coli*, enterococcus, *Bacteroides*, *Streptococcus*, and sometimes *Actinomyces*. Choice of appropriate antibiotics on the basis of the culture and sensitivity studies is of paramount importance. Because of the frequent interposition and adherence of bowel loops CT is the method of choice to identify the optimal drainage route. Complications have been reported to occur in 50%–70% of cases with ultrasound guidance but in no cases with CT guidance (TYRREL et al. 1990). Transvaginal, transabdominal, or transrectal access is recommended.

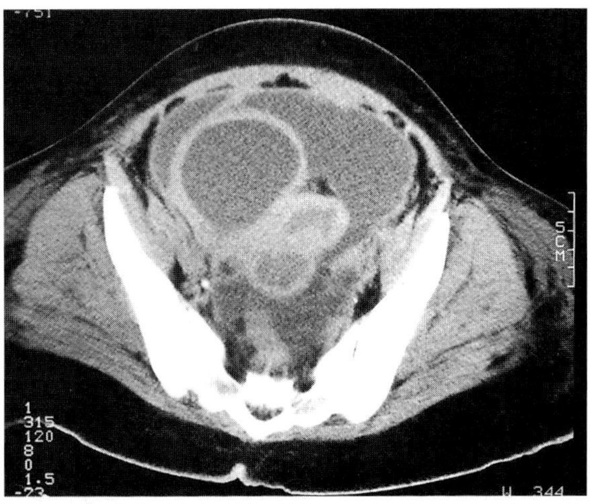

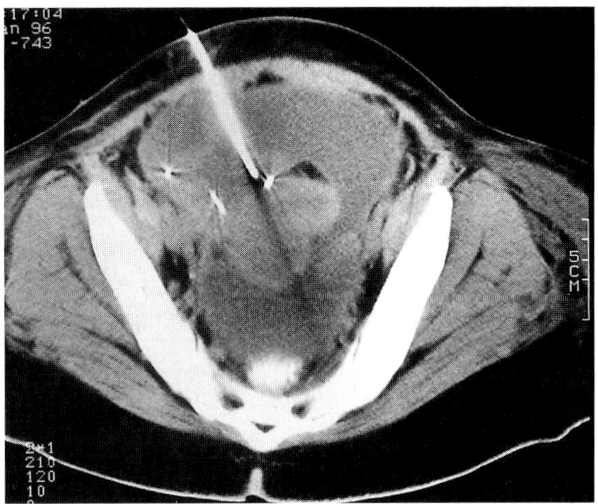

**Fig. 14.6.** **a** The hugely dilated and thick-walled segment of the fimbriated end of the right fallopian tube enveloped by a tubo-ovarian abscess is demonstrated on CT. **b** A CT-guided anterior drainage approach resulted in defervescence and salutary evacuation of the abscess. However, laparoscopic surgical removal of the remaining pyosalpinx was carried out at a later date

## 14.2 Drainage of Lymphatic Cysts

Lymphatic cysts occur after radical node dissection for pelvic neoplasms or with transplanted kidneys and are usually most easily drained under CT guidance (VANSONNENBERG et al. 1986). Thin-needle aspiration will provide an adequate sample for cytologic and biochemical assessment. Treatment by single aspiration is usually unsuccessful in eradicating or preventing recurrence of such cysts. After near-complete evacuation of fluid, alcohol, tetracycline, or doxycycline powder is introduced into the cysts to promote sclerosis of the cysts and prevent recurrence. Often up to ten cycles of treatment are necessary to accomplish this aim (VANSONNENBERG et al. 1986; WHITE et al. 1985).

## 14.3 Other Pelvic Drainage Procedures

Pelvic hematomas likewise can be treated via these access routes (ELCHALAL et al. 1993) (Fig. 14.7). However, the advantage of drainage must be weighed against the risk of secondary infection of the hematoma. Instillation of 100 000 to 200 000 units of urokinase will hasten liquefaction and hence speed up the drainage and evacuation of such hematomas (Fig. 14.8).

Urinomas associated with dehiscence of the ureter, fistulization from the ureters or the breakdown of tumor causing fistulae to the urinary bladder likewise can be drained via these routes (JOHNSON 1994; MUELLER et al. 1989; SANCHEZ et al. 1992). For successful eradication, bypass drainage of urine from the kidneys is mandatory. This can be achieved by percutaneous nephrostomy or, in cases of partial or complete dehiscence of the ureters, by placement of stents bridging the defect and seated in the renal pelvis and bladder respectively (LANG 1985, 1987, 1997a; VANSONNENBERG et al. 1994) (see Sect. 14.6).

Pyometra and hematometra can be drained transcervically (FELD et al. 1994; SANCHEZ et al. 1992). Dilation of the cervical canal is usually necessary to initiate satisfactory drainage. This is accom-

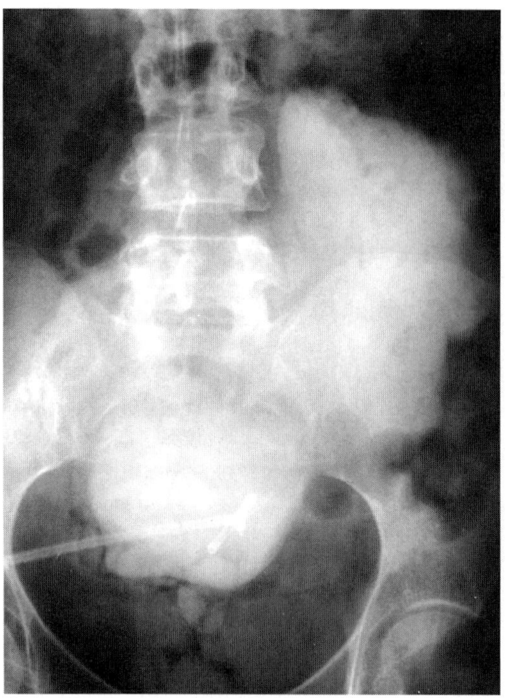

**Fig. 14.7.** A large pelvic hematoma and seroma is drained via an anterior abdominal approach

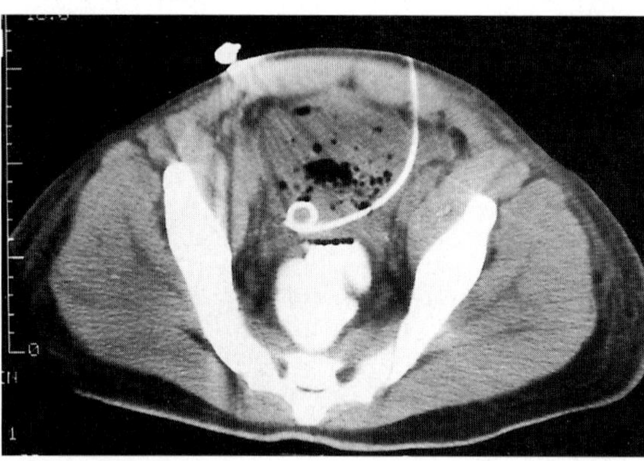

**Fig. 14.8.** After instillation of 200 000 units of urokinase there is liquefaction of a large infected hematoma which can now be drained percutaneously utilizing an approach through the anterior abdominal wall

plished by dilation of the endocervical canal with Hegar dilators or more recently by placing an 8-mm Olbert balloon into the cervical canal and dilating it (DICKEY et al. 1996). Indwelling drainage catheters in the uterine cavity are used to augment drainage and lavage necrotic debris. Hematocolpos is best drained via the vagina.

Necrosis, which is a frequent occurrence in extensive pelvic neoplasms, provides an excellent culture medium for bacteria. The open communication via the vagina explains the frequency of infected and necrotic cervical carcinomas. Drainage is the most important treatment modality (MUELLER et al. 1989). Management by antibiotic therapy alone may not be able to control the process because of the poor vascular perfusion of such necrotic and infected tumors and hence the inability to establish therapeutic levels of antibiotics. Drainage is, of course, of particular importance in the presence of anaerobic infections (Fig. 14.8). Depending on the location of the infected tumor, transvaginal, transrectal, perianal, paracoccygeal, or transabdominal drainage may be pursued (GAZELLE et al. 1991; LOMAS et al. 1992; LONGO et al. 1993; MAURO et al. 1985; MUELLER et al. 1989). Coexisting enteric fistulas, a complication of tissue breakdown of neoplasms invading adjacent organs, mandate specific and prolonged drainage (PAPANICOLAOU et al. 1987; SCHUSTER et al. 1992). Unfortunately, transcatheter embolization of necrotic and bleeding neoplasms can increase the probability of infection. Mere presence of gas in tumors after transcatheter embolization, however, does not necessarily herald the presence of a gas-forming organism but in fact may merely indicate the release of nitrogen in occluded vessels (HARIMA et al. 1995; KIM et al. 1995).

## 14.4 Transcatheter Embolization of Pelvic Vessels

Transcatheter embolization has gained widespread acceptance for controlling extraperitoneal hemorrhage due to pelvic trauma as well as intractable hemorrhage from pelvic neoplasms (AYELLA et al. 1978; GOLDSTEIN et al. 1975; KATZ et al. 1992; LANG et al. 1979). The method has been found equally effective in the management of hemorrhage resulting from orthopedic procedures or genitourinary surgery (particularly transurethral resection of the prostate), bleeding from arteriovenous malformations, bleeding as a late complication of radiation therapy, and even spontaneous puerperal hemorrhage (AYELLA et al. 1978; GOLDSTEIN et al. 1975; HESTON et al. 1979; HENDRICKX et al. 1995; KATZ et al. 1992; LANG et al. 1979; LANG 1981, 1989; MILLER et al. 1976; PISCO et al. 1989; VAN ALLEN and PENTECOST 1992; VOGELZANG et al. 1991; YAMASHITA et al. 1994). The intent in all instances is to curtail bleeding on a temporary, or preferably permanent basis while assuring continued collateral perfusion to prevent ischemic necrosis and sloughs (HENDRICKX et al. 1995).

The occasional failure to control hemorrhage by ligation of one or both hypogastric arteries is explained by data reported by BURCHELL (1968), indicating a drop in pulse pressure of 77% on the ipsilateral side of ligation but of only 14% on the contralateral side, with blood flow decreasing to 49% on the ipsilateral side. Even after bilateral ligation the blood flow rate is reduced to only 48%. An extensive network of precapillaries maintains perfusion and pulse pressure. Therefore occlusion must be carried out at a more peripheral level to be effective (BURCHELL 1968).

Selective and superselective transcatheter embolization techniques permit placement of embolic material at a peripheral location, thus limiting the volume of affected tissue. Moreover, a variety of embolic materials make possible occlusion at a capillary, precapillary, or muscular artery level on a permanent or temporary basis (LANG 1986, 1989, 1997a; YAMASHITA et al. 1994). Judicious selection of the site of embolization and the embolic material will ensure optimal results in curtailing hemorrhage and protecting tissues against avascular necrosis.

## 14.4.1 Technique

In general a Seldinger approach via the femoral or sometimes axillary artery is advocated. For superselective embolization a coaxial system consisting of a 5- or 4-French RC1 and tracker 18 catheters is favored for the femoral approach. The entry is on the contralateral side with the catheter being advanced across the bifurcation into the ipsilateral hypogastric artery. A digital arteriogram is then generated to identify the bleeding site or sites of tumor blush held responsible for the bleed (Fig. 14.9). Superselective catheterization with a tracker 18 system and a 0.015-in. platinum guidewire with a 7-cm flexible tip limits the injection to a restricted volume. The appropriate position of the tracker catheter is verified by a repeat injection of contrast medium recorded in digital format (LANG 1981, 1986; PISCO et al. 1989).

Embolization may proceed at this point. Depending on the volume of tissue supplied from the specific vascular location and the type of process addressed, different embolic materials are utilized (LANG 1981, 1986, 1989, 1997a; YAMASHITA et al. 1994).

Microcoils of 3 × 20 mm can be deployed through the tracker catheter and tend to occlude the embolized vessel, usually at the level above muscular branches. A permanent occlusion will result; however, some collateral circulation to the region may be maintained at the level of precapillaries (LANG 1986). Small Gelfoam particles of approximately 1 $mm^3$ occlude vessels of a slightly larger diameter. Once again, collateral circulation via precapillaries tends to maintain some perfusion of the involved tissues. Moreover occlusion with Gelfoam particles has a propensity for revascularization within about a 3-week period (Fig. 14.10). Ivalon (dehydrated polyvinyl alcohol) particles are available in various sizes from 30 to 500 μm. Depending on the particle size, occlusion at the level of arteries of different size or muscular arterioles will result. A very small particle size results in occlusion at the precapillary level and hence precludes collateral reconstitution of flow. Embolization with Ivalon particles is semipermanent. 6-Cyanoacrylate tends to result in a permanent occlusion not prone to revascularization. Depending on the mixture with contrast medium, the compound will set at different speeds (LANG 1997a). Hence occlusion will occur at a level from branch arteries to the capillary bed. At the dilution level of 1 to 3 with contrast medium, the compound remains liquid until it reaches the capillary bed and will totally occlude the same (LANG 1981, 1986). The occlusion is permanent and no revascularization occurs. Hence tissue sloughs may result. Autologous blood clot or Amicar-reinforced autologous blood clot (aminocaproic acid) provides temporary occlusion. Such clots tend to lyse within 24–96 h, reestablishing flow to the region (AYELLA et al. 1978; LANG 1989).

If restitution of flow is desired, autologous blood clot, Amicar-reinforced autologous blood clot, or Gelfoam particles are preferable. For permanent occlusion coils, microcoils, microspindle, Ivalon particles, and in rare instances 6-cyanoacrylate are the materials of choice (LANG 1989, 1997a).

In some instances selective engagement of the offensive vessel group may be technically impossible. Pharmacologic manipulation of blood flow by intraarterial administration of epinephrine hydrochloride in doses of 5–20 μg will result in constriction of the normal vascular bed but uninhibited flow to the bleeding site. Thus a preferential flow to an area of lower peripheral resistance, i.e. the bleeding site, is created and can be exploited for embolization from a nonselective catheter position (LANG 1981, 1986; PISCO et al. 1989; VAN ALLEN and PENTECOST 1992).

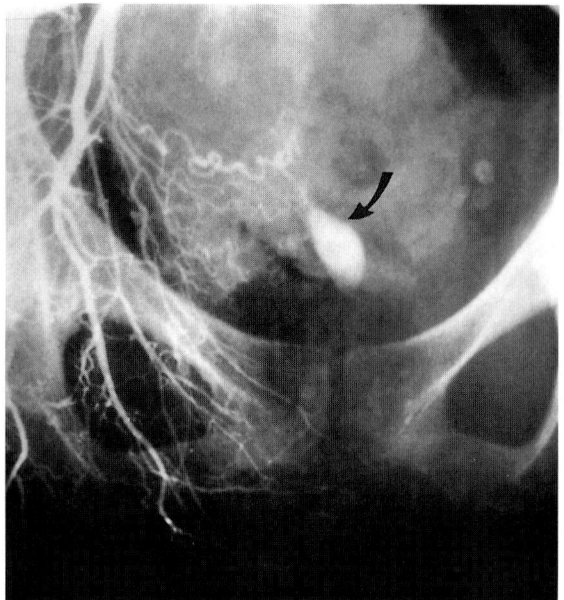

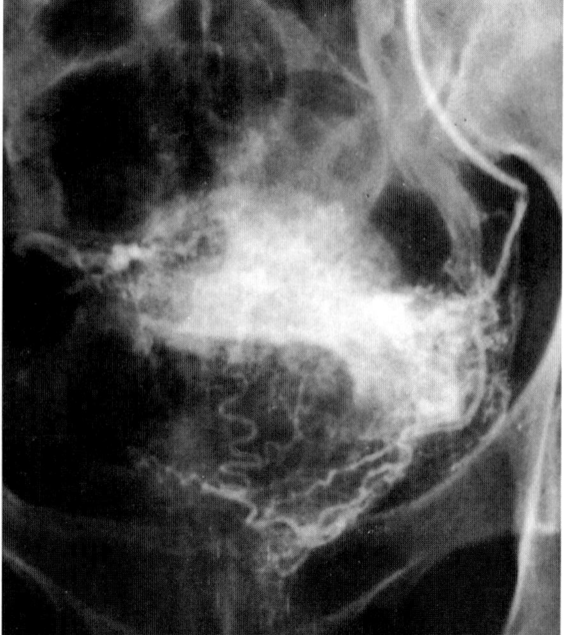

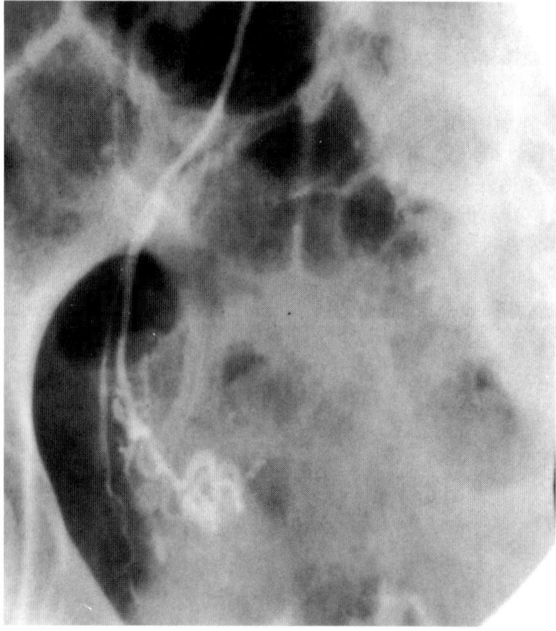

**Fig. 14.9. a** An arteriogram of the right hypogastric artery anterior division demonstrates active bleeding (*arrow*). **b** Superselective embolization with Gelfoam particles has successfully occluded the bleeding branches. **c** In another patient selective injection of the superior and inferior vesicle artery demonstrates a dense tumor blush in the vesicovaginal septum. This tumor extension of a carcinoma of the cervix appeared to be responsible for intractable hemorrhage from the bladder

### 14.4.2 Transcatheter Embolization for Control of Hemorrhage Following Pelvic Trauma

Both arterial and venous bleeding may be responsible for massive blood loss in patients with pelvic trauma. Immediate surgical exploration is fraught with the risk of increasing diffuse venous bleeding after losing the compression effect of fascial compartments. Therefore active arterial bleeding sites should be controlled by transcatheter embolization. Bleeding from small vessels can be satisfactorily controlled by temporary occlusion with autologous blood clot, Amicar-reinforced autologous blood clots, or Gelfoam particles (Ayella et al. 1978; Katz et al. 1992; Lang 1981, 1986, 1997a). Later restitution of flow will minimize ischemic injuries to muscles. In general fibrocytes will seal the bleeding site after occlusion with a clot within 24h.

The presence of bleeding from large vessels or evidence of severance of large vessels, even though they may be occluded by clot at the time of the

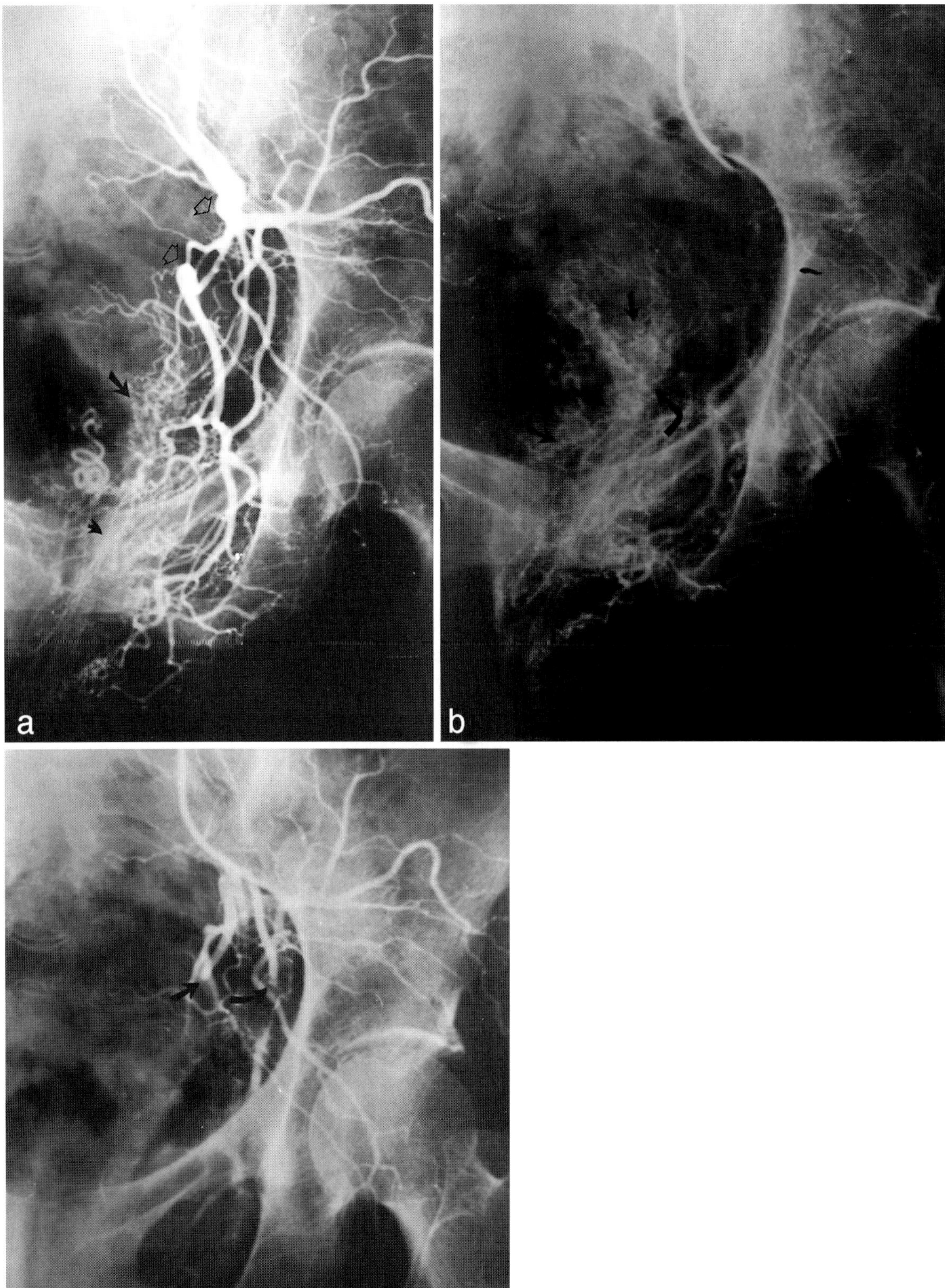


**Fig. 14.10.** **a** The main trunk of the left internal pudendal artery is occluded from prior embolization (*lucent arrows*). Note reconstitution via collaterals and continued massive supply to the tumor-bearing area in the vaginal fornix and parametrium (*black arrows*), resulting again in bleeding. **b** A later phase arteriogram demonstrates the tumor vascularity and dense stain in the parametrium and upper and lower vagina (*curved arrows*). **c** To control recurrent hemorrhage the collateral supply vessels are embolized

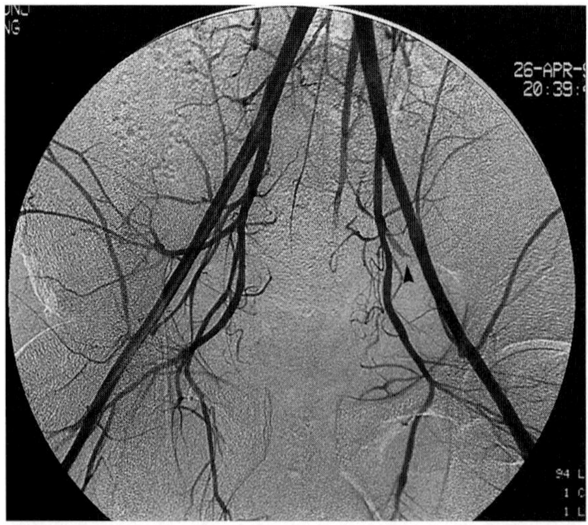


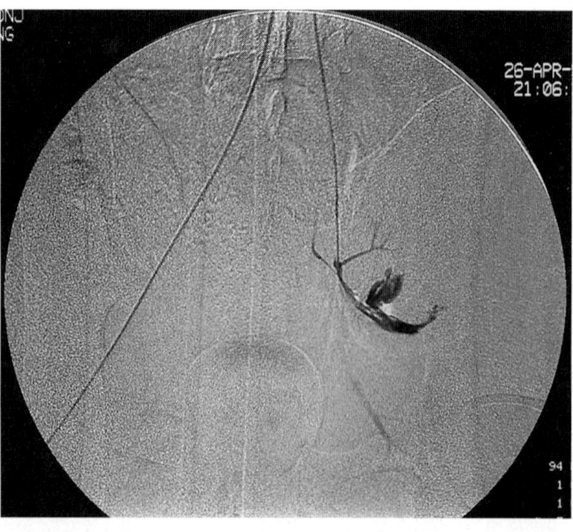


**Fig. 14.11. a** A digital arteriogram demonstrates occlusion of the first segment of the posterior division of the left hypogastric artery (*arrowhead*). **b** A selective injection through a tracker catheter in the first segment of the posterior division of the left hypogastric artery demonstrates extravasation of contrast medium, indicating severance or dehiscence of the vessel which was initially occluded by blood clot. To prevent late hemorrhage embolization with microcoils was carried out

examination, calls for permanent occlusion of the vessels (Fig. 14.11). Coils or microspindles, sometimes in conjunction with Ivalon particles, are favored for this purpose (Carmody et al. 1993). Despite the lack of identifiable bleeding at the time of the examination, permanent occlusion of a larger severed vessel must be carried out since otherwise there is a risk of late hemorrhage after lysis of the clot (Fig. 14.11b). Digital angiography is mandatory to minimize the amount of contrast medium used. Large amounts of contrast medium in conjunction with myoglobin released from muscular injury predispose to renal shutdown.

### 14.4.3 Embolization in Patients with Iatrogenic Hemorrhage

Intractable iatrogenic hemorrhage sometimes occurs after transurethral resection of the prostate and particularly after extensive orthopedic procedures such as total hip replacement. Selective transcatheter embolization is particularly useful in the management of bleeding after extensive orthopedic procedures (Lang 1986). Embolization with short-lived Amicar-reinforced blood clots has been successfully deployed in the management of diffuse bleeding from a TUR site. In general salutary long-term results can be expected.

### 14.4.4 Transcatheter Embolization for Control of Intractable Hemorrhage from Pelvic Neoplasms

Advanced stage female pelvic organ neoplasms not infrequently present with intractable hemorrhage from the primary organ (Lang 1997b). However, intractable hemorrhage may also occur at sites of contiguous extension of such neoplasms, particularly the bladder and rectum. Cautious embolization is advocated. Because of the large volume of tissue usually involved it is prudent to embolize at a level at which some collateral circulation via the precapillaries is preserved (Lang 1997a), otherwise viability of a large tissue volume may be compromised, resulting in later sloughs and repeated episodes of bleeding at times worse than the initial episode.

Not infrequently a precise bleeding site is not identifiable. In this case embolization of staining tumor components suspected to be the source for the bleeding is undertaken (Fig. 14.12). Embolization of ipsi- and contralateral supply vessels, such as the uterine, cervicovaginal, internal pudendal and even obturator group, may be necessary to adequately reduce the pulse pressure and curtail bleeding (Rosenthal and Colapinto 1985). However, in these instances embolization at the level of major vessels of the contralateral group is recommended to allow for some collateral flow (Fig. 14.12c). Semipermanent occlusive material such as Gelfoam particles

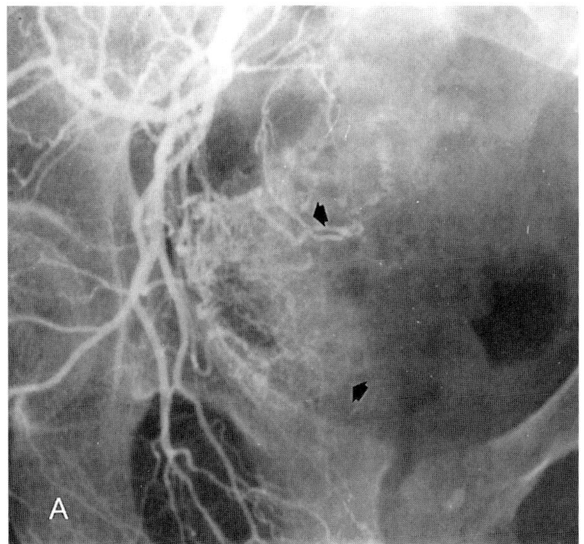


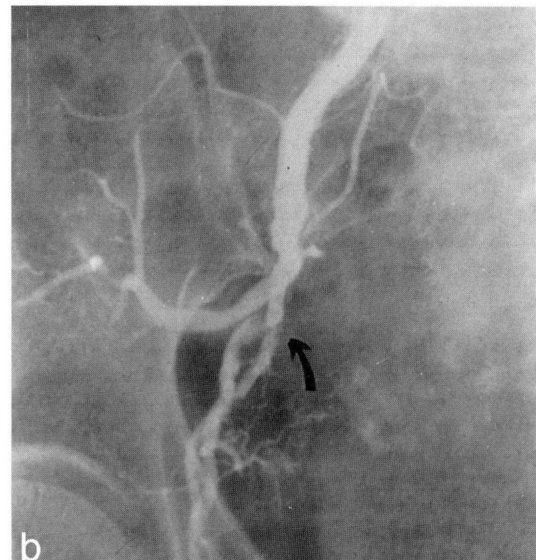


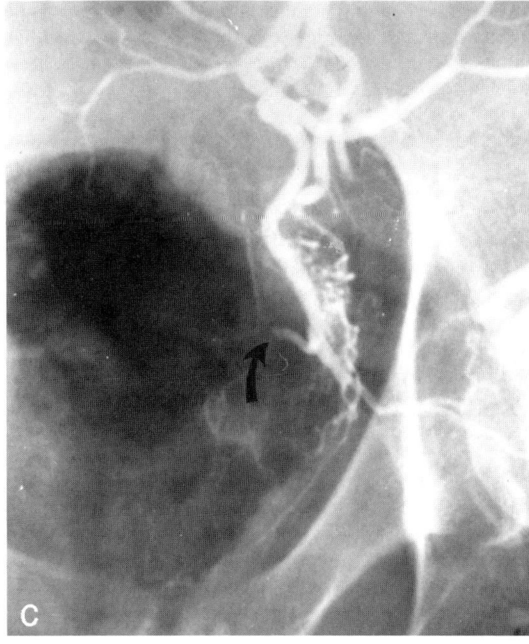


**Fig. 14.12.** **a** A prominent tumor stain is seen in the posterior and right lateral bladder wall. This was attributed to a carcinoma of the cervix contiguously involving the vesicovaginal septum and bladder wall (*arrows*). **b** Selective embolization with Gelfoam particles of the branches of the anterior division of the right hypogastric artery was carried out (*curved arrow*). **c** A similar diffuse involvement of the bladder by neoplasm was demonstrated on the left side. Embolization of the vessels of the contralateral side was carried out to a limited degree (*curved arrow*) to ensure some collateral perfusion of the bladder. (From LANG et al. 1979)

is generally favored. With identifiable bleeding sites, superselective catheterization and placement of microcoils is the procedure of choice (Fig. 14.9b). Occlusion with 6-cyanoacrylate at a distal site is fraught with a high degree of late complications and has been largely abandoned (LANG 1997a).

Technical success of the catheterization procedure can be expected in 98% of patients. Initial control of bleeding is reported to occur in 90%–95% of cases (GOLDSTEIN et al. 1975; GRACE et al. 1976; LANG 1981, 1986, 1997a; MILLER et al. 1976; PISCO et al. 1989; VAN ALLEN and PENTECOST 1992; YAMASHITA et al. 1994). Recurrent bleeds, however, are not infrequent and are reported in the literature to occur in 20%–60% of patients. Depending on the embolic material used and the extent of embolization, complications occur at a rate from 5% to 30% (LANG 1986, 1997a; MILLER et al. 1976; YAMASHITA et al. 1994).

In addition to limiting the amount of tissue affected, embolization of branches of the posterior division of the hypogastric artery should be kept to a minimum. Ischemic damage to the sciatic nerve is one of the dreaded complications of this procedure, extensive muscle necrosis of the gluteal muscle with release of myoglobin and renal shutdown being the other (LANG 1986, 1997a; VAN ALLEN and PENTECOST 1992; YAMASHITA et al. 1994).

### 14.4.5 Selective Arterial Chemotherapy

Selective arterial chemotherapy has been advocated to increase the concentration of the chemotherapeutic agent in tumor-bearing tissues while hopefully decreasing systemic effects (Harima et al. 1995). To some degree this is governed by the percentile extraction of the chemotherapeutic agent during the first passage through the tumor. However, superselective delivery of the chemotherapeutic agents makes the agent available first to the tumor and only after recirculation to other tissues, thus improving binding and extraction at the first tissue barrier. Moreover, combination with embolization can further improve retention of the chemotherapeutic agent in the tumor.

Chemotherapeutic perfusion can be carried out in bolus form, intermittently or continuously. For the latter the catheter is attached to a perfusion pump.

Percutaneous transfemoral catheters can be left in position for 7–10 days (Fig. 14.13). However, position of the catheter must be verified prior to each infusion cycle. Preferably this is done by introducing radioactive microembolic material or radioactive material circulating in the vascular bed such as RISA or tagged red cells in order to verify the perfused tissue on scintiscans. Intermittent flushing of the catheter is necessary to maintain patency when it is not in use. For long-term perfusions over many months, surgical placement of a perfusion catheter and connection to a subcutaneously placed pump reservoir is preferable (Yamada et al. 1996).

Embolization for control of bleeding and superselective arterial chemotherapy as well as chemoembolization are commonly performed for neoplasms of the uterine fundus, cervix, and ovary, and sometimes for neoplasms of the bladder (Harima et al. 1995; Hata et al. 1995; Lang 1997b). In addition to definitive therapeutic intervention, superselective chemotherapy can be used in conjunction with radiation therapy to enhance the radiation therapeutic effect. Particularly in the treatment of bladder neoplasms, salutary experience has been recorded for such protocols.

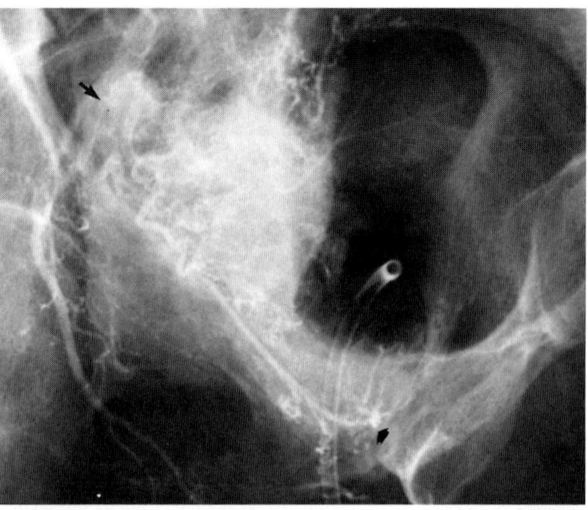

**Fig. 14.13.** A selective injection in the anterior division of the right hypogastri artery demonstrates a prominent tumor stain involving the wall of the bladder as well as staining tumor in the hypogastric lymph nodes (*thin arrow*). Tumor neovascularity is also demonstrated in the urethra (*thick arrow*). Selective arterial chemotherapy was initiated with the catheter in this position

### 14.4.6 Radioactive Infarct Implant

On occasions ulcerated carcinoma of cervix extending to the vulva may become refractory to control by methods such as packing or superficial sclerosing by radium sources. Selective embolization of such vascularized tumors with iodine-125 particles can rapidly deliver a massive dose to the tumor-bearing area and result in sclerosing of the tumor (Lang 1997a) (Fig. 14.14). However, overzealous embolization compromising the vascular supply may have the contrary effect by producing massive sloughs and thence again uncontrollable bleeding.

### 14.4.7 Embolization in the Management of Benign Neoplastic Conditions of the Pelvis

#### *14.4.7.1 Embolization of Uterine Fibroids*

Control of bleeding and pain, as well as shrinkage of uterine fibroids, can be achieved by transcatheter embolization of their vascular supply (Vedantham et al. 1997). The method is advocated in the presence of multiple or extremely large uterine fibroids that would pose technical difficulties for transabdominal leiomyomectomy, laparoscopic myomectomy, or hysteroscopic myomectomy. The method is an attractive alternative to surgical procedures, being highly effective in reducing the size of such leiomyomas and being tolerated by the patient without seeming adverse effects. A variety of techniques

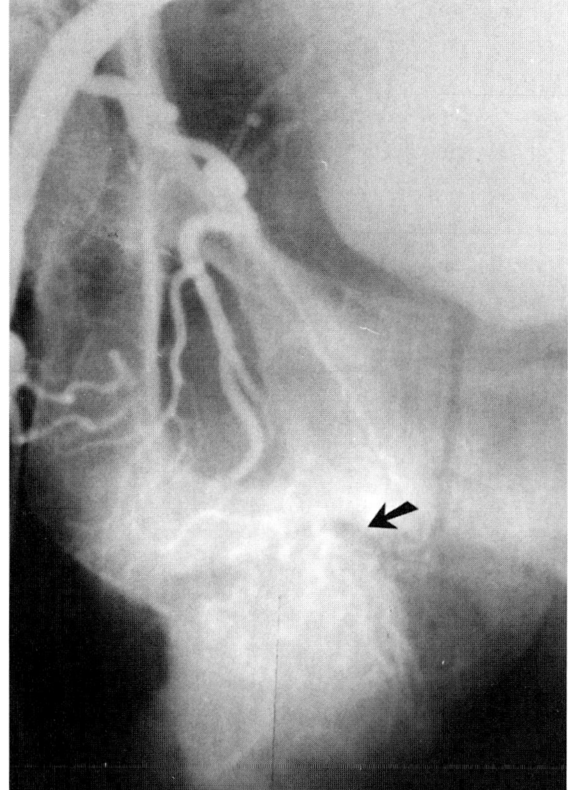

a

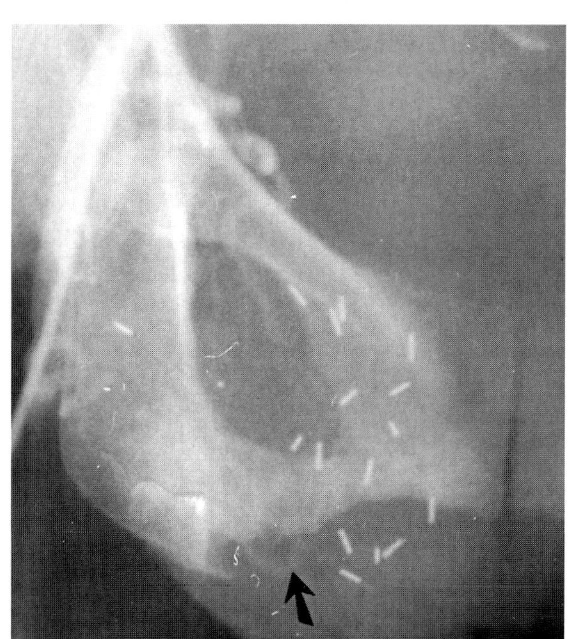

b

Fig. 14.14. **a** Arteriogram demonstrating massive tumor neovascularity (*arrow*) in the region of the vulva and distal third of the vagina. **b** Intractable hemorrhage was controlled by interstitial radiation therapy, the sources being delivered by transcatheter embolization of vessels supplying the tumor-bearing area (*arrow*)

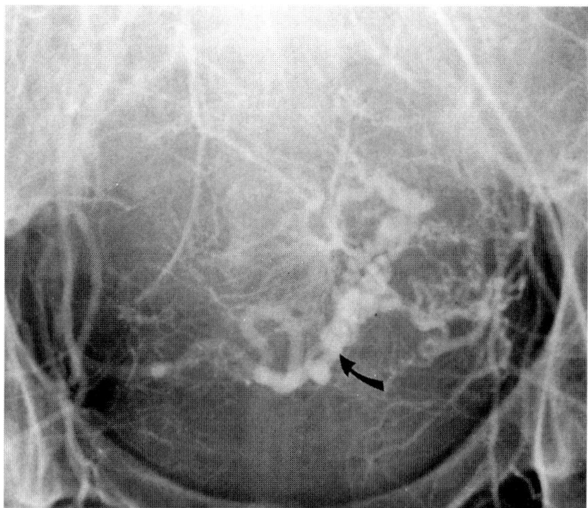

a

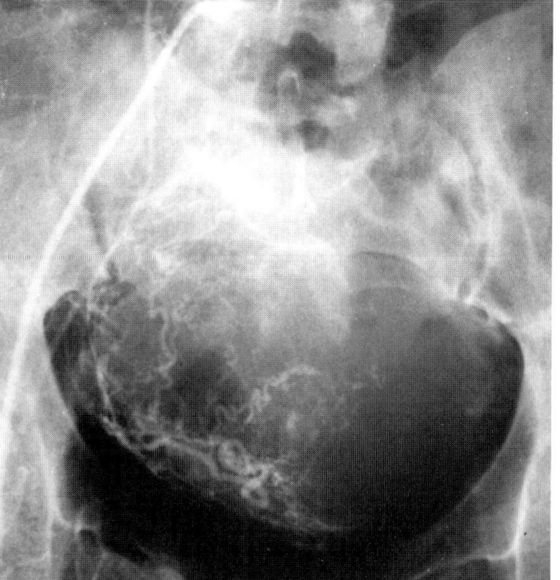

b

Fig. 14.15. **a** The survey arteriogram demonstrates a hugely dilated feeding vessel to a uterine fibroid (*arrow*). **b** Superselective embolization of the feeding vessel to the fibroid has been carried out. The vascular supply to the fundus and cervix is not compromised

have been advocated, ranging from release of embolic particles in both the right and left uterine arteries to superselective catheterization with tracker 18 catheters limiting embolization to the supply of the uterine fibroid (Fig. 14.15). Commonly such fibroids derive supply from both the right and the left uterine artery. Hence, if superselective techniques are used, bilateral superselective catheterization should be carried out. Embolization from a point in the main uterine artery but after pharmacological manipulation of flow by intra-arterial injection of 50 µg of epinephrine hydrochloride has been proposed, with the rationale that vessels of the fibroid do not show a pharmacologic response to epinephrine hydrochloride, while contraction of myometrial vessels protects the normal uterine myometrium against embolic material.

Dehydrated polyvinyl alcohol particles (Ivalon) of 50–500 µm have been successfully used, as have 1 $mm^3$ particles of Gelfoam and Ethiodol. Reproductive function does not appear to be impeded by prior embolization of the vascular bed of the uterus (LANG 1997b; McIVOR and CAMERON 1996; SALIKEN et al. 1994). Good reduction in the size of fibroids as well as cessation of bleeding and control of pain have been reported following embolization (VEDANTHAM et al. 1997).

#### 14.4.7.2
#### Embolization of Arteriovenous Malformations

Pelvic arteriovenous malformations may be of congenital or traumatic etiology. Frequently, there is involvement of pelvic organs such as the bladder, uterus, and rectosigmoid colon, and also extension into muscles (LANG 1986, 1997a).

Congenital arteriovenous malformations may present with hemihypertrophy of one of the lower extremities. Left heart failure is a classic presenting symptoms of large arteriovenous malformations. Hematuria and clot retention may herald the presence of arteriovenous malformations involving the bladder (LANG et al. 1979; LANG 1981) (Fig. 14.16).

Recruitment of vascular supply from vessels of abutting organs makes difficult surgical eradication of such arteriovenous malformations. Staged arterial embolization, sometimes in conjunction with surgical skeletonization of the venous structure (Fig. 14.17e), is the procedure of choice to eradicate extensive pelvic arteriovenous malformations (LANG et al. 1979; VOGELZANG et al. 1991) (Fig. 14.17c). Intervals of 6–8 weeks between embolization series are recommended to permit enlargement of collateral pathways, which can then be embolized (Fig. 14.17). Initially coils and Gelfoam particles are the favored occlusive materials (Fig. 14.17a,b). After the majority of the large arterial collateral connections have been occluded, superselective embolization and placement of microcoils, spindles, and dehydrated polyvinyl alcohol particles of 500 µm are generally favored to occlude small residual arteriovenous malformations (Fig. 14.17d). The frequent need to embolize presacral arteries has to be weighed against the risk of resultant damage to nerves, causing erectile impotence (Fig. 4.17d). Use of 6-cyanoacrylate diluted with contrast medium at a 1 : 1 ratio and therefore prone to set at the level of muscular arteries or arterioles is particularly advocated for embolization of

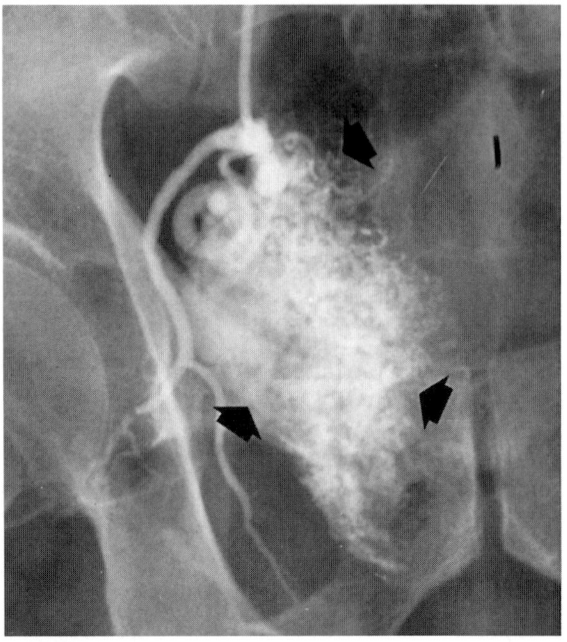
a

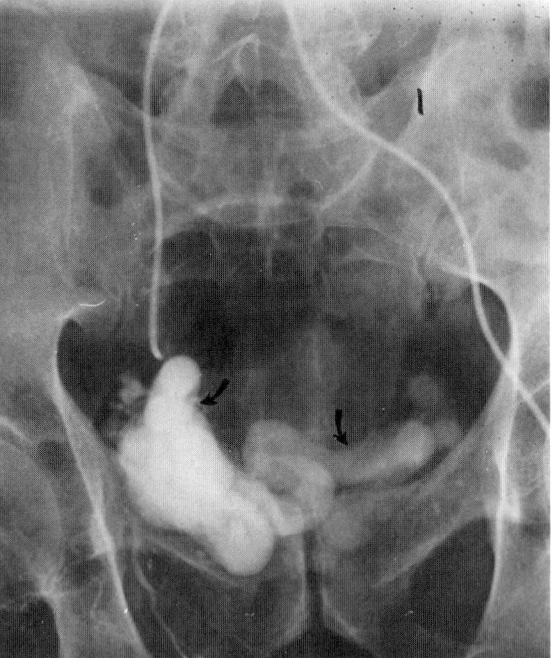
b

**Fig. 14.16.** **a** A selective injection of the right superior vesical artery demonstrates a huge racematous angioma involving the bladder (*arrows*). **b** A 14-s delayed film demonstrates huge draining veins (*arrows*). The patient presented with left heart failure and clot retention. (From LANG et al. 1979)

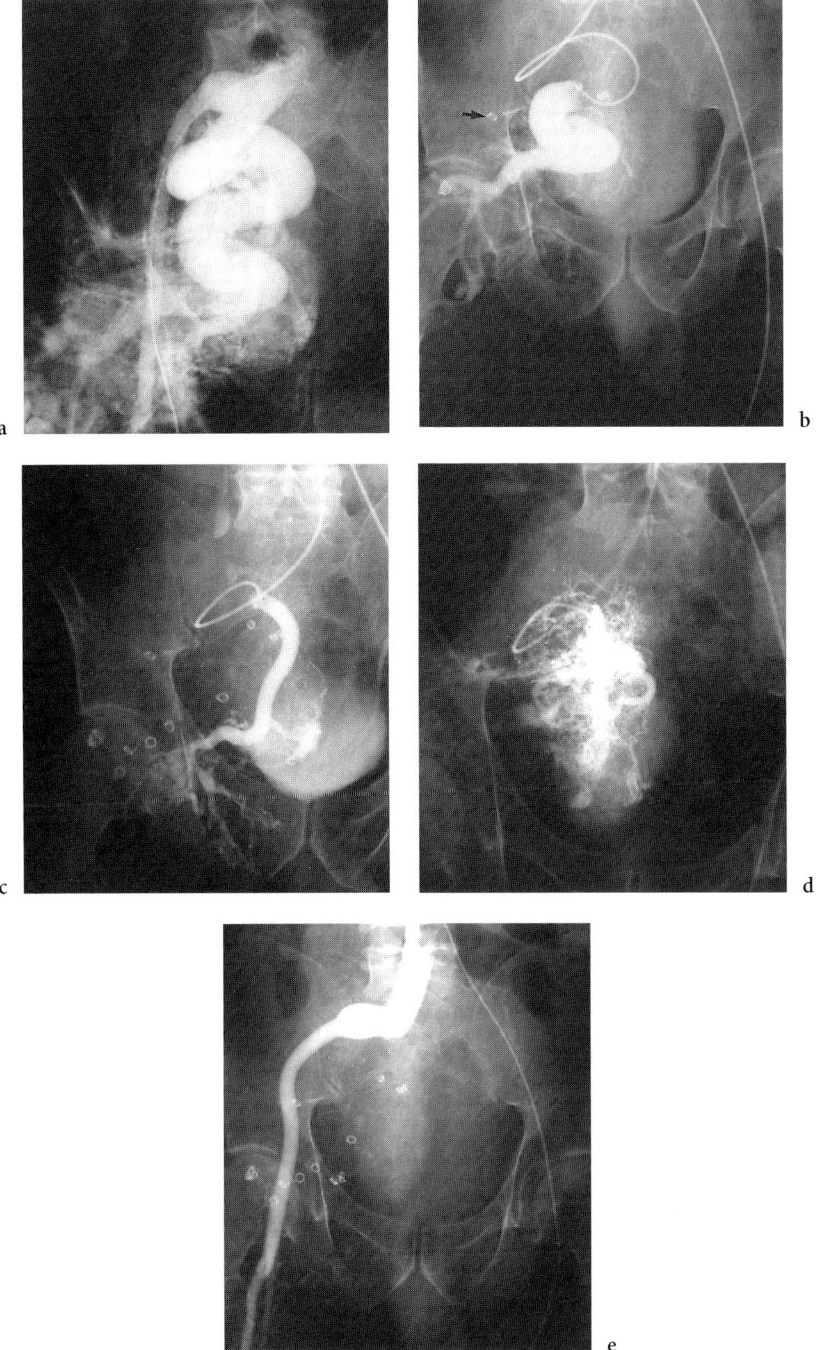

**Fig. 14.17. a** Arteriogram demonstrating an enormous arteriovenous malformation predominantly fed by the right hypogastric artery (*arrow*). **b** Superselective embolization of branch arteries was carried out with coils. **c** After numerous branches of both the anterior and the posterior division of the right hypogastric artery had been occluded, selective engagement of the obturator artery was carried out and remaining arteriovenous malformations feeding from this vessel were embolized. **d** A selective injection of the midsacral artery also demonstrates racematous arteriovenous malformations which were embolized with microcoils and Ivalon. **e** Following occlusion of the arterial feeders to the malformation, skeletonization of the venous system was carried out to prevent recurrence

small-caliber arteriovenous malformations. However, care must be exercised so as not to deprive an organ of its entire vascular supply. Overzealous embolization has resulted in severe complications such as gangrene of the bladder (Braf and Koontz 1977; Hietala 1978).

#### *14.4.7.3 Embolization of Trophoblastic Disease*

Chemoembolization with methyltrexate, cisplatinum, and Ethiodol has been successfully used in the treatment of high-risk metastatic gestational trophoblastic disease (both primary and metastatic tumors), particularly in the liver (Lang 1997b). Repeat embolizations are carried out at 3- to 4-weekly intervals until normalization of the β-human chorionic gonadotropin (β-hCG) level is achieved and maintained (Lang 1997b). Chemoembolization is particularly advocated for patients who have failed standard intravenous therapy such as the CHAMOMA or MAC protocol. Embolization may also be useful in the preparation to terminate advanced pregnancies (Saliken et al. 1994).

Residual placental tissue in the uterus or after incomplete expression of a tubal pregnancy can be opportunely treated by transcatheter embolization (Kerr et al. 1993; Lang 1997b; Vogelzang et al. 1991). This technique is useful as a preoperative preparatory measure, particularly in patients with abdominal pregnancy (Kerr et al. 1993; McIvor and Cameron 1996). However, it can also be utilized as definitive therapy for uterine arteriovenous malformations (Vogelzang et al. 1991). In combination with methyltrexate, it can be used as definitive treatment for retained placental tissue with hydatidiform degeneration of an incompletely expressed tubal pregnancy (Fig. 4.18).

## 14.5 Biopsy of Pelvic Mass Lesions

Biopsies guided by CT, fluoroscopy, or transabdominal, transvaginal, or transrectal ultrasound are advocated for histopathologic diagnosis of abdominal masses and particularly for improving staging criteria for neoplasms (Bret et al. 1992; Kim et al. 1995; Savader et al. 1990; Shipley et al. 1994; Triller et al. 1991; Zanetta et al. 1996) (Figs. 14.19, 14.20). Biopsy techniques have been proven to be safe and effective for categorization of lesions (Graham and Sanders 1982; Zanetta et al. 1996). Ultrasound-guided techniques are lauded for their cost-effectiveness. CT-guided techniques have a higher acceptance rate among clinicians and make a negative histologic/cytologic diagnosis more meaningful since the precise location of the origin of the biopsy is recorded. Spiral CT techniques generating 4-mm-thick slices that can be reconstructed at 2-mm intervals are particularly useful for this purpose and can identify the precise tip of the biopsy needle with great accuracy.

Biopsies of bladder or parametria can be undertaken safely via a transvesical route. Transrectal or transvaginal routes are equally safe (Cohen and Kucera 1992; Savader et al. 1990; Triller et al.1991; Zanetta et al. 1996). Coaxial biopsy needle systems have been developed to allow multiple consecutive biopsies and to protect overlying tissues against implantation of tumor cells. While these coaxial systems are of great importance in the diagnosis of renal, adrenal, lung, and breast neoplasms, the problem of tumor cell implantation in the tract is of less importance with pelvic neoplasms of the urogenital tract. Cytologic diagnosis can be rendered from aspirates from a 22-gauge biopsy needle. For histopathologic diagnosis 21- to 14-gauge biopsy needles are recommended. Spring biopsy needles tend to have the advantage of providing solid core samples, facilitating histopathologic and electron microscopic evaluation.

On rare occasions, assessment of normal-size lymph nodes for presence of neoplasm may be important to establish a definitive stage. Lymphangiography may reveal architectural changes in the lymph node implying the presence of small neoplastic implants; fluoroscopically guided biopsy is then the procedure of choice.

## 14.6 Urinary Diversion, Stents of the Ureter, Ureteroneocystostomy

Contiguous extension of female genital neoplasms, particularly carcinoma of the cervix, to the bladder and involving the ureters is a common occurrence in late and advanced stage disease. Invasion of the bladder and urethra may give rise to intractable hemorrhage. Involvement of the ureters and/or the bladder may result in obstruction, progressive hydronephrosis, and uremic conditions. Surgical bypass procedures such as cutaneous ureterostomies, ileal loop bladder, Koch's pouch, or Indiana pouch can bypass

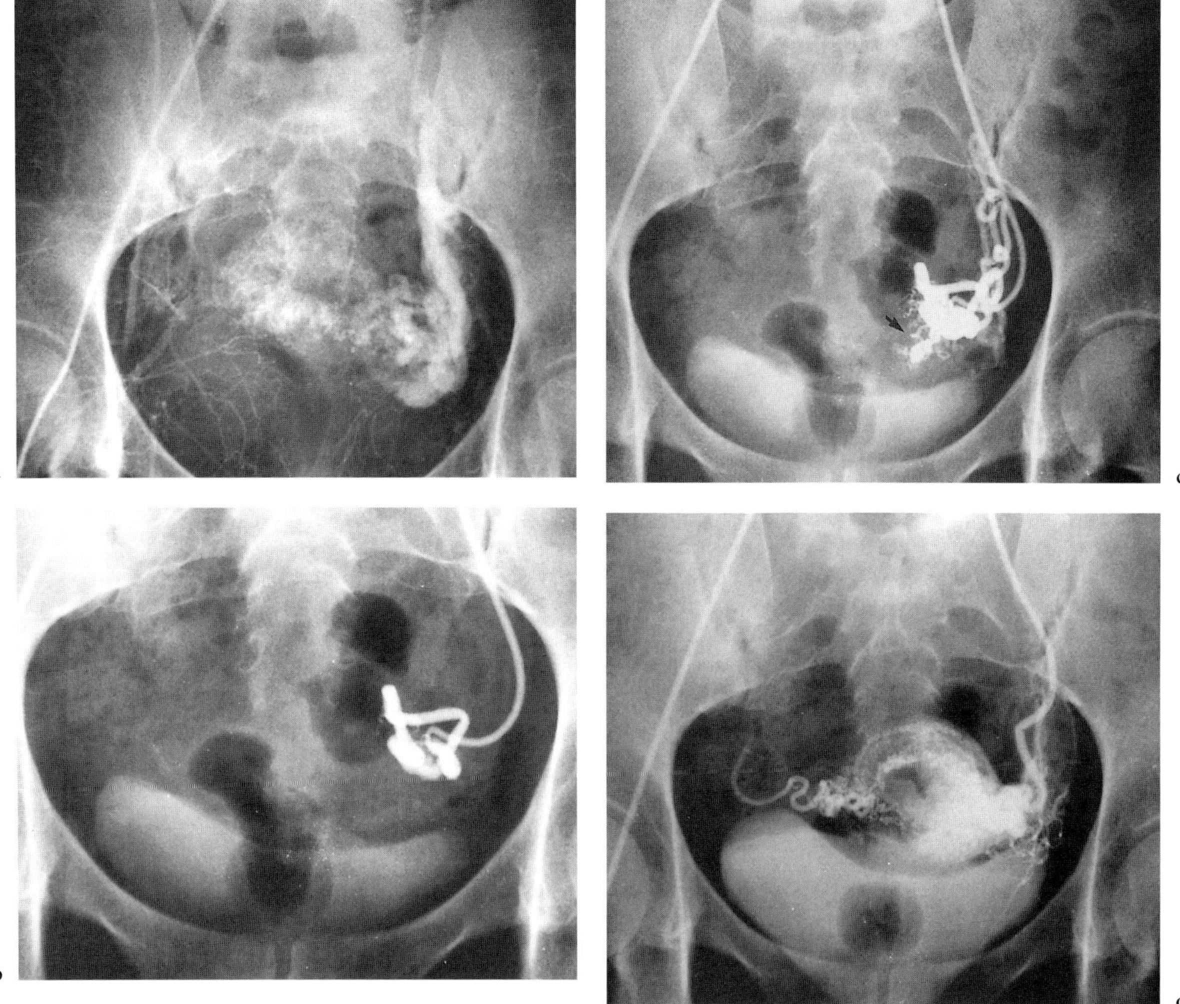


**Fig. 14.18.** **a** A hypervascular mass is demonstrated in the left parametrium. Note prominent opacified draining veins indicating the presence of arteriovenous shunts. Rising β-hCG levels 5 weeks after the expression of a tubal pregnancy prompted the investigation. **b** Superselective engagement of the feeder vessel arising from the uterine artery was carried out. **c** Note the abnormal vascularity in the distal portion of the left tube and parametrium, indicating residual placental tissue with hydatidiform degeneration (*arrow*). **d** After superselective embolization there is no longer evidence of a hypervascular mass in the left parametrium. Vascular supply to the uterus is unaffected. The patient experienced an uncomplicated pregnancy and normal delivery some 18 months later

the obstructions and reestablish normal urine drainage from the kidney. Percutaneous nephrostomy, stenting of the obstructed ureter, and antegrade ureteroneocystostomy can accomplish the same by radiologic intervention. However, prior to undertaking these corrective measures the physician, patient, and family should assess the implications for quality of life of the patient. In some patients with a very short life expectancy and in whom there is no hope of correcting the underlying process, uremic death may be preferable over death secondary to metastatic and primary disease complications. If, however, chemotherapy or radiation therapy is still an option and particularly if chemotherapy is contemplated, maintenance of renal function is a sine qua non. Particularly the use of cisplatinum and 5-fluorouracil requires good renal function.

On a temporary basis improvement in renal function can be accomplished by percutaneous nephrostomy. On a more permanent basis retrograde or antegrade placement of stents through the compromised ureters can reestablish flow into the bladder and thus safeguard renal function (Lang 1985, 1987). More recently metallic stents (wallstents) have

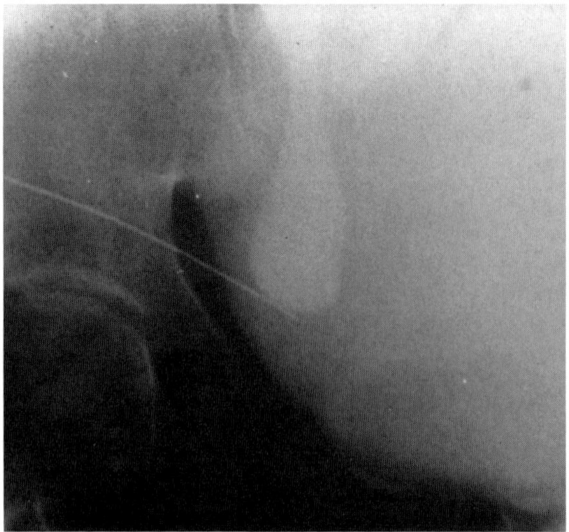

**Fig. 14.19.** Fluoroscopically guided biopsy obtained at a point of obstruction of the right ureter. Carcinoma of the cervix extending into the parametrium was identified

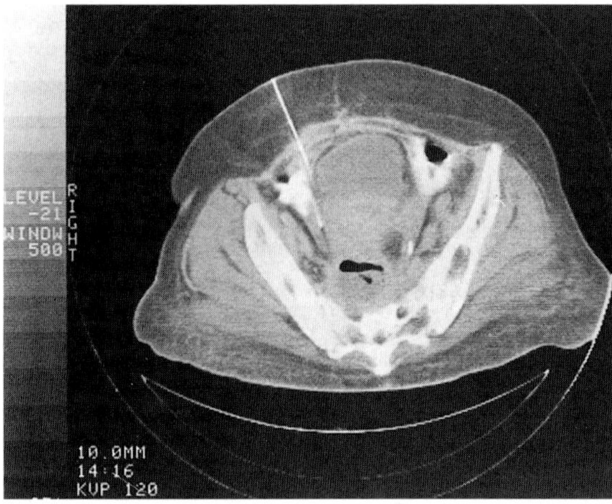


**Fig. 14.20.** Transabdominal CT-guided biopsy of hypogastric nodes, which confirmed neoplastic involvement

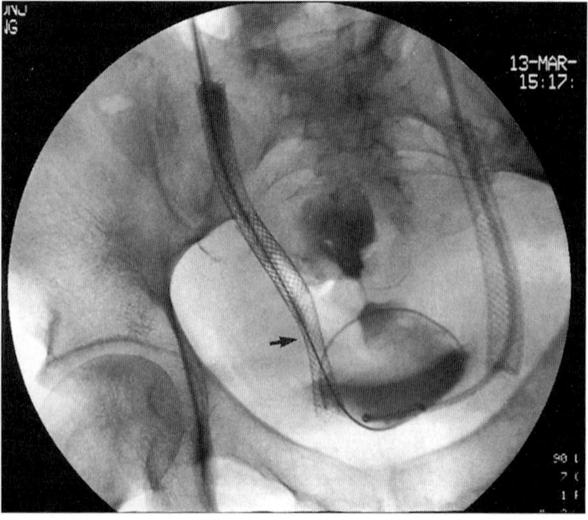


**Fig. 14.21.** Metallic wallstents have been placed in the distal right and left ureter. Note the residual waste effect upon the distal right wallstent caused by pressure of the tumor (*arrow*). A double "J" stent has been advanced through the left wallstent with the upper coil in the renal pelvis and the lower coil in the bladder

been placed via an antegrade approach through the interpolar calyx to ensure maintenance of the lumen of the ureter compromised by tumor (Lang et al. 1997; vanSonnenberg et al. 1994).

The metallic stent is seated with its distal end in the muscularis of the bladder and its rostral end at least 1 inch above the compromised ureter. Telescopic seating of multiple stents is an alternative if very long segments of the ureter are involved (Fig. 14.21). Because of tumor growth through the struts of the metal stent, double "J" endostents may be placed from the renal pelvis to the bladder. They can easily be exchanged cystoscopically once the lumen of the ureter is safeguarded by a seated metal stent (Lang et al. 1997; vanSonnenberg et al. 1994).

Particularly after alleviating an acute bilateral obstruction, careful clinical follow-up of the patient is indicated. A massive reactive diuresis may result in electrolyte imbalance and in particular in marked lowering of the potassium level, which must then be corrected.

If metallic stents are placed in patients subsequently subjected to external radiation therapy these stents may loosen due to regression of tumor encasing the ureter. Secondary radiation emitted from the metal of the stent bombarded by high-energy external radiation can result in a very high, though low energy and locally defined dose rate to the ureter (Lang et al. 1997).

In advanced neoplasms, often filling the entire pelvis and permeating the ureter over long segments, passage of a guidewire via a retrograde or antegrade approach may be impossible. A percutaneous ureteroneocystostomy is the procedure of choice in such patients (Lang 1988). For this purpose the posterior interpolar calyx is accessed percutaneously. The ureteropelvic junction is engaged with a renal curve 5-French catheter and a stiff Amplatz guidewire advanced downstream as far as possible. Over this guidewire the sheath of a transseptal needle, Colapinto transjugular needle, or TIPS needle is introduced and advanced. Thereafter the perforating trocar replaces the guidewire and the

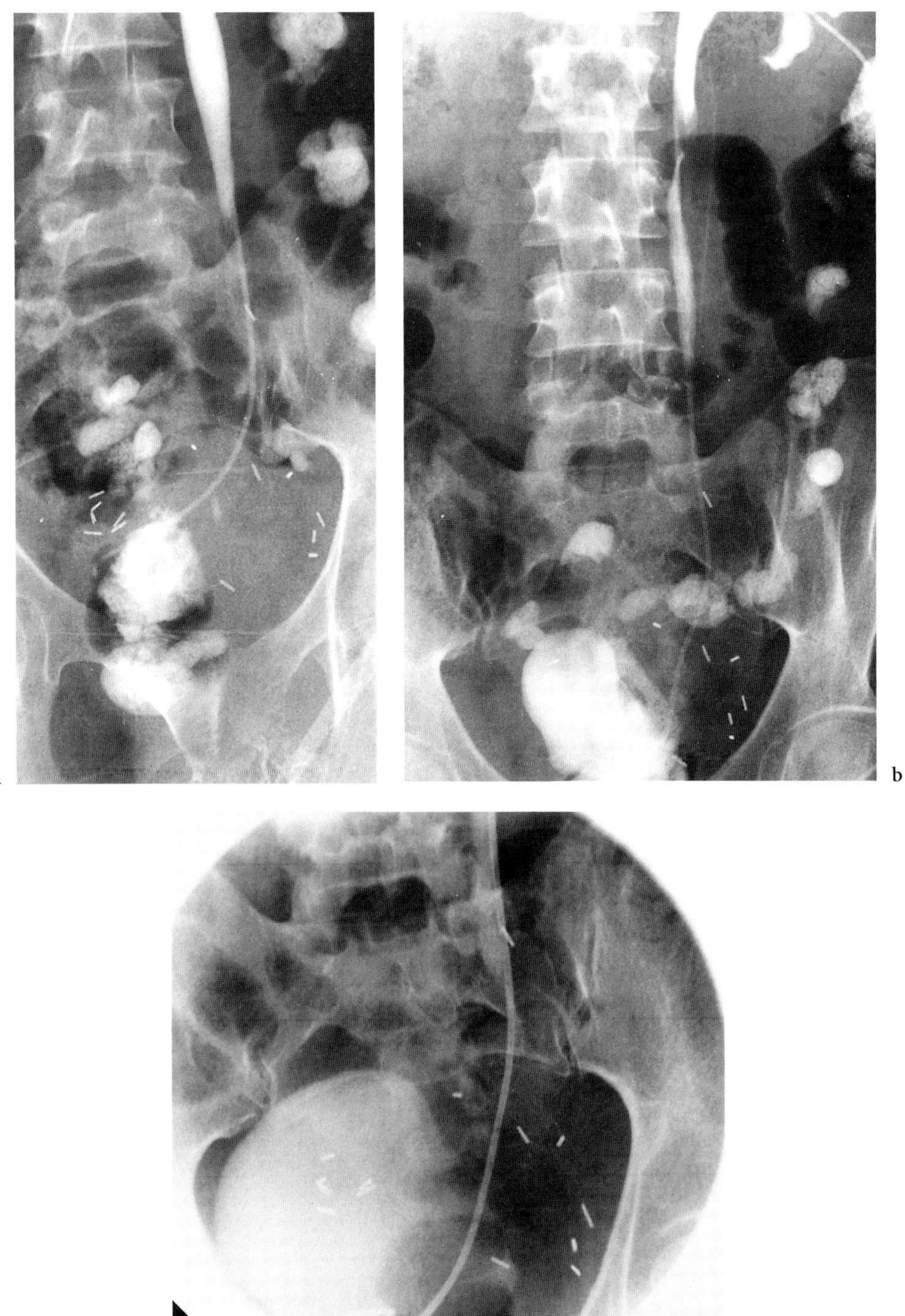


**Fig. 14.22.** **a** The sheath of a Colapinto needle has been advanced through a massive tumor. An injection, however, fails to show opacification of the bladder but rather extravasation along fistula tracts into the vagina. **b** The bladder is distended with dilute contrast and a repeat puncture with the trocar through the anteriorly directed Colapinto sheath successfully enters the bladder. **c** Finally, a double "J" stent is advanced over a stiff Amplatz guidewire through massive amounts of tumor into the bladder displaced to the right

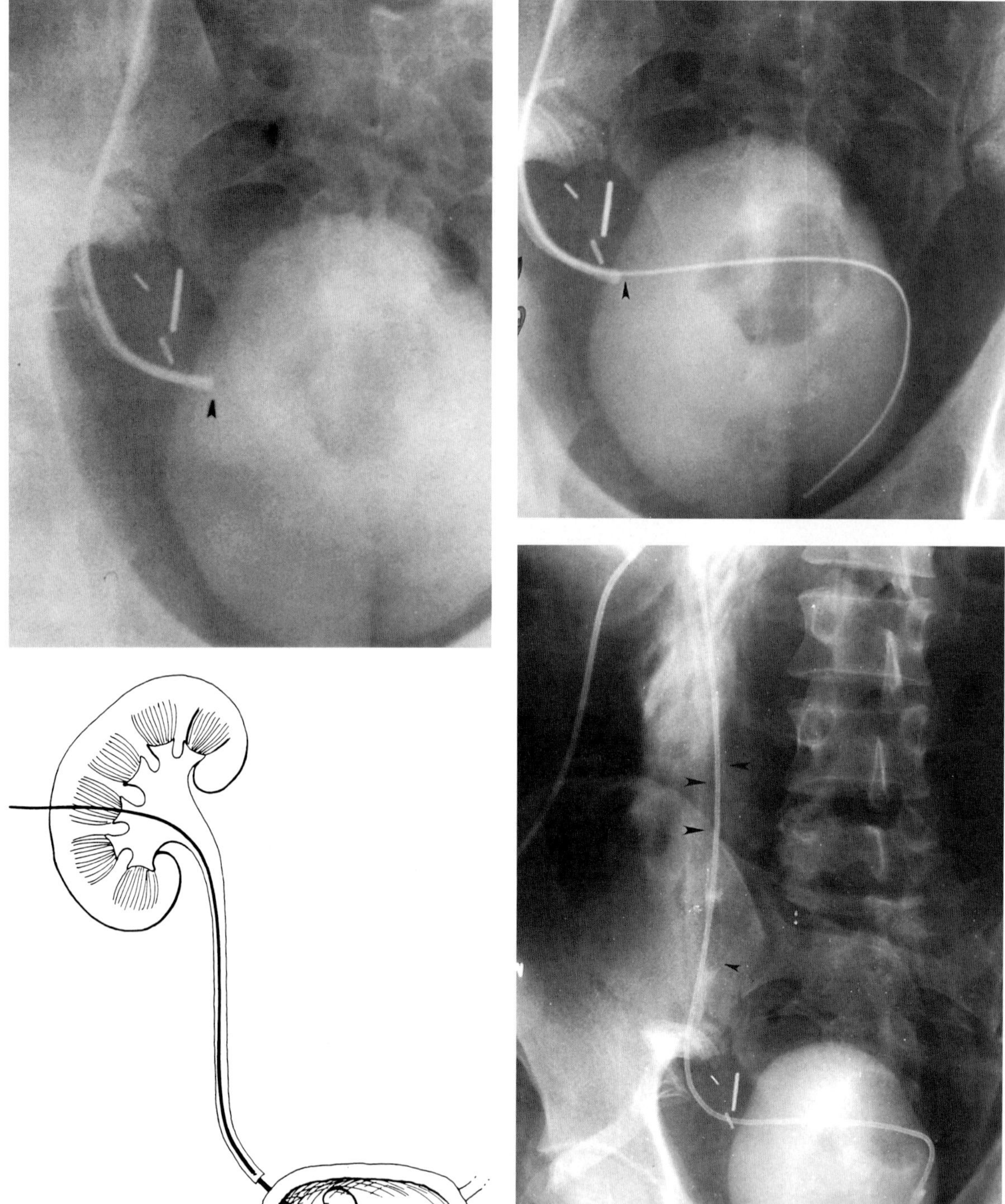

**Fig. 14.23.** **a** The sheath of a transseptal needle has been advanced through the severed end of the right ureter to come into apposition to the posterior wall of the distended bladder. **b** A schematic drawing demonstrates the position of the sheath and perforating trocar. **c** A stiff guidewire is advanced into the bladder after entry has been gained by trocar puncture and advancement of the sheath over the trocar. **d** Finally, an externalized stent is placed with the lower coil in the bladder. An externalized or double "J" stent is retained for 4–6 weeks until fibrous healing and reepithelialization with uroepithelium has occurred at the ureteroneocystomy site. (From LANG 1988)

curvature of the sheath is directed anteriorly. The trocar needle then perforates through the tumor into the bladder, which has been maximally distended by infusion of dilute contrast medium through a Foley catheter. Once the bladder has been entered, a stiff guidewire is advanced into the bladder and, after dilation of the newly formed tract with Olbert balloons, metallic or plastic stents are placed (Lang 1985, 1987, 1988, 1997a) (Fig. 14.22). The same technique can be utilized to create a percutaneous ureteroneocystostomy in patients in whom the distal ureter has been severed, a complication seen with hysterectomies and particularly vaginal hysterectomies (Lang 1988). Defects of up to 3 cm of distal ureter are amenable to this corrective intervention, benefiting from the propensity of uroepithelium to bridge stented defects (Lang 1988) (Fig. 14.23).

## References


Alexander AA, Eschelman DJ, Nazarian LN, et al. (1994) Transcervical sonographically guided drainage of deep pelvic abscesses. AJR 162:1227–1230

Ayella RJ, DuPriest RW Jr, Khaneja SC, et al. (1978) Transcatheter embolization of autologous clot in the management of bleeding associated with fractures of the pelvis. Surg Gynecol Obstet 147:849–852

Bennett JD, Kozak RI, Taylor BM, Jory TA (1992) Deep pelvic abscesses: transrectal drainage with radiologic guidance. Radiology 185:825–828

Braf ZF, Koontz WW Jr (1977) Gangrene of bladder, complication of hypogastric artery embolization. Urology 9:670–671

Bret PM, Guibaud L, Atri M, Gillet P, Seymour FJ, Senterman MK (1992) Transvaginal US-guided aspiration of ovarian cysts and solid pelvic masses. Radiology 185:377–380

Burchell RC (1968) Physiology of internal iliac artery ligation. J Obstet Gynaecol Br Comm 75:642–651

Butch RJ, Mueller PR, Ferrucci JT Jr, et al (1968) Drainage of pelvic abscesses through the greater sciatic foramen. Radiology 158:487–491

Carmody E, Thurston W, Yeung E, et al. (1993) Transrectal drainage of deep pelvic collections under fluoroscopic guidance. Can Assoc Radiol J 44:429–433

Casola G, vanSonnenberg E, D'Agostino HB, Harker CP, Varney RR, Smith D (1992) Percutaneous drainage of tubo-ovarian abscesses. Radiology 182:399–402

Cohen DJ, Kucera PR (1992) Percutaneous biopsy of pelvic masses. Semin Intervent Radiol 9:138–144

Dickey KW, Zreik TG, Hsia HC, et al. (1996) Transvaginal uterine cervical dilation with fluoroscopic guidance: preliminary results in patients with infertility, Radiology 200:497–503

Elchalal U, Caspi B, Manor Y, et al. (1993) Ultrasound directed diagnosis and treatment of pelvic hematoma after therapeutic abortion. JCU 21:55–59

Eschelmann DJ, Sullivan KL (1993) Use of a Colapinto needle in US-guided transvaginal drainage of pelvic abscesses. Radiology 186:893–894

Feld R, Eschelman DJ, Sagerman JE, et al. (1994) Treatment of pelvic abscesses and other fluid collections: efficacy of transvaginal sonographically guided aspiration and drainage. AJR 163:1141–1145

Gazelle GS, Haaga JR, Stallato TA, et al. (1991) Pelvic abscesses: CT guided transrectal drainage. Radiology 181: 49–51

Goldstein HM, Medellin H, Ben-Menachem Y, et al. (1975) Transcatheter arterial embolization in the management of bleeding in the cancer patient. Radiology 115:603–608

Grace DM, Pitt DF, Bold RE (1976) Vascular embolization and occlusion by angiographic techniques as an aid or alternative to operation. Surg Gynecol Obstet 143:469–482

Graham D, Sanders RC (1982) Ultrasound-directed transvaginal aspiration biopsy of pelvic masses. J Ultrasound Med 1:279–280

Harima K, Harima Y, Hasegawa T, et al. (1995) Transcatheter arterial embolization as a method of cisplatin retention enhancement on the VX2 tumor uterus transplants. Cardiovasc Intervent Radiol 18:30–35

Hata K, Hata T, Fujiwaki R, et al. (1995) Hypertensive intra-arterial chemotherapy for endometrial carcinoma assessed by transvaginal Doppler ultrasound and magnetic resonance imaging. JCU 23:407–411

Heston DK, Mineau DE, Brown BJ, et al. (1979) Transcatheter arterial embolization for control of persistent massive puerperal hemorrhage after bilateral surgical hypogastric artery ligation. AJR 133:152–154

Hendrickx P, Orth G, Grunert J-H (1995) Long-term survival after embolization of potentially lethal bleeding malignant pelvic tumors. Br J Radiol 68:1336–1340

Hietala SO (1978) Urinary bladder necrosis following selective embolization of the internal iliac artery. Acta Radiol Diagn 19:316–320

Johnson CM (1994) Drainage of retroperitoneal and pelvic abscesses and fluid collections. In: Kadir S (ed) Current practice of interventional radiology. Dekker, Philadelphia, pp 727–734

Kastan DJ, Nelsen KM, Shetty PC, et al. (1996) Combined transrectal sonographic and fluoroscopic guidance for deep pelvic abscess drainage. J Ultrasound Med 15:235–341

Katz MD, Teitelbaum GP, Pentecost MJ (1992) Diagnostic arteriography and therapeutic transcatheter embolization for post-traumatic pelvic hemorrhage. Semin Intervent Radiol 9:4–10

Keller FS (1992) Hemorrhagic complication of transgluteal pelvic abscess drainage: successful percutaneous treatment: invited commentary. J Vasc Intervent Radiol 3: 327

Kerr A, Trambert J, Mikhail M, Hodges L, Runowicz C (1993) Preoperative transcatheter embolization of abdominal pregnancy: report of three cases. J Vasc Intervent Radiol 4:733–735

Kim SH, Kim HD, Son YS, et al. (1995) Detection of deep myometrial invasion in endometrial carcinoma: comparison of transvaginal ultrasound, CT and MRI. J Comput Assist Tomogr 19:766–771

Kopechy KK (1992) Hemorrhagic complication of transgluteal pelvic abscess drainage: successful percutaneous treatment: invited commentary. J Vasc Intervent Radiol 3: 327

Kuligowska E, Keller E, Ferrucci JT (1995) Treatment of pelvic abscesses: value of one-step sonographically guided transrectal needle aspiration and lavage. AJR 164:201–206

Lang EK (1981) Transcatheter embolization of pelvic vessels for control of intractable hemorrhage. Radiology 140:331–339

Lang EK (1985) Antigrade ureteral stenting for dehiscence, strictures and fistulae. AJR 143:795–801

Lang EK (1986) Transcatheter embolization in the management of intractable hemorrhage from pelvic organs. In: Lang EK (ed) Percutaneous and interventional urology and radiology. Springer, Berlin Heidelberg New York, pp 201–210

Lang EK (1987) Nonsurgical management of ureteral fistulae. Semin Intervent Radiol 4:53–69

Lang EK (1988) Percutaneous ureterocystostomy and ureteroneocystostomy. AJR 150:1065–1068

Lang EK (1989) Management of hemorrhagic pelvic neoplasms by transcatheter embolization. J Intervent Radiol 4:113–117

Lang EK (1997a) The role of interventional radiology in emergency medicine. Emerg Radiol

Lang EK (1997b) Reduced systemic toxicity from superselective chemoembolization compared with systemic chemotherapy in patients with high-risk metastatic gestational trophoblastic disease. Cardiovasc Intervent Radiol 20:280–284

Lang EK, Deutsch JS, Goodman JR, Barnett T, Lanasa JA, Duplessis GH (1979) Transcatheter embolization of hypogastric branch arteries in the management of intractable bladder hemorrhage. J Urol 121:30–36

Lang EK, Lopez R, Watson RA (1997) Wallstents in treatment of ureteral obstructions secondary to residual or recurrent carcinoma of the cervix. AJR 168(Suppl):42

Lomas DJ, Dixon AK, Thomsom HJ, et al. (1992) CT guided drainage of pelvic abscesses: the perianal transrectal approach. Clin Radiol 45:246–249

Longo JM, Bilbao JI, de Villa VH, et al. (1993) CT-guided paracoccygeal drainage of pelvic abscesses. J Comput Assist Tomogr 17:909–914

Malden ES, Picus D (1992) Hemorrhagic complication of transgluteal pelvic abscess drainage: successful percutaneous treatment. J Vasc Intervent Radiol 3:323–328

Mauro MA, Jaques PF, Mandell VS, et al. (1985) Pelvic abscess drainage by the transrectal catheter approach in men. AJR 144:477–479

McDowell RK, Mueller PR (1995) Pelvic fluid collections: anatomy for interventional procedures. Semin Intervent Radiol 12:177–185

McGahan JP, Brown B, Jones CD, Stein M (1996) Pelvic abscesses: transvaginal US-guided drainage with the trocar method. Radiology 200:579–581

McIvor J, Cameron EW (1996) Pregnancy after uterine artery embolization to control hemorrhage from gestational trophoblastic tumor. Br J Radiol 69:624–627

Miller FJ Jr, Mortel R, Mann WJ, et al. (1976) Selective artery embolization for control of hemorrhage in pelvic malignancy: femoral and brachial catheter approaches. AJR 126:1028–1032

Mueller PR, Saini S, Wittenberg J, et al. (1987) Sigmoid diverticular abscesses: percutaneous drainage as an adjunct to surgical resection in 24 cases. Radiology 164: 321–325

Mueller PR, White EM, Glass-Royal M, et al. (1989) Infected abdominal tumors: percutaneous catheter drainage. Radiology 173:627–629

Nosher JL, Needell GS, Amorosa JK, et al. (1986) Transrectal pelvic abscess drainage with sonographic guidance. AJR 146:1047–1048

Nosher JL, Winchman HK, Needell GS (1987) Transvaginal pelvic abscess drainage with US guidance. Radiology 165:872–873

Nunez D, Huber JS, Yrizarry JM, et al. (1986) Nonsurgical drainage of appendiceal abscesses. AJR 146:587–589

Papanicolaou N, Mueller P, Ferrucci JT, et al. (1987) Abscess-fistula association: radiologic recognition and percutaneous management. AJR 143:811–815

Pereira JK, Chait PG, Miller SF (1996) Deep pelvic abscesses in children: transrectal drainage under radiologic guidance. Radiology 198:393–396

Pisco JM, Martins JM, Correia MG (1989) Internal iliac artery embolization to control hemorrhage from pelvic neoplasms. Radiology 172:337–342

Rosenthal DM, Colapinto R (1985) Angiographic arterial embolization and management of postoperative vaginal hemorrhage. Am J Obstet Gynecol 75:642–651

Saliken JC, Normore WJ, Pattinson HA, et al. (1994) Embolization of the uterine arteries before termination of a 15 week cervical pregnancy. Can Assoc Radiol J 45:399–342

Sanchez RB, vanSonnenberg E, D'Agostino HB, et al. (1992) Transvaginal drainage of pelvic fluid collections. Semin Intervent Radiol 9:152–155

Savader BL, Hamper UM, Sheth S, Ballard RL, Sanders RC (1990) Pelvic masses: aspiration biopsy with transrectal US guidance. Radiology 176:351–353

Schuster MR, Crummy AG, Wojtowycz MM, et al. (1992) Abdominal abscesses associated with enteric fistulas: percutaneous management. J Vasc Intervent Radiol 3:359–363

Shipley CF III, Simmons CL, Nelson GH (1994) Comparison of transvaginal sonography with endometrial biopsy in asymptomatic postmenopausal women. J Ultrasound Med 13:99–102

Triller J, Maddern G, Kraft P, et al. (1991) CT-guided biopsy of pelvic masses. Cardiovasc Intervent Radiol 14:63

Tyrrel RT, Murphy FB, Bernadino ME (1990) Tubo-ovarian abscesses: CT-guided percutaneous drainage. Radiology 175:87–89

Van Allen RJ, Pentecost MJ (1992) Transcatheter control of hemorrhage in the cancer patients. Semin Intervent Radiol 9:38–43

Van DerKolk HL (1991) Small deep pelvic abscesses: definition and drainage guided with an endovaginal probe. Radiology 181:283–284

van Sonnenberg E (1992) Hemorrhagic complication of transgluteal pelvic abscess drainage: successful percutaneous treatment: invited commentary. J Vasc Intervent Radiol 3:328

vanSonnenberg E, Wittich GR, Casola G, et al. (1986) Lymphoceles: imaging characteristics and percutaneous management. Radiology 161:593–596

vanSonnenberg E, D'Agostino HB, Casola G, et al. (1991a) US-guided transvaginal drainage of pelvic abscesses and fluid collections. Radiology 181:53–56

vanSonnenberg E, D'Agostino HB, Casola G, Goodacre BW, Sanchez RG, Taylor B (1991b) US-guided transvaginal drainage of pelvic abscesses and fluid collections. Radiology 181:53

vanSonnenberg E, D'Agostino HB, O Laoide RM, Donaldson JS, Sanchez RB, Hoyt A, Pittman CC (1994) Malignant ureteral obstruction: treatment with metal stents – technique, results, and observations with percutaneous intraluminal US. Radiology 191:765–768

vanSonnenberg E, Ali S, Goodacre B, et al. (1997) Making undrainable abscesses and fluid collections drainable – preliminary laboratory and clinical experience. AJR 168(Suppl):121

Vedantham S, Goodman SG, McLucas B, Forno AE (1997) Uterine artery embolization for uterine fibroids: results of pilot study. AJR 168(Suppl):41

Vogelzang RL, Nemcek AA Jr, Skrtic Z, Gorrell J, Lurain JR (1991) Uterine arteriovenous malformations: primary treatment with therapeutic embolization. J Vasc Intervent Radiol 2:517–522

White M, Mueller PR, Ferrucci JT Jr, et al. (1985) Percutaneous drainage of postoperative abdominal and pelvic lymphoceles. AJR 145:1065–1069

Yamada T, Ujita M, Ishii C, et al. (1996) Long term results of extended intra-arterial cisplatin infusion. Therapy to treat locally advanced cervical carcinoma. Cardiovasc Intervent Radiol 19:596

Yamashita Y, Harada M, Yamamoto H, et al. (1994) Transcatheter arterial embolization of obstetric and gynecological bleeding: efficacy and clinical outcome. Br J Radiol 67:530–536

Zanetta G, Lissoni A, Franchi D, et al. (1996) Safety of transvaginal fine needle puncture of gynecological masses: report after 500 consecutive procedures. J Ultrasound Med 15:401–405

# Subject Index

# List of Contributors


Susan M. Ascher, MD
Associate Professor of Radiology
Director of Body MRI
Department of Radiology
Georgetown University Medical Center
3800 Reservoir Road NW
Washington, DC 20007-2197
USA

Mostafa Atri, MD
Associate Professor of Radiology, McGill University
Associate Professor,
Department of Obstetrics and Gynecology
Director, Ultrasound Division
Department of Radiology
Montreal General Hospital
1650 Cedar Avenue
Montréal, Québec H3G 1A4
Canada

Philip Baharamipour, MD
Assistant Professor of Radiology
Department of Radiology
UMDNJ – New Jersey Medical School
150 Bergen Street
Newark, NJ 07103
USA

Gianpaolo Biti, MD
Unit of Radiation Therapy
Department of Clinical Physiopathology
Careggi Hospital – University of Florence
Viale Morgagni 85
I-50134 Florence
Italy

Cynthia I. Caskey, MD
Division of Ultrasound
Department of Radiology and Radiological Sciences
The Johns Hopkins Medical Institutions
600 North Wolfe Street
Baltimore, MD 21287, USA
*current address:* Department of Radiology,
University of Texas – Houston, LBJ General Hospital
5656 Kelly Street, Houston, TX 77026, USA

Francesco De Cobelli, MD
Department of Radiology
Scientific Institute S. Raffaele
University Hospital
Olgettina 60
I-20132 Milan
Italy

Alessandro Del Maschio, MD
Director, Department of Radiology
Scientific Institute S. Raffaele
University Hospital
Olgettina 60
I-20132 Milan
Italy

Heber H. Dunaway Jr., MD, FACOG
Fertility Center of Louisiana
4720 SI/O Service Rd.
Metaire; LA 70001
USA

Ulrike M. Hamper, MD
Division of Ultrasound
Department of Radiology and Radiological Sciences
The Johns Hopkins Medical Institutions
600 North Wolfe Street
Baltimore, MD 21287
USA

Paolo Innocenti, MD
Professor of Radiology
Unit of Radiodiagnostics
Department of Clinical Physiopathology
Careggi Hospital
University of Florence
Viale Morgagni 85
I-50134 Florence
Italy

Nabet G. Kasabian, MD
Director of Female Urology and Neurourology
Assistant Professor of Surgery
Division of Urology
Department of Surgery
UMDNJ – New Jersey Medical School
150 Bergen Street
Newark, NJ 07103-2406, USA
*current address:* Urologic Associates P.C.
535 Plandome Road, Manhasset, NY 11030, USA

Kie Hwan Kim, MD
Director
Department of Diagnostic Radiology
Korea Cancer Center Hospital
215-4 Gongneung-dong, Nowon-gu
Seoul, 139-706
KOREA

Erich K. Lang, MD
Professor of Radiology and Urology
Department of Radiology School of Medicine
Louisiana State University Medical Center
1543 Tulane Avenue
New Orleans, LA 70122-2822
USA

Gerald C. Mingin, Jr., MD
Resident, Division of Urology
Department of Surgery
UMDNJ - New Jersey Medical School
150 Bergen Street
Newark, NJ 07103-2406
USA

Kumar R. Mullangi, MD
Chief Resident, Division of Urology
Department of Surgery
UMDNJ - New Jersey Medical School
150 Bergen Street
Newark, NJ 07103-2406; USA
*current address:* 517 North 3rd Street
Burlington, IA 52601, USA

Jacopo Nori, MD
Unit of Radiodiagnostics
Obstetric and Gynecological Clinic
Careggi Hospital
University of Florence
Viale Morgagni 85
I-50134 Florence
Italy

Yashwan D. Patel, MD
Associate Professor of Clinical Radiology
Director, Division of Vascular and Interventional Radiology
UMDNJ - New Jersey Medical School
150 Bergen Street
Newark, NJ 07103-2406
USA

Caroline Reinhold, MD
Assistant Professor of Radiology
Director of Body MRI
Montreal General Hospital
McGill University
1650 Cedar Avenue
Montréal, Québec H3G 1A4
Canada

Riccardo Santoni, MD
Unit of Radiation Therapy
Department of Clinical Physiopathology
Careggi Hospital
University of Florence
Viale Morgagni 85
I-50134 Florence
Italy

Sheila Sheth, MD
Division of Ultrasound
Department of Radiology and Radiological Sciences
The Johns Hopkins Medical Institutions
600 North Wolfe Street
Baltimore, MD 21287
USA

Alvin Silva, MD
Clinical Instructor
Department of Radiology
Georgetown University Medical Center
3800 Reservoir Road NW
Washington, DC 20007-2197
USA

Sandro Sironi
Department of Radiology
Scientific Institute S. Raffaele
University Hospital
Olgettina 60
I-20132 Milan
Italy

Daniele Spagnolo, MD
Department of Radiology
Scientific Institute S. Raffaele
University Hospital
Olgettina 60
I-20132 Milan
Italy

David B. Spring, MD
Director GU Radiology
Kaiser Permanente Medical Center
280 West McArthur Blvd.
Oakland, CA 94611
USA

Mutsumasa Takahashi, MD
Professor and Chairman
Department of Radiology
Kumamoto University School of Medicine
1-1-1 Honjo
Kumamoto, 860
JAPAN

Angelo Vanzulli, MD
Department of Radiology
Scientific Institute S. Raffaele
University Hospital
Olgettina 60
I-20132 Milan
Italy

Natale Villari, MD
Unit of Radiodiagnostics
Department of Clinical Physiopathology
Careggi Hospital
University of Florence
Viale Morgagni 85
I-50134 Florence
Italy

Yasuyuki Yamashita, MD
Associate Professor
Department of Radiology
Kumamoto University School of Medicine
1-1-1 Honjo
Kumamoto, 860
JAPAN

# Medical Radiology
## Diagnostic Imaging and Radiation Oncology

*Titles in the series already published*

### Diagnostic Imaging

**Innovations in Diagnostic Imaging**
Edited by J.H. Anderson

**Radiology of the Upper Urinary Tract**
Edited by E.K. Lang

**The Thymus - Diagnostic Imaging, Functions, and Pathologic Anatomy**
Edited by E. Walter, E. Willich, and W.R. Webb

**Interventional Neuroradiology**
Edited by A. Valavanis

**Radiology of the Pancreas**
Edited by A.L. Baert, co-edited by G. Delorme

**Radiology of the Lower Urinary Tract**
Edited by E.K. Lang

**Magnetic Resonance Angiography**
Edited by I.P. Arlart, G.M. Bongartz, and G. Marchal

**Contrast-Enhanced MRI of the Breast**
S. Heywang-Köbrunner and R. Beck

**Spiral CT of the Chest**
Edited by M. Rémy-Jardin and J. Rémy

**Radiological Diagnosis of Breast Diseases**
Edited by M. Friedrich and E.A. Sickles

**Radiology of the Trauma**
Edited by M. Heller and A. Fink

**Biliary Tract Radiology**
Edited by P. Rossi

**Radiological Imaging of Sports Injuries**
Edited by C. Masciocchi

**Modern Imaging of the Alimentary Tube**
Edited by A. R. Margulis

**Diagnosis and Therapy of Spinal Tumors**
Edited by P. R. Algra, J. Valk, and J. J. Heimans

**Interventional Magnetic Resonance Imaging**
Edited by J. F. Debatin and G. Adam

**Abdominal and Pelvic MRI**
Edited by A. Heuck and M. Reiser

**Orthopedic Imaging**
Edited by A.M. Davies and H. Pettersson

**Radiology of the Female Pelvic Organs**
Edited by E.K.Lang

### Radiation Oncology

**Lung Cancer**
Edited by C.W. Scarantino

**Innovations in Radiation Oncology**
Edited by H.R. Withers and L.J. Peters

**Radiation Therapy of Head and Neck Cancer**
Edited by G.E. Laramore

**Gastrointestinal Cancer – Radiation Therapy**
Edited by R.R. Dobelbower, Jr.

**Radiation Exposure and Occupational Risks**
Edited by E. Scherer, C. Streffer, and K.-R. Trott

**Radiation Therapy of Benign Diseases - A Clinical Guide**
S.E. Order and S.S. Donaldson

# Medical Radiology
## Diagnostic Imaging and Radiation Oncology

*Titles in the series already published*

### Radiation Oncology

**Interventional Radiation Therapy Techniques - Brachytherapy**
Edited by R. Sauer

**Radiopathology of Organs and Tissues**
Edited by E. Scherer, C. Streffer, and K.-R. Trott

**Concomitant Continuous Infusion Chemotherapy and Radiation**
Edited by M. Rotman and C.J. Rosenthal

**Intraoperative Radiotherapy – Clinical Experiences and Results**
Edited by F.A. Calvo, M. Santos, and L.W. Brady

**Radiotherapy of Intraocular and Orbital Tumors**
Edited by W.E. Alberti and R.H. Sagerman

**Interstitial and Intracavitary Thermoradiotherapy**
Edited by M.H. Seegenschmiedt and R. Sauer

**Non-Disseminated Breast Cancer**
**Controversial Issues in Management**
Edited by G.H. Fletcher and S.H. Levitt

**Current Topics in Clinical Radiobiology of Tumors**
Edited by H.-P. Beck-Bornholdt

**Practical Approaches to Cancer Invasion and Metastases**
**A Compendium of Radiation Oncologists' Responses to 40 Histories**
Edited by A.R. Kagan with the Assistance of R.J. Steckel

**Radiation Therapy in Pediatric Oncology**
Edited by J.R. Cassady

**Radiation Therapy Physics**
Edited by A.R. Smith

**Late Sequelae in Oncology**
Edited by J. Dunst and R. Sauer

**Mediastinal Tumors. Update 1995**
Edited by D.E. Wood and C.R. Thomas, Jr.

**Thermoradiotherapy and Thermochemotherapy**
**Volume 1: Biology, Physiology, and Physics**
**Volume 2: Clinical Applications**
Edited by M.H. Seegenschmiedt, P. Fessenden, and C.C. Vernon

**Carcinoma of the Prostate**
**Innovations in Management**
Edited by Z. Petrovich, L. Baert, and L.W. Brady

**Radiation Oncology of Gynecological Cancers**
Edited by H.W. Vahrson

**Carcinoma of the Bladder**
**Innovations in Management**
Edited by Z. Petrovich, L. Baert, and L.W. Brady

**Blood Perfusion and Microenvironment of Human Tumors**
**Implications for Clinical Radiooncology**
Edited by M. Molls and P. Vaupel

**Radiation Therapy of Benign Diseases. A Clinical Guide**
2nd revised edition
S.E. Order and S.S. Donaldson